Occupation-centred
Practice with Children

2 4 MAY 2024

WITHDRAWN

Occupation-centred Practice with Children

A Practical Guide for Occupational Therapists

Edited by

Sylvia Rodger

Associate Professor
Division of Occupational Therapy
School of Health and Rehabilitation Sciences
The University of Queensland, Australia

WILEY-BLACKWELL

A John Wiley & Sons, Ltd., Publication

Library of Congress Cataloging-in-Publication Data

Rodger, Sylvia.
Occupation-centred practice with children: a practical guide for occupational therapists/
Sylvia Rodger.
     p. ; cm.
   Includes bibliographical references and index.
   ISBN 978-1-4051-8427-4 (pbk. : alk. paper) 1. Occupational therapy for children. I. Title.
   [DNLM: 1. Occupational Therapy–methods. 2. Child. WS 368 R723o 2010]
   RJ53.025R63 2010
   618.92'89165–dc22   2009033619

A catalogue record for this book is available from the British Library.

Set in 9/12.5pt Interstate Light by MPS Limited, A Macmillan Company
Printed and bound in Singapore by Ho Printing Singapore Pte Ltd

2 2013

Contents

Contributors

Jill Ashburner BOccThy, PhD
Principal Research and Development
Officer
437 Hellawell Road, Sunnybank Hills
PO Box 354
Sunnybank, Brisbane, Qld 4109
Australia

Rebecca Banks BOccThy (Hons 1)
PhD Candidate
Division of Occupational Therapy
School of Health and Rehabilitation
Sciences
The University of Queensland
St. Lucia, Brisbane
Qld 4072
Australia

Sally Bennett BOccThy (Hons), PhD
Division of Occupational Therapy
School of Health and Rehabilitation
Sciences
The University of Queensland
St. Lucia, Qld 4072
Australia

Ted Brown, PhD, MSc, MPA, BScOT (Hons),
OT(C), OTR, AccOT
Senior Lecturer
Department of Occupational Therapy
School of Primary Health Care
Faculty of Medicine, Nursing and Health
Sciences
Monash University, Peninsula Campus
Frankston, Vic., Australia

Imelda Burgman PhD
Lecturer
School of Health Sciences
University of Newcastle
Callaghan, NSW 2304
Australia

Christine Chapparo, PhD, MA, Dip OT
(NSW)
Senior Lecturer
Discipline of Occupational Therapy
Faculty of Health Sciences
The University of Sydney
PO Box 170, Lidcombe
NSW, Australia

Chi-Wen Chien, MEd (Hons), BScOT, OTR
PhD Candidate
Department of Occupational Therapy
School of Primary Health Care
Faculty of Medicine, Nursing and Health
Sciences
Monash University, Peninsula Campus
Frankston, Vic., Australia

Jodie Copley BOccThy (Hons), PhD
Division of Occupational Therapy
School of Health and Rehabilitation
Sciences
The University of Queensland
St. Lucia, Qld 4072
Australia

Fiona Graham BOccThy
Doctoral Candidate
Division of Occupational Therapy

School of Health and Rehabilitation
Sciences
The University of Queensland
St. Lucia, Brisbane
Qld 4072
Australia

Elizabeth A. Hinder BOccThy (Hons)
Senior Occupational Therapist
Disability Services Support Unit
Education Queensland
Brisbane, Qld, Australia

Michael Iwama
Associate Professor
Department of Occupational Science and
Occupational Therapy
University of Toronto
University Avenue
Toronto, Canada

Desleigh de Jonge BOccThy, MOccThy
Lecturer
Division of Occupational Therapy
School of Health and Rehabilitation
Sciences
The University of Queensland
Brisbane, Qld, Australia

Deb Keen PhD, MA, BSpecEd, DipEdPsych,
BSc
Associate Professor
Deputy Dean (Research), Faculty of
Education
Lecturer, School of Education and
Professional Studies (Brisbane, Logan)
Faculty of Education Executive, Mt.
Gravatt Campus, Griffith University
176 Messines Ridge Road
Mt. Gravatt
Qld 4122
Australia

Rachael McDonald BAppSc, PGDip, PhD
Senior Lecturer
Department of Occupational Therapy
School of Primary Health Care

Faculty of Medicine, Nursing and Health
Sciences
Monash University, Peninsula Campus
Frankston, Vic., Australia

Cheryl Missiuna, PhD, OT Reg (Ont)
Associate Professor, School of
Rehabilitation Science
Director, CanChild Centre for Childhood
Disability Research
McMaster University
Hamilton, ON, Canada

Alison Nelson
Clinical Educator and Lecturer
School of Human Movement Studies and
Division of Occupational Therapy
School of Health and Rehabilitation
Sciences
The University of Queensland
St. Lucia, Brisbane
Qld 4072
Australia

Helene Polatajko BOT, MEd, PhD
Professor
Department of Occupational Science and
Occupational Therapy
Graduate Department of Rehabilitation
Science
Dalla Lami School of Public Health
Science
University of Toronto
Toronto
Canada

Nancy Pollock MSc, OT Reg (Ont)
Associate Clinical Professor, School of
Rehabilitation Science
Investigator, CanChild Centre for
Childhood Disability Research
McMaster University
Hamilton, ON, Canada

Anne Poulsen BOccThy (Hons), PhD
Lecturer
Division of Occupational Therapy

School of Health and Rehabilitation
Sciences
The University of Queensland
St. Lucia, Brisbane
Qld 4072
Australia

Sylvia Rodger BOccThy, MEdSt, PhD
Associate Professor
Division of Occupational
Therapy
School of Health and Rehabilitation
Sciences
The University of Queensland
St. Lucia, Brisbane
Qld 4072
Australia

Merrill Turpin BOccThy (Hons), PhD
Division of Occupational Therapy
School of Health and Rehabilitation
Sciences
The University of Queensland
St. Lucia, Qld 4072
Australia

Jenny Ziviani BOccThy, MEd, PhD
Associate Professor
Division of Occupational Therapy
School of Health and Rehabilitation
Sciences
The University of Queensland
St. Lucia, Brisbane
Qld 4072
Australia

Foreword

As Rodger correctly describes, a focus on occupation in our profession has re-emerged over past 20–30 years. These developments have led to a lack of fit between the centrality of occupation in the profession, our current knowledge and the way in which occupational therapists have provided assessment and intervention to children and families.

This book, edited by Sylvia Rodger, is an excellent resource to support the development and implementation of occupation-based practice with children and families. Figure 1.4 clearly and comprehensively illustrates the factors influencing these changes in occupational therapy knowledge and practice. Information in the first several chapters outlines the conceptual foundations of occupation-based practice.

The book addresses the issue of the type of occupational therapy practice that fits with society, as well as what is best practice, and interventions that provide best outcomes at least cost. From the broadest perspective, this book centres on children in our society who are limited in participation in occupations for various reasons (e.g. disability, poverty, war and discrimination).

In reading this volume, I have been impressed by the focus on practical strategies, the 'how to' of occupation-based assessment and intervention based on sound theoretical foundations. The material fits well with current occupational therapy theoretical models as well, with a focus on children and youth in the context of their families, the occupations they do and their environments.

There are several highlights of this book that enhance its utility for students and practitioners. Early in the book (Chapter 2), the authors outline a client-centred practice framework that can be used in occupation-based practice with children. Sharing similarities with other frameworks such as CPPF and AOTA practice profile, the framework provides an excellent tool for therapists to organise the processes of assessment and intervention. The fundamental principles underpinning occupation-based practice are clearly discussed.

The book outlines the conceptual background for client- and family-centred practice and the importance of the goal-setting process as a key to effective collaboration and shared decision-making. Issues of cultural relevance, children's spirituality and the complexity of decision-making are discussed in depth. Several chapters in this volume provide examples of innovative intervention models that illustrate an occupation-based therapy approach. Additional chapters outline strategies that can guide therapists in specific practice settings.

The occupational therapy profession, students, practitioners, educators and researchers will benefit from the wonderful compilation of material in this book. Thanks to Sylvia Rodger for bringing these authors together in one volume.

Professor Mary Law
Ph.D., OT Reg. (Ont.), FCAOT, Associate Dean, School of Rehabilitation
Science, McMaster University, Hamilton, ON, Canada

Preface

The origin of this edited book arose from an awareness of the need for more practical information addressing occupation-centred practice for children and families. The previous book I co-edited (Rodger & Ziviani, 2006) provided some of the theoretical underpinnings of occupation-centred practice in terms of supporting children's occupational mastery and participation in their life contexts, in light of significant changes in contemporary society. This book aims to be more practical in providing examples of the 'how to' undertake occupation-centred practice; however, it draws extensively from the extant theoretical and empirical literature. In particular, I argue that occupational therapists need a strong theoretical basis to explain 'why' they do what they do. In Chapter 1, I address changes in the occupational therapy profession and health/human services environments as well as international trends in advocating for children's rights. In Chapter 2, I propose an occupational therapy process that focuses on information gathering, intervention and evaluation of outcomes within the context of child- and family-centred practice. Throughout the book, examples of the use of the occupational therapy process with individual children as clients, families as clients and organisations (such as schools) as clients are provided to demonstrate the potential impact of occupational therapy at individual as well as organisational and systems levels. In Chapter 3 with Deb Keen, I address child- and family-centred practice in detail at the levels of the individual therapist, family and organisation/system.

The next two chapters look at cultural influences on children's occupational performance and participation (Chapter 4) and call for therapists to be culturally sensitive in working with children and families from different cultural backgrounds to their own. Nelson and Iwama introduce the Kawa Model (Iwama, 2006) as a theoretically and culturally sound occupational performance model for addressing cultural differences. In Chapter 5, Burgman describes children's spiritual qualities and ways in which occupational therapists can nurture children's spirituality, a central feature of who they are as occupational beings.

Next, Chapters 6 and 7 address the information-gathering process. Chapter 6 by Pollock, Missiuna and Rodger focuses on the importance of client-centred goal setting and tools for goal setting with children and families and Chapter 7 by Brown and Chien describes a range of assessments of children's occupations, performance and participation. The next stage of the occupational therapy process is intervention and this is illustrated over three chapters that highlight three occupation-centred intervention approaches. Polatajko and I discuss Cognitive Orientation for daily Occupational Performance (CO-OP) in Chapter 8, Chapparo describes the Perceive, Recall, Plan and Perform (PRPP) system in Chapter 9, and Graham and I discuss occupational performance coaching (OPC) that enables parents to act as change agents for their own and their children's occupational performance in Chapter 10.

The book then turns to various children's occupations, namely those of school work and leisure. In Chapter 11, Hinder and Ashburner highlight an occupation-centred approach in school settings, demonstrating interventions at an individual student, whole of class and whole of school level. Chapter 12 illustrates practice that supports children's engagement and mastery of leisure skills. In this chapter, Poulsen and Ziviani describe how occupation-centred practitioners can facilitate children's engagement in discretionary leisure pursuits out of school hours using leisure coaching and mapping. Chapter 13 tackles hospital contexts in which the focus is on acute medical care, hence making it difficult at times to be occupation-centred. In Chapter 14, deJonge and McDonald illustrate how assistive technology (AT) can enable children's mastery of meaningful occupations and enhance their participation in relevant life situations.

In the final chapter, Copley, Bennett and Turpin describe the complex process of bringing together the evidence, therapists' clinical experience, their reasoning processes and other salient features to ensure sound decision making when working with children and families.

It is my hope that this book will provide practical information that can guide occupational therapy students and clinicians in becoming more occupation-centred in their practice.

Sylvia Rodger
Associate Professor
Division of Occupational Therapy
School of Health and Rehabilitation Sciences
The University of Queensland
Australia

Acknowledgements

In writing this book, I wish first to acknowledge some of the master clinicians (Mrs Moira Boyle and Dr Angie Mandich) who have mentored me at various times in my clinical practice with children and the occupational therapy theoreticians and researchers who have influenced my thinking about occupation-centred practice (Professors Carolyn Baum, Mary Law, Helene Polatajko and Wendy Coster).

Second, I wish to acknowledge the research higher degree students I have supervised and continue to supervise who stretch my thinking, challenge my ideas and whose projects and enthusiasm for researching various aspects of occupational therapy practice with children continue to energise me (Fiona Graham, Craig Greber, Ted Brown, Jenny Sturgess, May Lim, Kate Miller, Belinda Kipping, Fiona Jones, Karen Hanna, Lyndal Franklin and Michele Cheng).

Third, I would like to thank my husband John and children Elise and Sam who continue to encourage my writing endeavours, despite the fact that these inevitably take time away from them.

Finally, thanks to my sister Nicky who has let me share in many of her joys in parenting her daughter Bronte. The experience of becoming an aunty and reconnecting with our shared childhood experiences reminds me of the blessings brought by children, the awe and wonder of discovery, the exquisite joy of mastering new tasks and activities, and the success that inevitably builds confidence and self-efficacy.

Chapter 1

Introduction to Occupation-centred Practice with Children

Sylvia Rodger

Learning objectives

The primary aim of this chapter is to set the scene for this book and in doing so to fulfill the following objectives, namely to:

- Briefly describe the resurgence of occupation within the occupational therapy profession.
- Outline some other global trends, which have occurred in parallel with the refocusing of the profession.
- Describe some of the challenges to traditional developmental theory that has historically informed occupational therapy practice with children, as well as emerging views and theories of occupational development that have the potential to better inform our practice with children and their families.
- Identify the impact of these professional and more global trends on occupational therapy practice for children.

Introduction

Children engage in many social and occupational roles every day. They are variously grandchildren, children, nieces/nephews, siblings, friends, peers and playmates. In addition, they are school or kindergarten students, players and self-carers/maintainers, albeit they are developing independence and autonomy in these latter roles (Rodger & Ziviani, 2006). Healthy active children engage in occupations relevant to these roles all the time: they play, dress, eat and manage their personal care needs; engage in household chores and schoolwork tasks; and extracurricular activities such as soccer, ballet, scouts, tae kwon do and playing musical instruments. Children engage in these occupations in a range of environments such as with their families at home and friends at school, and in their

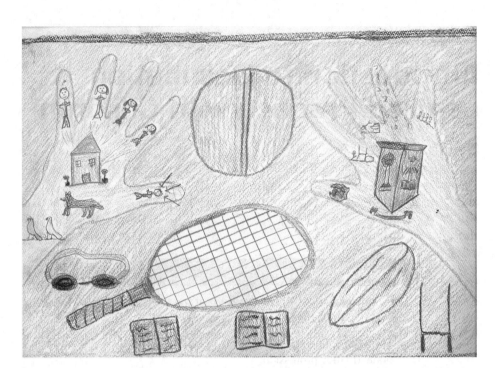

Figure 1.1 Daily life and occupations of a boy aged 11 years in metropolitan Brisbane. Copyright Thomas Beirne. Reproduced with permission

communities (e.g. church, neighbourhoods, local parks and sports clubs) (Rodger & Ziviani, 2006).

The children's artworks in Figures 1.1 and 1.2 illustrate the daily occupations of two boys, one growing up in metropolitan Brisbane, Australia, and the other in a village in East Timor. Figure 1.1 illustrates the boy's daily life with family, friends and his occupations of schoolwork, playing sports, ball games, listening to music and the importance of school. By contrast, Figure 1.2 illustrates the outdoor environment in which this Timorese boy lives, his home, the hills, his village and his role in tending crops. These drawings demonstrate some of the many cultural differences in children's occupations and daily lives.

Typically, occupational therapists come into contact with children when there are concerns about their occupational performance (e.g. ability to engage fully in their roles, issues with performance of tasks or activities associated with various occupations, or environmental hindrances to their performance and participation). However, it has been previously proposed (Rodger & Ziviani, 2006) that as a profession, we also have a role in advocating for children's place and rights in society, their need for health-promoting occupations, and safe, supportive and healthy environments that can optimise their occupational performance and participation. This may be through supporting campaigns promoting healthy lifestyle choices such as having smoking banned in children's playgrounds, lobbying for traffic calming and

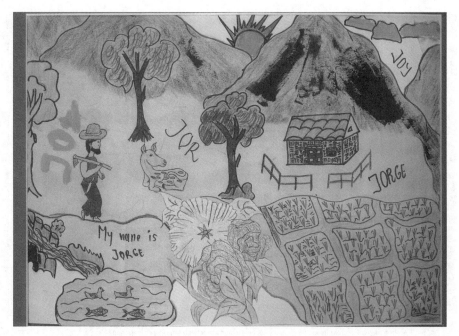

Figure 1.2 Daily life and occupations of a boy aged 15 years in East Timorese village. Copyright Jorge do Rosario. Reproduced with permission

pedestrian footpaths/sidewalks to enable safe walking to school, advocating for more green spaces such as parks and raising awareness about excessive involvement in virtual environments (e.g. computers and hand-held games) which may lead to decreased engagement in physical activity and social isolation.

There are many advocacy and professional groups that provide information for parents about children's health and well-being issues such as The Parents' Jury (http://www.parentsjury.org.au/index.asp) and the American Academy of Pediatrics (n.d., http://www.aap.org/healthtopics/parenting.cfm). The Parents' Jury organisation promotes activity-friendly communities (The Parents' Jury, 2008). It provides information about how to advocate at a local level for activity-friendly communities that readily support active living and family recreation as an essential part of a healthy lifestyle for both children and adults (see Figure 1.3). Such sites provide parent information as well as avenues for personal and professional advocacy regarding healthy neighbourhoods and communities for children.

In addition, we have a role as both individuals, health professionals and occupational therapists to advocate for children, whose lives are deprived of health-giving occupations and safe environments as a result of war, natural disasters, dislocation, social disadvantage, poverty and neglect/abuse (e.g. World Federation of Occupational Therapists Position Statement on Human Rights (WFOT, 2006) and Occupational Opportunities for Refugees and Asylum Seekers (OOFRAS), n.d.).

The Parents Jury's

☑Active
☑Community
☑Checklist

the **parents** jury

Your voice on food and activity

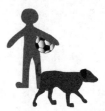

How activity-friendly is your community?

Use this assessment tool to determine how activity friendly your community is and find areas for improvement.

Tick the boxes that apply and tally up your responses. If your community is lacking in adequate activity and recreation areas, we've provided some suggestions to help you advocate for improvement.

Active transport   Yes:

+ Are the footpaths in your community well maintained, with adequate street lighting and shade?

+ Does your community have scenic walking/cycling tracks, which are well maintained, with adequate lighting, shade and rest stops?

+ Does your community have designated bikes lanes, on the footpath or road?

Recreation areas*

+ Are the recreation areas in your community kept clean and attractively landscaped/designed?

+ Are there enough well maintained amenities in these recreation areas, such as public toilets, seating, shade/shelter, public phones?

+ Do the recreation areas have well maintained age-appropriate playgrounds, which attract and engage children?

+ Are the recreation areas in your community easily accessible via walking or cycling?

+ Is dog-walking permitted in these recreation areas, and if so, are the areas kept clean with dog-litter facilities provided?

Community and safety

+ Do you feel that your local recreation areas and streets are safe for you and your family? Consider how open or secluded they are, street lighting, public phones and visible vandalism.

+ Are there enough pedestrian crossings at appropriate places in built-up areas of the community?

+ Does your community have sufficient and safe bike parking facilities at schools, shopping centres, recreation areas and public transport stations?

*Recreation areas can include parks, beaches, sporting grounds, skate parks, etc.   **Tally   /11**

Scores

0-4
Your community seems to be lacking in activity-friendly town planning. Which areas are in most need of improvement? How can you be part of creating change? Check out The Parents Jury's Activity Friendly Communities campaign for advocacy tips and suggestions to get you started – www.parentsjury.org.au.

5-7
Your community has a moderate amount of facilities to promote active living, but residents could always benefit from more. Are there some aspects that could do with improvement? Be active in creating change! Check out The Parents Jury's Activity Friendly Communities campaign for advocacy tips and suggestions to get you started – www.parentsjury.org.au.

8-11
It seems like you live in a very activity-friendly area, congratulations. Be an 'active living family' by making use of these facilities with your children regularly. Daily physical exercise sets a good example for children and benefits their health now and into the future.

Figure 1.3 Active community checklist. www.parentsjury.org.au. Reproduced by permission

While this book focuses primarily on the occupational therapy practitioner engaging with children and their families at an individual, group or family level, it also addresses occupation-centred practice in school environments (Chapter 11), and in the context of community-based leisure pursuits (Chapter 12). The broader benefits of occupational engagement for children who are deprived of occupations are not specifically addressed; however, readers are encouraged to consider the opportunities they may have for advocacy and engagement at a societal and political level in instances where children experience poor health (Spencer, 2008), occupational deprivation, alienation and injustice (see Kronenberg, Simo Algado, & Pollard, 2005; Whiteford & Wright-St Clair, 2005).

Re-affirming occupation: the core of occupational therapy

Over the past several decades, there has been a major focus within occupational therapy on the provision of client-centred services, with its counterparts in child- and family-centred practice. Emanating from Canada, the emphasis on guidelines for enabling occupation- and client-centred practice has spread throughout the occupational therapy profession internationally (Baum & Law, 1997; Canadian Association of Occupational Therapists (CAOT), 1991; Sumsion, 1996). This will be discussed at length in Chapter 3.

There has also been a resurgence of interest in occupation at the core of occupational therapy. This occurred in response to critical reflection by a number of occupational therapy theorists and researchers (e.g. Clark, 1993; Fisher, 1998; Kielhofner, 2007; Molineux, 2004; Pierce, 2001; Yerxa, 1998). This has led to the reclamation of occupation as the defining feature of our profession and practice focused on occupation, its meaning for individuals, its importance for health and well-being (Kielhofner, 2007; Molineux, 2001; Wilcock, 1998) and the importance of an individual's occupational identity as a way of defining self within relevant social and cultural contexts (Christiansen, 1999). The centrality of occupation to occupational therapy practice has been referred to by some as the 'renaissance' of occupation (Whiteford, Townsend, & Hocking, 2000).

This has in turn resulted in a call for the use of occupation-based assessment (Coster, 1998; Hocking, 2001) as a key way of focusing our resulting interventions on the healing power of occupations (e.g. particular schoolwork or play activities), rather than focusing specifically on performance components (e.g. fine motor or visual perceptual skills) that may not lead to significant changes in an individual's occupational functioning. Assessments that facilitate goal setting and those that are occupation-centred will be addressed in detail in Chapters 6 and 7. Paediatric frames of reference have also been developed that specifically enhance children's occupations such as Synthesis of Child, Occupational Performance and Environment in Time (SCOPE-IT) (Haertl, 2009; Poulsen & Ziviani, 2004).

There has also been an increased interest in scholarship about occupation and the growth of a body of research in the field of occupational science. Since the start of the new millennium, there has been an emphasis on meeting the needs of underserved groups with seminal books by Kronenberg et al. (2005) and the writing of advocates of occupational justice (Townsend & Whiteford, 2005; Townsend & Wilcock, 2004; Whiteford, 2002). Townsend and colleagues described occupational alienation (where occupational choice is limited by external forces), occupational apartheid (where individuals are denied access to meaningful occupation due to organised political or social agendas) and occupational deprivation (prolonged blocking of access to meaningful occupation due to environmental restrictions) (Polatajko et al., 2007; Townsend & Whiteford, 2005; Townsend & Wilcock, 2004). Children may be caught up in war zones and refugee camps where they experience occupational alienation or are victims of neglect and impoverished environments. Coinciding with these trends within occupational therapy, a number of global influences and other changes within health/social care systems have occurred which have also impacted on our practice.

External influences impacting occupational therapy practice

Changes in health and social care impacting on occupational therapy practice include: (1) the emergence of evidence-based practice (Sackett, Rosenberg, Gray, Haynes, & Richardson, 1996; Taylor, 2007; Whiteford, 2005); (2) managed health care (Pierce, 2003) and health care reform (Trombly, 1993); (3) increased incidence of lifestyle-related diseases (e.g. Rippe, Crossley, & Ringer, 1998; Sokol, 2000); (4) diseases of meaning such as mental illness (Christiansen, 1999); (5) increasingly informed consumers; and (6) increased global awareness of human rights' abuses amongst marginalised groups, refugees and asylum seekers (many of whom are children) (Kronenberg et al., 2005). Figure 1.4 illustrates the influences both external to and within the profession that have led to the evolution of occupation-centred practice with children and families.

Several recent newspaper headlines in Brisbane, Queensland, in 2008 suggest there is a lot to be concerned about, such as adult beauty treatments for children: 'Making princesses: Beauty treats for girls aged 5–14 years' (*Courier Mail*, 4 May 2008), the impact of busy lives on children: 'We're more selfish – Busy stressful lives leave little time for others' (*Courier Mail*, 4 May 2008), and others. Such societal concerns reinforce the importance of vigilance and for our profession to contribute to the enhancement of children's health and well-being.

Furthermore, in service contexts, reduced funding, mergers and new models of care (e.g. clinical pathways, diagnostic-related groups and managed care) have changed the way allied health services are delivered in the health/human service sectors (Layman & Bamberg, 2003). From a health sector

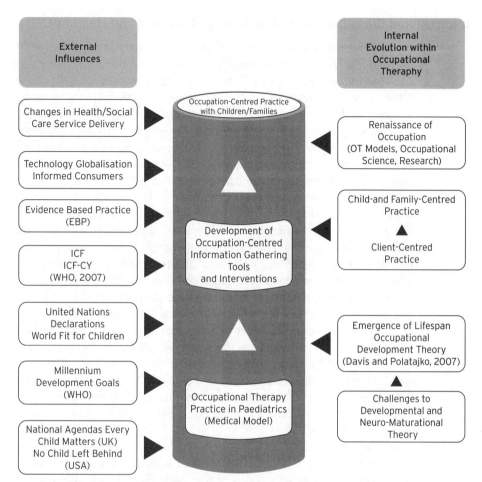

Figure 1.4 External influences and internal evolution within the profession leading to occupation-centred practice with children and families

perspective, significant changes have occurred with respect to financing and the organisation of health care (such as programme management and regionalisation) and service delivery such as technological advances impacting on life span, quality of life and the shift of care from institutions to the community (Layman & Bamberg, 2003).

According to Wood (1998), occupational therapists have not easily implemented occupation-centred and evidence-based practices. Wood, Towers, and Malchow (2000) have challenged us to think outside the box to fully meet the occupational wants and needs of persons receiving our services. Chapter 15 highlights how professional reasoning can be utilised along with evidence-based and occupation-centred practice to better meet the needs of the children and families. The next section turns to international classifications/frameworks and declarations that have impacted on our practice.

International Classification of Functioning, Disability and Health (ICF)

On the international stage, the World Health Organisation (WHO, 2001) released the *ICF* which evolved from earlier iterations – *International Classification of Impairments, Disabilities and Handicaps* (ICIDH) (Wood, 1980). It was proposed as a scientific framework for understanding and studying health and health-related states, outcomes and determinants. Its authors also argued that it would enhance communication between health care workers, researchers and the public by providing a classification system for a person with a given health condition (WHO, 2001) (see Figure 1.5). This re-conceptualisation outlined the impact of a health condition on an individual's functioning at the levels of body structures and functions, activities and participation. The domains of activity and participation are of special interest to occupational therapists and include: learning and applying knowledge, general tasks and demands, communication, mobility, self-care, domestic life, interpersonal interactions and relationships, major life areas, and community, social and civic life (WHO, 2001). Equally it illustrates the importance of understanding the personal characteristics and environmental factors that impact on how a health condition may be experienced and how these may help or hinder the person's engagement in activities and participation in life situations. Under environmental factors, one needs to consider the physical, social and attitudinal environment in which people live and conduct their lives. Personal factors, though not classified in the ICF, comprise features such as a person's gender, race and age, which are features of an individual but not part of a health condition or health states.

In adopting a 'biopsychosocial' approach (WHO, 2001), the ICF acknowledges not only the bi-directional impact of body functions on the ability to perform activities and hence enable participation, but also the fact that environmental factors can impact on the performance and even modify body function and structures. The *International Classification of Functioning, Disability and Health for Children and Youth* (ICF-CY) (WHO, 2007) recently became available for the purpose of recording characteristics

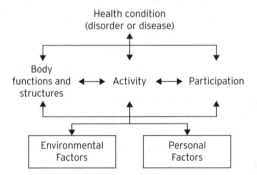

Figure 1.5 Interactions between the components of ICF (WHO, 2001). Reproduced with permission from the World Health Organization.

of the developing child and the influence of his/her environment. For children, the mediating roles of environment and development are highly significant as their environments change across the stages of infancy, early childhood, middle childhood and adolescence. In addition, adults, usually parents/ carers or teachers, exercise significant control over children's environments and opportunities for engagement. There are a number of assessments available for children that are compatible with the components of the ICF (see Simeonsson et al., 2003); however, there is still a need for more assessment tools to address the developmental needs of children, particularly at the level of participation. These will be discussed further in Chapter 7.

The ICF classification system and framework have proven useful for occupational therapists and other health team members in conceptualising where they provide the most input/expertise in assisting the individual manage and promote his/her health and well-being. In contrast to its predecessor, it provides a more global view of health and well-being that is highly consistent with occupational therapy philosophy and practice (Baum & Baptiste, 2002), particularly with its emphasis on participation (Christiansen, Baum, & BassHaugen, 2005). Health professionals endorse best practice interventions that effectively support a person's meaningful and satisfactory participation in real life activities and situations (Law & Baum, 1998; WHO, 2001). With the availability of ICF-CY, occupational therapists working with children and their families can use this version to consider a child's development in health, education and social sectors (WHO, 2007).

United Nations declarations

World fit for children

Other global declarations have also developed in parallel with the work of the WHO, such as the United Nations' (2002) declaration of a *World Fit for Children* (WFFC), an action plan with 21 goals and targets for improving children's welfare (e.g. eradicating poverty, caring for every child, educating, protecting from harm and war, combating HIV/AIDS, listening to children and ensuring their participation, and environmental protection). Most pertinently, the declaration acknowledges the rights of children and young people for self-expression and participation in all matters relating to themselves according to their age and maturity. Consistent with this declaration, the Canadian Association of Occupational Therapists (CAOT) produced a position statement on Healthy Occupations for Children and Youth (CAOT, 2004). This position paper recognises that children and youth have the right for opportunities to develop healthy patterns of occupations and outlines CAOT's approach to advocacy for children and youth to protect and fulfil this right. In addition, the statement recognises the inequities and occupational injustices that limit children's and young people's opportunities for engagement in healthy occupations (e.g. indigenous youth, immigrants, refugees, children with disabilities and those living in poverty or care/protection). The role of occupational therapists – in advocacy and taking collective action at multiple levels (systems, provincial/state and national raised in this document) – is exemplary.

Millennium development goals

Another important United Nations' declaration is the *Millennium Development Goals* (MDGs; United Nations, 2000). The MDGs agreed to in 2000 range from halving extreme poverty to halting the spread of HIV/AIDS and providing universal primary education, by the target date of 2015. These have been agreed to by all the world's countries and leading development institutions. They have spurred international efforts to meet the needs of the world's poorest citizens, many of them being vulnerable children. The eight goals are to:

(1) eradicate extreme poverty and hunger
(2) achieve universal primary education
(3) promote gender equality and empower women
(4) improve child mortality (by two-thirds for children under 5 years)
(5) improve maternal health
(6) combat HIV/AIDS, malaria and other diseases
(7) ensure environmental sustainability
(8) develop a global partnership for development.

A recognition of these goals taps into occupational therapy's interest in social justice and preventing occupational deprivation and alienation (Townsend & Whiteford, 2005; Townsend & Wilcock, 2004) experienced by individuals, especially children, in countries affected by war, natural disasters and occupation forces, where issues of extreme poverty, lack of education, poor health outcomes due to sanitation issues, lack of clean water, low rates of immunisation and infectious diseases are pervasive. While in Western developed countries we do not face these issues on a daily basis, there continue to be examples of children who are disadvantaged through poverty, domestic violence, child abuse and neglect, and lack of appropriate housing in many large cities and rural locations where there are large indigenous communities. See Chapter 4 for a discussion of the cultural implications of occupation-centred practice. As a profession and as individuals, we still have an obligation to reflect and take action to improve the situations in which future generations of children grow and develop.

The evolution of occupational therapy practice with children

Paediatric occupational therapy researchers have supported the renaissance of occupation and have made very strong calls for a better understanding of the essence of children's occupations and their optimal participation. Some examples are illustrative. Lawlor (2003) called for a better understanding of the significance of 'being occupied' and the social construction of childhood occupations, given that children do so many things 'with' significant others (e.g. parents, siblings, peers and teachers). She argued that occupations are socially co-constructed and negotiated with others. Hence, how children interpret and engage in their everyday social worlds is pivotal to our under-standing of human development and childhood occupations. Understanding the social engagement of children during their 'doing' of occupations is critical so that we can optimise their participation. More recently, specific frames of reference have been described that focus on enhancing social participation (Olson, 2009) in recognition of the social nature of many occupations.

Equally Segal and Hinojosa (2006) argued that we need to better appre-ciate the contexts or settings in which childhood occupations occur. They researched the 'doing of homework' as an example of a productive occupation that occurred at home. In order to better assist children and parents with this, at times stressful occupation, we need to understand the activities, tasks, values and goals of children and their parents and the social inter-actions that occur around the task performance. Further, Larson (2004) called for an understanding of children's work/productivity occupations and children's decisions about whether activities are work or play. Her qualitative study explored chores and schoolwork tasks and how parents graded children's participation in household tasks with age. She also docu-mented the scaffolds, supports and supervision provided to enable task completion. The application of such occupational science research focus-ing on understanding occupations helps occupational therapy clinicians to better support parents and children with issues related to a broad range of occupations.

Changing views of child development and maturation

A decade ago, Coster (1998) proposed that one of the largest obstacles to practitioners becoming more occupation-centred (especially in assessment) was the dominance of the developmental model. This model promulgates development as linear and emphasises performance components and abili-ties and was seen as a critical determinant of children's behaviour. Major criticisms of this model are that it: (1) lacks extensive consideration of the context (environment) and the characteristics of the child (person) such as a focus on personal goals, motivation and temperament; and (2) ignores multiple developmental pathways (Horowitz, 2000). The pervasive use of standardised developmental tests and interventional approaches aiming to normalise underlying developmental processes continues to feature strongly in paediatric practice 10 years later. Coster (1998) argued for a focus on the primacy of tasks/activities and occupations and the environmental context in organising a person's behaviour.

Alternate theories of development such as dynamical systems theory (Thelen, 1995) and motor behaviour/motor relearning theories (Mathiowetz &

Bass Haugen, 1994) challenge occupational therapists to reconsider their views about children's developmental progress as being reflex orientated, neuro-maturational and hierarchical in nature. They also challenge the previously accepted linear nature of development expressed as genetically pre-determined ages and stages. The traditional models also failed to address the role of the environment in motor control.

Systems models such as dynamical systems theory (Mathiowetz & Bass Haugen, 1994) have been proposed based on a heterarchical model that focuses on the interaction of a person with his/her environment and also emphasises task performance as well as the unique task and environmental constraints. Both functional tasks and the environmental context are used to organise behaviour. Use or modification of personal and environmental constraints leads to optimal strategy development for functional task performance. This approach arose from an ecological view of perception and action by Gibson (1966) and Bernstein (1967) cited in Mathiowetz and Bass Haugen (1994). This ecological approach focuses on studying the person–environment interaction during daily functional tasks. Some occupational therapy models related to these concepts include the Ecological Model of Human Performance (Dunn, Brown, & McGuigan, 1994), Person-Environment-Occupation Model (Law et al., 1996) and the Person-Environment-Occupation-Performance Model (Christiansen & Baum, 1997; Christiansen et al., 2005).

Dynamical systems (Thelen, 1995) acknowledge that order and patterns emerge from the interaction and cooperation of many systems that lead to self-organisation. This model explains the relative stability of movement patterns in the face of efficient movement requiring the least amount of energy (attractor states). The reciprocity between person and environment is also emphasised. Mathiowetz and Bass Haugen (1994) proposed a systems model of motor control for occupational therapy, illustrating the interaction between the personal characteristics or systems of the person (sensorimotor, cognitive and psychosocial) and the environment (physical, socioeconomic and cultural) that leads to occupational performance (ADL, work and play/leisure) enabling role performance. This illustrates the role of many systems in determining occupational performance outcomes (see Figure 1.6).

The traditional view of development incorporating invariable stages guided therapists' intervention using developmental milestones to mark progress and led to the extensive use of reflex testing and developmental assessment, with normal developmental sequences being the organising framework for therapy. While the emphasis was on working at the child's developmental level, it has lacked a focus on functional tasks. These were considered to result in splinter skills that would not generalise and might interfere with developmental sequences. However, contemporary theories of motor learning view nervous system maturation as only one influence with other systems having important roles to play. Motor learning relies on practice or experience leading to changes in the capabilities of the learner using random rather

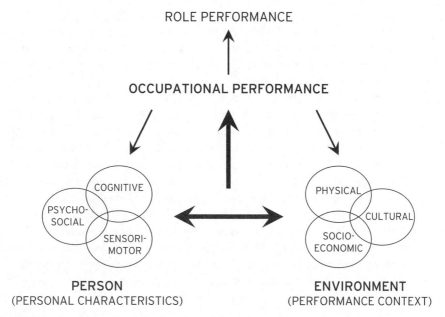

ROLE PERFORMANCE

OCCUPATIONAL PERFORMANCE

COGNITIVE

PSYCHO-SOCIAL

SENSORI-MOTOR

PHYSICAL

CULTURAL

SOCIO-ECONOMIC

PERSON
(PERSONAL CHARACTERISTICS)

ENVIRONMENT
(PERFORMANCE CONTEXT)

Figure 1.6 A systems model of motor control emphasising that occupational perform-ance emerges from an interaction of personal characteristics and performance contexts. In addition, any occupational performance affects the environment and the person. From Mathiowetz and Bass Haugen (1994) 48(8): 738). Reproduced with permission from the American Occupational Therapy Association

than blocked practice and practice of the whole rather than parts of the task. It also focuses on the use of physical and verbal guidance during practice and the use of feedback (e.g. intermittent, random and after multiple trials) (Mathiowetz & Bass Haugen, 1994).

Ongoing research with individuals with disabilities and in naturalistic versus lab/clinic-based settings is needed. Cognitive Orientation to daily Occupational Performance (CO-OP) (Polatajko & Mandich, 2004) is an example of an occupation-centred intervention based on contemporary views of development and motor control that has been evaluated with chil-dren with a range of occupational performance problems (see Chapter 8). The contemporary approaches to motor skill acquisition focus on the goal of helping clients to become competent problem solvers when they engage in functional tasks within relevant performance contexts. Similarly, Perceive, Recall, Plan and Perform (PRPP) (Chapparo & Ranka, 1997a, b) and Occupational Performance Coping (Graham, Rodger, & Ziviani, 2009) provide other examples of occupation-centred interventions discussed in this book (Chapters 9 and 10, respectively).

Occupational therapists such as Humphry (2002) claimed that we know little about the role of occupational engagement as both a process for and outcome of development, nor about children as developing occupational beings. She challenged us to research occupation and to foreground our occupational knowledge with respect to how early childhood health and educational professionals are learning to view children's developmental progress. Humphry (2002) argued that there has been an over-reliance by occupational therapists on other disciplines such as psychology for our understanding of child development and maturation processes, and a lack of reliance on understanding the impact of context and dynamical systems theory. She also proposed that occupational engagement leads to the enhancement of developmental processes, skill acquisition and performance refinement. Through occupation or children's 'doing' their development progresses, skills are acquired and tasks/activities are mastered; hence, occupation is regarded as a crucible for development. Further, she cogently posited a conceptual model that development of the occupational being does not just occur within the child. Participation in family life and sharing activities with significant others have been proposed as crucial developmental mechanisms. Hence, the importance of context and social interaction are highlighted as critical to children's learning about and doing of occupations (Muhlenhaupt, 2009; Olson, 2009). These are congruent with family- and child-centred practice and the use of naturalistic settings involving the child's natural social partners.

Emerging views about occupational development

Only in the past 5 years has there been a significant focus on occupational development across the life span as distinct to traditional views of the linear stages of child and adolescent development. Davis and Polatajko (2006) described occupational development as a 'systematic process of change in occupational behaviours across time, resulting from growth and maturation of the individual in interaction with the environment' (p. 138). This development results in a life course occupational repertoire that is marked by changes in the specific occupations that individuals perform across the life course. They argued that infants are occupational beings from the outset and that the occupations engaged in develop and change over time. They are unique to the individual as they result from the interaction of the person and his/her skills, talents and interests with the opportunities and events that life presents. Typically these occupations change gradually and predictably over the course of development and as a result of transitions but change may be sudden due to loss, disease or injury (Polatajko et al., 2007). Davis and Polatajko (2006) postulated that occupational development occurs at micro, meso and macro levels.

Micro-occupational development focuses on developing occupational competence along a continuum of novice to mastery for a specific occupation (Davis & Polatajko, 2006) and is repeated for each new occupation. While the trajectory and speed is individual, it is dependent on the child's ability, capacity, growth and maturation as well as the supports and opportunities in place to enable competency development. *Meso-occupational development* focuses on developing an occupational repertoire. This repertoire of developing competence and mastery changes across the life span expanding and shrinking. Innate drive, exposure, resources, opportunities and values influence the development of this repertoire (Wiseman, Davis, & Polatajko, 2005). *Macro-occupational development* or development of occupations results from exposure and opportunities. This development occurs across time with species evolution (Davis & Polatajko). This may be exemplified by the development of new occupations in recent years such as listening to iPods® and Nintendo Wii® activities which did not exist a decade ago. *Occupational transitions* occur when there is shift from one set of occupations to an alternative set as a result of life events or developmental processes such as moving from preschool/kindergarten to school. These occur at individual, group (e.g. nuclear to single-parent family) or societal levels (e.g. unemployment in a small town due to a particular industry closing down) (Polatajko et al., 2007).

Gender, cultural, socioeconomic, societal and other factors influence occupations across the life course such as the required time in the armed forces for young men at age 18 years, the increased age of women having their first child, leaving the labour force for child-raising purposes, etc. (Polatajko et al., 2007). Occupational loss is described as an imposed or unanticipated transition which typically results from environmental factors (e.g. parental unemployment leading to children not being able to continue with extra-curricular activities) or permanent or temporary loss of body functions due to illness/injury (e.g. child who acquires a head injury after a bicycle accident or is disfigured as a result of burns). Macro-environmental losses may occur as a result of natural disasters such as destruction after a tsunami, bushfire or earthquake leading to relocation and issues with basic survival needs (e.g. food, water, shelter and basic care routines) (Polatajko et al.). It is important for occupational therapists working with children and adults to keep abreast of this growing theoretical understanding of development from an occupational perspective, focusing on occupational roles, associated occupations and the environmental impacts on development. Further theoretical and research work in this area will enhance our capacity to be more occupation-centred in our practice.

Refocusing occupational therapy with children

Arguably in the past, the occupational therapy profession has failed to realise that one of our most significant contributions is our focus on children's roles, their occupations, the contexts in which they live, work and play, as well as our interest in their priorities and goals. Occupational therapy as a profession offers a unique approach to intervention which focuses on occupational performance and participation when children's lives are impacted by illness, disability and social or environmental deprivation or disadvantage. This book promotes an occupation-centred approach to practice with children and their families. It introduces an occupation-centred occupational therapy process for working with children based on existing processes utilised with adults.

Conceptually, occupation-centred practice for children allows occupational therapists to focus appropriately on the child (and family), the child's and family's occupations, and environments during the stages of information gathering, intervention and evaluation within a client-centred practice framework. This process is described in detail in Chapter 2.

By focusing on the person, his/her environment and occupations, the therapist is able to optimise the child's and family's participation in relevant life situations, the latter being the critical outcome of any occupational therapy intervention. One of the key messages of this book is that to be *relevant*, occupational therapy intervention must extend beyond the acquisition of skills and occupations to the optimisation of children's engagement in their life roles (Case-Smith, 2007). The ultimate aim of occupational therapy is to promote children's competence and participation at home, school and in their communities. An individual child's level of participation reflects the child's capacities, the opportunities available, the social and physical supports present (environmental affordances) and the family's and society's values about participation. Drawing from the literature, key characteristics of occupation-centred practice for children are introduced in Chapter 2. Knowing these characteristics will enable occupational therapists to evaluate whether their daily practice with children is truly occupation-centred, enabling practitioners to make informed choices about what they do and how they do it.

Conclusion

In conclusion, in applying an occupation-centred approach to practice with children, it is important that therapists are cognisant of contemporary frameworks in health care such as the ICF, concepts such as evidence-based practice and child- and family-centred practice, and are aware of the global trends that have impacted service delivery in health/ human services sectors. In addition, such practice focuses on the activities and participation levels of the ICF and on occupations related to children's social and occupational roles. Therapists must also consider the evidence suggesting the theoretical limitations of traditional views of child development and neuro-maturation and be open to contemporary theories of motor behaviour and learning, occupational development and child- and family-centred practice. This chapter has also challenged occupational therapists to act as individuals as well as members of a profession to advocate for societies that better enable children's participation in safe and supportive environments and developmentally appropriate life situations. This requires a global consciousness that recognises the impacts of natural disasters, poverty, ill health, and social, cultural and temporal environmental stressors on children's optimal development and participation.

References

American Academy of Pediatrics. (n.d.). *Children's health topics: Parenting*. Retrieved 13 March 2009 from http://www.aap.org/healthtopics/parenting.cfm.

Baum, C., & Baptiste, S. (2002). Reframing occupational therapy practice. In M. Law, C. Baum, & S. Baptiste (Eds.), *Occupation-based practice: Fostering performance and participation* (pp. 3–15). Thorofare, NJ: SLACK Incorporated.

Baum, C. M., & Law, M. (1997). Occupational therapy practice: Focusing on occupational performance. *American Journal of Occupational Therapy, 51*(4), 277-288.

Canadian Association of Occupational Therapists (CAOT). (1991). *Occupational therapy guidelines for client centred practice*. Toronto, ON: CAOT Publications ACE.

Canadian Association of Occupational Therapists (CAOT). (2004). Health occupations for children and youth. CAOT Position Statement. *Canadian Journal of Occupational Therapy, 71*(3), 182–183.

Case-Smith, J. (2007). Deriving practice implications from this issue's sample of pediatric occupational therapy research literature. *American Journal of Occupational Therapy, 61*, 375–377.

Chapparo, C., & Ranka, J. (1997a). *Occupational Performance Model – Australia monograph*. Sydney, NSW: Unpublished manuscript.

Chapparo, C., & Ranka, J. (1997b). The perceive, recall, plan and perform system of task analysis. In C. Chapparo, & J. Ranka (Eds.), *Occupational performance model (Australia): Monograph 1* (pp. 189–198). Sydney: Total Print Control.

Christiansen, C. (1999). Defining lives: An essay on competence, coherence and the creation of meaning. *American Journal of Occupational Therapy, 53*, 547-558.

Christiansen, C., & Baum, C. (1997). Person–environment–occupational performance: A conceptual model for practice. In C. Baum, & C. H. Christiansen (Eds.), *Occupational therapy: Enabling function and well-being* (2nd ed., pp. 47–70). Thorofare, NJ: SLACK Incorporated.

Christiansen, C., Baum, C., & Bass-Haugen, J. (Eds.). (2005). *Occupational therapy: Performance, participation and well-being* (3rd ed.). Thorofare, NJ: SLACK Incorporated.

Clark, F. (1993). Occupation embedded in a real life: Interweaving occupational science and occupational therapy. *American Journal of Occupational Therapy, 47*, 1067-1077.

Coster, W. (1998). Occupation-centred assessment of children. *American Journal of Occupational Therapy, 52*, 227–344.

Davis, J. A., & Polatajko, H. J. (2006). The occupational development of children. In S. Rodger, & J. Ziviani (Eds.), *Occupational therapy for children: Understanding children's occupations and enabling participation* (pp. 136–157). Oxford, UK: Blackwell Science.

Dunn, W., Brown, C., & McGuigan, A. (1994). The ecology of human performance: A framework for considering the effect of context. *American Journal of Occupational Therapy, 48*, 595–607.

Fisher, A. G. (1998). Uniting practice and theory in an occupational framework. *American Journal of Occupational Therapy, 52*, 509–521.

Graham, F., Rodger, S., & Ziviani, J. (2009). Coaching parents to enable children's participation: An approach to working with parents and their children. *Australian Occupational Therapy Journal, 56*(1), 16-23.

Haertl, K. (2009). A frame of reference to enhance children's occupations: SCOPE-IT. In P. Kramer, & J. Hinojosa (Eds.), *Frames of reference for pediatric occupational therapy* (2nd ed., pp. 266-305). Philadelphia, PA: Lippincott Williams & Wilkins.

Hocking, C. (2001). Implementing occupation-based assessment. *American Journal of Occupational Therapy, 55*(4), 463-469.

Horowitz, E. D. (2000). Child development and the PITS: Simple questions, complex answers and developmental theory. *Child Development, 71,* 1-10.

Humphry, R. (2002). Young children's occupations: Explicating the dynamics of developmental processes. *American Journal of Occupational Therapy, 56,* 171-179.

Kielhofner, G. (2007). *The model of human occupation: Theory and application* (4th ed.). Baltimore, MD: Lippincott Williams & Wilkins.

Kronenberg, F., Simo Algado, S., & Pollard, N. (Eds.). (2005). *Occupational therapy without borders: Learning from the spirit of survivors.* London, UK: Elsevier, Churchill Livingstone.

Larson, E. A. (2004). Children's work: The less considered occupation. *American Journal of Occupational Therapy, 58,* 369-379.

Law, M., & Baum, C. (1998). Evidence based practice. *Canadian Journal of Occupational Therapy, 65*(3), 131-135 (Special Issue).

Law, M., Cooper, B., Strong, S., Stewart, D., Rigby, P., & Letts, L. (1996). The person-environment-occupation model: A transactive approach to occupational performance. *Canadian Journal of Occupational Therapy, 63,* 9-23.

Lawlor, M. C. (2003). The significance of being occupied: The social construction of childhood occupations. *American Journal of Occupational Therapy, 57,* 424-434.

Layman, E. J., & Bamberg, R. (2003). Coping with a turbulent health care environment: An integrative literature review. *Journal of Allied Health, 35,* 50-60.

Mathiowetz, V., & Bass Haugen, J. (1994). Motor behavior research: Implications for approaches to CNS dysfunction. *American Journal of Occupational Therapy, 48,* 733-745.

Molineux, M. (2001). Occupation: The two sides of popularity. *Australian Occupational Therapy Journal, 48,* 92-95.

Molineux, M. (2004). Occupation in occupational therapy: A labour in vain? In M. Molineux (Ed.), *Occupation for occupational therapists* (pp. 17-31). Oxford, UK: Blackwell Science.

Muhlenhaupt, M. (2009). The perspective of context as related to frame of reference. In P. Kramer, & J. Hinojosa (Eds.), *Frames of reference for pediatric occupational therapy* (3rd ed., pp. 67-95). Philadelphia, PA: Lippincott Williams Wilkins.

Occupational Opportunities for Refugees and Asylum Seekers (OOFRAS). (n.d.). *Occupational opportunities for refugees and asylum seekers.* Retrieved 13 March 2009 from http://www.oofras.com/rs/7/sites/177/user_uploads/File/OOFRAS%20Brochure.pdf (brochure).

Olson, L. J. (2009). A frame of reference to enhance social participation. In P. Kramer, & J. Hinojosa (Eds.), *Frames of reference for pediatric occupational therapy* (3rd ed., pp. 306-348). Philadelphia, PA: Walters Kluwer, Lippincott Williams & Wilkins.

Pierce, D. (2001). Occupation by design: Dimensions, therapeutic power and creative process. *American Journal of Occupational Therapy, 55,* 249-259.

Pierce, D. (2003). How can the occupation base of occupational therapy be strengthened? *Australian Occupational Therapy Journal, 50,* 1-2.

Polatajko, H. J., & Mandich, A. D. (2004). *Enabling occupation in children: The cognitive orientation to daily occupational performance (CO-OP) approach.* Ottawa, ON: CAOT Publications ACE.

Polatajko, H. J., Molke, D., Baptiste, S., Doble, S., Caron Santha, J., Kirsh, B., et al. (2007). Occupational science: Imperatives for occupational therapy. In E. Townsend, & H. Polatajko (Eds.), *Enabling occupation II: Advancing an occupational therapy vision for health, well-being and justice through occupation* (pp. 63–86). Ottawa, ON: CAOT Publications ACE.

Poulsen, A. A., & Ziviani, J. M. (2004). Health enhancing physical activity: Factors influencing engagement patterns in children. *Australian Occupational Therapy Journal, 51*, 69–79.

Rippe, J. M., Crossley, S., & Ringer, R. (1998). Obesity as a chronic disease: Modern medical and lifestyle management. *Journal of the American Dietetic Association, 98*, S9–S15.

Rodger, S., & Ziviani, J. (2006). Children, their occupations and environments in contemporary society. In S. Rodger, & J. Ziviani (Eds.), *Occupational therapy for children: Understanding children's occupations and enabling participation* (pp. 3–21). Oxford, UK: Blackwell Science.

Sackett, D. L., Rosenberg, W. M., Gray, J. A., Haynes, R. B., & Richardson, W. S. (1996). Evidence based medicine: What is it and what it isn't. *British Medical Journal, 312*(7023), 71–72.

Segal, R., & Hinojosa, J. (2006). The activity setting of homework: An analysis of three cases and implications for occupational therapy. *American Journal of Occupational Therapy, 60*, 50–59.

Simeonsson, R. J., Leonardi, M., Lollars, D., Bjorck-Akesson, E., Hollenweger, J., & Martinuzzi, A. (2003). Applying the international classification of functioning, disability and health (ICF) to measure childhood disability. *Disability and Rehabilitation, 25*(11–12), 602–610.

Sokol, R. J. (2000). The chronic disease of childhood obesity: The sleeping giant has awakened. *Journal of Pediatrics, 136*, 711–713.

Spencer, N. (2008). European Society for Social Pediatrics and Child Health position statement. *Child: Care, Health & Development, 34*, 631–634.

Sumsion, T. (1996). Implementation issues. In T. Sumsion (Ed.), *Client-centred practice in occupational therapy: A guide to implementation* (pp. 27–37). London, UK: Churchill Livingstone.

Taylor, C. M. (2007). *Evidence based practice for occupational therapists* (2nd ed.). Oxford, UK: Wiley Blackwell.

The Parents' Jury. (2008). *Active communities checklist.* Retrieved 13 March 2009 from http://www.parentsjury.org.au/tpj_article.asp?ContentID=afc_advocacy.

Thelen, E. (1995). Motor development: A new synthesis. *American Psychologist, 50*(2), 79–95.

Townsend, E., & Whiteford, G. (2005). A participatory occupational justice framework: Population based processes of practice. In F. Kronenberg, S. Simo Algada, & N. Pollard (Eds.), *Occupational therapy without borders: Learning from the spirit of survivors* (pp. 110–127). London, UK: Elsevier, Churchill Livingstone.

Townsend, E., & Wilcock, A. (2004). Occupational justice and client centred practice: A dialogue in progress. *Canadian Journal of Occupational Therapy, 71*(2), 75–87.

Trombly, C. (1993). Anticipating the future: Assessment of occupational function. *American Journal of Occupational Therapy, 47*(3), 253–257.

United Nations. (2000). *Millennium development goals: End poverty 2015.* Retrieved 13 March 2009 from http://www.un.org/millenniumgoals/.

United Nations. (2002). *World fit for children*. New York: United Nations Children's Fund. Retrieved 13 March 2009 from http://www.worldfitforchildren.com/.

Whiteford, G. (2002). Occupation: The essential nexus between philosophy, theory and practice. *Australian Occupational Therapy Journal, 49*, 1-2.

Whiteford, G. (2005). Knowledge, power, evidence: A critical analysis of key issues in evidence based practice. In G. Whiteford, & V. Wright-St Clair (Eds.), *Occupation and practice in context* (pp. 34-50). Merrickville, NSW: Elsevier Australia.

Whiteford, G., Townsend, E., & Hocking, C. (2000). Reflections on the renaissance of occupation. *Canadian Journal of Occupational Therapy, 67*(1), 61-69.

Whiteford, G., & Wright-St Clair, V. (2005). *Occupation and practice in context*. Merrickville, NSW: Elsevier Australia.

Wilcock, A. (1998). *An occupational perspective of health*. Thorofare, NJ: SLACK Incorporated.

Wiseman, J. O., Davis, J., & Polatajko, H. J. (2005). Occupational development: Understanding why children do the things they do. *Journal of Occupational Science, 12*(1), 26-35.

Wood, P. H. N. (1980). Appreciating the consequences of disease: The International Classification of Impairments, Disabilities, and Handicaps. *WHO Chronicle, 34*, 376-380.

Wood, W. (1998). Is it jump time for occupational therapy? *American Journal of Occupational Therapy, 52*, 403-411.

Wood, W., Towers, L., & Malchow, J. (2000). Environment time use and adaptedness in prosimians: Implications for discerning behavior that is occupational. *Journal of Occupational Science, 7*, 5-18.

World Federation of Occupational Therapists (WFOT). (2006). *Position Statement on Human Rights*. Retrieved 13 March 2009 from http://www.wfot.org/office_files/Human%20Rights%20Position%20Statement%20Final%20NLH(1).pdf.

World Health Organisation (WHO). (2001). *International Classification of Functioning, Disability and Health (ICF)*. Geneva, Switzerland: WHO.

World Health Organisation (WHO). (2007). *International Classification of Functioning, Disability and Health (ICF): Children and youth version*. Geneva, Switzerland: WHO.

Yerxa, E. J. (1998). Health and the human spirit for occupation. *American Journal of Occupational Therapy, 52*, 413-418.

Chapter 2

Becoming more Occupation-centred When Working with Children

Sylvia Rodger

Learning objectives

The specific chapter objectives are to:

- Describe the theoretical underpinnings of practice with children in terms of relevant occupational therapy theories, models and frames of reference.
- Highlight the differences between 'top-down' and 'bottom-up' approaches to assessment and intervention.
- Outline the characteristics of occupation-centred practice with children.
- Describe an occupation-centred practice process for working with children and families.

Introduction

Occupation-based practice places enablement of occupation, namely individuals' meaningful performance of occupational roles and tasks in everyday contexts as the defining element of occupational therapy (Law, Baum, & Baptiste, 2002). The aim of this chapter is to assist occupational therapy students and practitioners to become more occupation-centred when working with children and their families.

In this chapter, I will not describe the range of models and frames of reference underlying occupation-centred practice. However, this does not mean that a detailed conceptual understanding of these is not important. Some of these theoretical models and frameworks for practice with children have been described recently elsewhere (e.g. Dunbar, 2007; Kramer & Hinojosa, 2009). However, what is critical to being an occupation-centred practitioner is having a deep understanding of the theory behind one's practice.

Theoretical underpinnings of occupational therapy with children

At the core of embarking on occupation-centred practice is the choice of a theoretical model that articulates the interaction of the person, the occupation and the environment and the impact of each of these on occupational performance. In this book, I do not expound the superiority of any one occupational performance model over another, but rather recommend that therapists choose one overarching occupational therapy model that is both culturally relevant and appropriate to their practice context. There are many such models to choose from such as Person-Environment-Occupation (Law & Dunbar, 2007), Occupational Performance Model (Australia) (OPM(A)) (Chapparo & Ranka, 1997a), the Model of Human Occupation (MOHO) (Kielhofner, 2007; Kramer & Bowyer, 2007), the Ecological Human Performance Model (Dunn, 2007), the Kawa Model (Iwama, 2006), Person-Environment-Occupation-Performance Model (Christiansen, Baum, & Bass-Haugen, 2005), or the Canadian Model of Occupational Performance - Enablement (CMOP-E) (Townsend & Polatajko, 2007). Their major role is to outline *what occupational therapy is about* and outline the scope or domain of occupational therapy practice, our concerns, values, beliefs and expectations. These models also delineate our expertise as occupational therapists, namely our depth of knowledge of person, environment and occupation, barriers and facilitators to occupational performance, and participation.

However, these models in isolation do not provide sufficient information about *how to go about doing occupational therapy* with any given client. Hence, there is also a need to employ what is commonly referred to in occupational therapy practice with children as frames of reference (Dunbar, 2007; Kramer & Hinojosa, 1999, 2009). Sometimes referred to as 'practice models', these provide more information about the *how*. Some frames of reference include sensory integration (Schaaf et al., 2009), neurodevelopmental treatment (Barthel, 2009; Blanche & Blanche Kiefer, 2007), visual perception (Schneck, 2009), biomechanical (Colangelo & Shea, 2009), acquisitional (Luebben & Brasic Royeen, 2009), psychosocial (Olson, 2009) and social participation (Olson, 2009). Each of these contains assumptions about practice, details of function and dysfunction, postulates regarding change, and assessments and treatment techniques or approaches that are conceptually consistent with the frame of reference (Dunbar, 2007; Kramer & Hinojosa, 2009). The therapist's choice of and combinations of these will depend on the child's and family's presenting concerns, stage of development, underlying condition, its aetiology (e.g. environmental deprivation versus acquired brain injury) (Copley, Turpin, & Bennett, in press), conceptual congruency of the frames of reference (Hinojosa & Kramer, 2009) and the therapist's past experience, clinical reasoning and practice setting (Copley et al., in press). These factors will be considered in detail in Chapter 15 in relation to reasoning, the evidence and decision making.

What is clear from our research is that occupational therapists working with a range of children's ages and conditions use an eclectic mix of frames of reference or models (Brown, Rodger, Brown, & Roever, 2007; Rodger, Brown, & Brown, 2005). This is also the case when they are working specifically with groups of children such as those with cerebral palsy (Berry & Ryan, 2002) or learning disabilities (LD) (Nelson, Copley, Flanigan, & Underwood, 2009). This eclecticism can lead to a conceptual mismatch between the frameworks or models that therapists report that they use and the assessments and techniques applied with various groups of children (Brown et al., 2007; Rodger et al., 2005) unless therapists are clear about the underlying theoretical assumptions regarding each framework (Hinojosa & Kramer, 2009). Nelson et al. (2009) reported that there were significant gaps in therapists' translation of theories and frames of reference to treatment techniques and their use of outcome measures when working with children with LD. These findings suggest that occupational therapists frequently use theoretical models and frameworks that are not conceptually congruent. At best, this practice is not theoretically sound and at worst this incongruence may lead to practice that is neither safe and appropriate, nor efficacious. In order to discuss practice approaches with children further, the terms 'top-down' and 'bottom-up' approaches need to be explored.

Top-down and bottom-up approaches to occupational therapy practice with children

The phrases 'top-down' and 'bottom-up' approaches have been used in the occupational therapy literature since the early to mid-1990s. The term 'top-down' was coined by Trombly (1993) who referred to 'top-down assessment' as inquiry into role competence and meaning, tasks that comprise roles and examination of barriers to task achievement. In this approach, foundational factors such as performance skills (motor, process, communication and interaction skills), patterns (habits, routines and rituals), activity demands and client factors (body structures/functions), also known as performance components, are only considered if required (Trombly, 1993; Weinstock-Zlotnick & Hinojosa, 2004). The American Occupational Therapy Association (AOTA) Occupational Therapy Practice Framework (AOTA Commission on Practice, 2008) specifies a 'top-down' approach that always begins with developing an occupational therapy profile and analysis of occupational performance. Similarly, occupational therapy models such as CMOP-E (Townsend & Polatajko, 2007) and PEO (Law & Dunbar, 2007) primarily support 'top-down' approaches to practice as these are occupation-centred. Frames of reference that are 'top-down' include the acquisitional and visual perception frames of reference as the intervention focus of the former is on skill learning or acquisition for optimal performance within the environment (Royeen & Duncan, 1999), and that of the latter is on enhancing information processing by intervening through enhancing learning or cognitive skills to improve visual output (Schneck, 2009).

In contrast 'bottom-up' approaches consider foundational factors first and foremost to understand a client's limitations and strengths. The focus is on assessment and treatment of components of function such as strength, tone, range of motion (ROM), balance and sensory functions/processing, etc., that are considered pre-requisites for successful occupational performance (Trombly, 1993). This approach is largely associated with acute care hospital settings and those using more traditional reductionist medical models (Weinstock-Zlotnick & Hinojosa, 2004). The assumption that the acquisition of motor, cognitive and affective components will lead directly to functional gains or successful occupational performance has not yet been empirically demonstrated.

Weinstock-Zlotnick and Hinojosa (2004) questioned whether one approach was better than the other. They argued that focusing at the 'bottom-up' level may lead to focusing on intricate details (e.g. grip strength and ROM gains as a result of casting/splinting or Botox® injections) without adequate emphasis on the functional consequences of these gains such as the child's ability to extend arms to don a sweater/pullover. Equally, occupation-centred practice does not easily address acute care situations that are time limited, such as managing a client with an acute burn. In this situation, positioning, ROM, pressure garments and splinting during surgery are critical, in order for a child to progress to long-term goals such as managing self-care with a burn-affected upper limb, re-integration to school and assuming meaningful life roles. It is in acute hospital practice settings where the implementation of occupation-centred practice is most challenging. These acute care practice contexts will be addressed in more detail in Chapter 13. The risk according to Weinstock-Zlotnick and Hinojosa (2004) of focusing exclusively on 'bottom-up' approaches lies in practitioners failing to connect their focus on occupational performance and make these explicit for clients as well as for themselves.

Missiuna, Malloy-Miller, and Mandich (1997) explored the feasibility of moving from a 'bottom-up' to a 'top-down' approach when working with children. They summarised that 'bottom-up' approaches focused on remediating children's skill deficits (impairments), based on the assumption that development of foundational motor skills would allow motor control and task performance to emerge. They exemplified the 'top-down' approach with children with cognitive approaches that were emerging at the time. These approaches focus on utilising cognitive strategies to help children manage daily tasks more effectively, given that the motor requirements for tasks are variable and that motor control becomes more efficient when children understand the task expectations. They claimed that meta-cognition (knowing about ones' cognition) is targeted in the emergent cognitive 'top-down' approaches (Missiuna et al., 1997). Using these interventions, children's motor experiences are organised and integrated with greater cognitive awareness on their part. In order to become more 'top-down' or cognitive in approach, Missiuna et al. (1997) concluded that therapists needed to:

(1) Think about the tasks and roles that a child wants, needs or has to perform rather than the foundational skills (e.g. riding a bike as a task in the child's role as playmate rather than improving balance or bilateral co-ordination as component skills);

(2) Use a general problem-solving structure that allows application of strategies;

(3) Use questioning to increase child's meta-cognitive awareness; and

(4) Plan for transfer and generalisation of learned skills to relevant contexts.

Some of these cognitive approaches are described further in this chapter and in Chapter 8.

Other proponents of a 'top-down' approach when working with children (Marr, 1999) purport that this way of working: (1) sends a message to parents, teachers and other team members about the full scope and depth of occupational therapy practice; (2) focuses assessment necessarily on a broad range of issues, roles and areas of performance, communicating that our scope of practice extends beyond components such as sensory processing and fine motor abilities and encompasses play, socialisation, self-care and classroom skills; and (3) manifests the uniqueness of occupational therapy intervention as practitioners routinely focus on the roles, contexts and priorities of clients. Further she argued that it is critical for occupational therapists to make their clinical reasoning explicit to others so that they understand that occupational therapists' capacity for effecting change goes beyond performance components. Such a 'top-down' approach also enables linking children's goals with school-based curriculum requirements and environmental demands within school settings (Marr, 1999). This will be further illustrated in Chapter 11.

Weinstock-Zlotnick and Hinojosa (2004) proposed that the key difference between the 'top-down' and 'bottom-up' approach lies in Schön's (1987) work about the way problems are framed. This is because the two approaches are based on differing philosophical assumptions resulting from the models or theories and frames of reference that are consistent with each. They proffered that rather than arguing about the supremacy of one approach over the other, both approaches were appropriate to help clients with different presenting issues in various contexts. They cautioned those using a 'top-down' approach to be cognisant of measurability issues such as the limited number of assessment tools that focus on roles, occupations and participation outcomes, and the limitations of this approach in acute care settings. They also posited that the isolated use of the 'bottom-up' approach is flawed due to its lack of focus on occupational and participation outcomes. A comparison of the strengths and limitations of each approach can be found in Table 2.1.

There is somewhat of a division in the profession that has been promoted by discussion of 'top-down approaches' versus 'bottom-up approaches'. While philosophically these approaches have arisen from very different theoretical parison of bottom-up and top-down approaches

ns	Bottom-up approaches	Top-down approaches
...s and frames of reference	*Models*: OPM(A) (Chapparo & Ranka, 1997a)	*Models*: MOHO (Kramer & Bowyer, 2007); PEO (Law & Dunbar, 2007); CMOP-E (Townsend & Polatajko, 2007); Kawa Model (Iwama, 2006); OPM(A) (Chapparo & Ranka, 1997a); OTIP Model (Fisher, 1998); Ecological Model of Human Performance (Dunn, 2007)
	Frames of reference: Sensory Integration (Ayres, 1972; Blanche & Blanche Kiefer, 2007; Kimball, 1999a,b; Parham & Mailloux, 1998); Neurodevelopmental Treatment (NDT) (Blanche & Blanche Kiefer, 2007; Schoen & Anderson, 1999; Stanton, 1997; Weston, Kinley, Hughes, & Fishwick, 1998)	*Frames of reference*: Motor Skill Acquisition (Kaplan & Bedell, 1999); Acquisitional (Luebben & Brasic Royeen, 2009); Visual Information Analysis (Schneck, 2009; Todd, 1999); 4QM (Greber et al., 2007); Conductive Education (Stanton, 1997; Todd, 1990); CO-OP (Polatajko & Mandich, 2004)
Strengths	Easily incorporated with all clients, even those with limited insight, cognition, language, and without family to provide information about roles and occupations	Consistent with the philosophical basis of the profession. Provides occupational therapists with knowledge of domain of concern/area of expertise – occupations
	Compatible with biomedical team philosophies (Law, 1998)	Focuses on the whole person in context
	Appropriate for time-limited physical impairments which require immediate interventions such as fractures/burns/ traumatic brain injury	Identifies clients with occupational dysfunction rather than medical conditions. Engenders professional autonomy
	Focus in detail on the ICF level of body structure and function (WHO, 2001)	Focus on the ICF levels of activities and participation (WHO, 2001)
	Emphasis on remediating impairments, problem focused	Emphasis on adaptation, compensation, prevention, accommodation, skill acquisition

Table 2.1 (Continued)

Considerations	Bottom-up approaches	Top-down approaches
	Deficit orientation	Strengths orientation
	Emphasis on occupation/activity as means	Emphasis on occupation as ends
	Directed by applied scientific inquiry appropriate and ready for clinical use	Directed by understanding client's narratives and increasing evidence of efficacy
	Compatible with acute health care settings	Compatible with community-based, long-term care
Limitations	Frames of reference utilise theory from other disciplines	Difficulties noted with assessment and implementation of this approach (Law, 1998)
	Empirical evidence still lacking	Lacks many valid and reliable measures of outcomes, participation
	Does not prioritise environment (decontextualised service provision)	Can be time consuming to implement
	Less client-centred	More challenging with clients who are culturally and linguistically diverse and those with cognitive limitations
		Requires explanation of abstract concepts (performance, satisfaction, roles and goals)

Adapted and expanded from Weinstock-Zlotnick and Hinojosa (2004, p. 597).

perspectives, there is little empirical evidence that has compared interventions associated with one approach in comparison with the other for particular children with specific occupational performance issues or in particular contexts. In the absence of evidence suggesting the superiority of one approach over the other, occupational therapy clinicians and students are left to make decisions based on their clinical reasoning, the existing evidence (albeit often inconclusive), their expertise, the context in which they work and their clients' and families' needs. The following section describes the characteristics of occupation-centred practice and an occupation-centred practice process that charts the course of therapists' engagement with children and their families from the beginning to the end of therapy engagement, which is more philosophically consistent with a 'top-down' approach.

Characteristics of occupation-centred practice for children

This chapter proposes that occupation-centred practice with children involves 11 characteristics. These are summarised in Table 2.2 and each will be briefly discussed in the following section. These will be expanded upon in subsequent chapters.

Client-centred orientation (child- and family-centred)

Pivotal to occupational therapy is the recognition that client-centredness pervades all stages of service delivery (e.g. Baum & Law, 1997; Fearing & Clark, 2000; Sumsion, 1996). McLaughlin Gray (1998) proposed that occupation-centred interventions must be purposeful and meaningful to the client. This reflects the orientation of occupation-centred interventions as being *client-centred*. When working with children, there is a need to acknowledge both the child and the parents (family) as clients. When practice is occupation-centred, all assessments and interventions need to focus on client-derived priorities with the assumption that children and their families will be active participants in these processes. The complexities of client- and family-centred service provision, the development of collaborative relationships with children and families and family involvement are discussed in detail in Chapter 3. As client-centredness is central to the way occupational therapists work when using an occupation-centred approach, there is also a need to consider the social and cultural contexts of both the client and the therapist. These considerations are addressed further in Chapter 4.

Table 2.2 Characteristics of occupation-centred practice for children

Client-centred orientation (child- and/or family-centred)
Based on collaborative partnerships with child and parents/caregivers
Client-chosen - child and/or parent/family chosen goals
Contextually relevant to child's circumstances
Active engagement of child and parent/s at all stages
Individualised intervention
Focus on occupational performance and participation - at all stages of OT Process (goal setting, assessment, intervention, evaluation)
Information gathering focuses on roles, occupations, occupational performance and environment
Intervention focuses on roles, occupations, occupational performance and environment
Interventions are 'whole' or 'finite' - have a beginning, middle and end.
Occupation-centred evaluation of intervention outcomes

Based on collaborative relationships

When being both child- and family-centred, there is a need to develop trusting partnerships or collaborative relationships with both children and their parents, and other family members as relevant. Occupational therapists' use of interactive reasoning supports the creation of collaborative relationships with clients that actively engage them in intervention processes by fostering motivation and commitment. Therapists employ a number of strategies to encourage the formation and maintenance of these productive, mutually engaging relationships (Mattingly & Fleming, 1994; Turpin, 2004) such as:

- *Creating choices*: Occupational therapists structure situations so that the client has to make a choice. A client's motivation to engage in treatment activities is enhanced through the opportunity to choose between options.
- *Individualising treatment*: Occupational therapists structure and adapt sessions to fit the unique interests and characteristics of their clients, their developmental and occupational status, stage in the intervention process and progress.
- *Structuring success*: This involves clinical judgement related to the capabilities of the client, his/her willingness to 'apply' him/herself and sensitivity to subtle cues about his/her involvement in activities. Validating the client's success is another important consideration as is facilitating a 'just right fit' between client, task complexity and environmental supports.
- *Exchanging stories*: Occupational therapists at times consciously and explicitly exchange personal stories or those of other clients (with due respect to confidentiality) with clients as a means of creating collaborative relationships. This involves careful consideration about how much of the self the therapist should reveal, the impact on the therapeutic alliance and outcomes and how they manage the momentary shift from the client to the therapist being the centre of attention.
- *Joint problem-solving*: Collaborative problem-solving empowers the client and focuses on the partnership acknowledging the clients' own expertise (Turpin, 2004).
- *Ensuring developmental, cultural and gender appropriateness.*

Client-chosen goals (child- and family-chosen goals)

Occupation-centred practice focuses on child- and/or family-chosen goals that emphasise skill acquisition, modification to occupations/tasks and/or environments to enhance the child's performance of meaningful and purposeful occupations and hence their participation. McLaughlin Gray (1998) described this as being goal-directed. This characteristic is detailed further in the information-gathering stage of the occupational therapy process described below and in Chapter 6.

Contextual relevance

McLaughlin Gray (1998) described contextual relevance as a characteristic of occupation-centred interventions, meaning that interventions emphasise people as occupational beings within their own environments. The ultimate objective is to enhance the child's participation in relevant life situations. Occupational therapists understand children's roles and occupations, as well as the environments that support or hinder their occupational performance. This emphasis on the person (child), occupation and environment is unique to occupational therapy. Occupational therapists are experts in understanding the environmental contexts (e.g. home, school, community and neighbourhoods) in which children engage in terms of their physical, cognitive, social, temporal and cultural dimensions and how to positively harness these to support children's participation.

Active engagement of children and parents

Because occupation-centred interventions are child- and family-centred and focus on child-chosen goals in relevant contexts, children (and their parents) are by necessity actively involved in the whole occupational therapy process of information gathering, goal setting, intervention and outcome evaluation. Occupational therapists have the requisite skills to actively involve children and their families in a meaningful way in such processes. This requires therapeutic use of self (e.g. excellent interpersonal skills and capacity to build collaborative relationships with children and families), a broad interest in the child's and family's well-being and knowledge about and skills in choosing appropriate occupation performance models and frames of reference to guide practice, as well as utilising assessment methods and intervention techniques that are conceptually congruent.

Individualisation of intervention

As with many interventions, individualising the process is central so that the child's and family's goals can be specifically addressed. It is acknowledged that each child's and family's context is unique and hence there will always be distinctive features such as the child's temperament/personality, strengths, preferences, interests, roles, occupations and occupational performance concerns. Additionally, the environmental context will vary based on the composition of the family, presence of siblings, the family routines and rituals, parents' engagement in paid employment, the needs of other family members, prior experiences with occupational therapy and the multiple demands on family members.

Focus on occupational performance and participation throughout the occupational therapy process

While many professions utilise a process of assessing, intervening and evaluating outcomes, our expertise related to occupation makes the profession's focus during this process unique (AOTA Commission on Practice, 2008). Irrespective of the type of models and frames of reference used, all occupational therapists engage in a similar occupational therapy process when working with clients (AOTA Commission on Practice, 2008; Baum & Law, 1997; Davis, Craik, & Polatajko, 2007; Sumsion, 1996). This incorporates the basic steps of initiating contact, discussions with the client regarding his/her concerns and goals for therapy, assessment, collabora- tive goal setting, treatment/intervention and evaluation of the outcomes of intervention. Variations on the occupational therapy process have been developed such as the Occupational Therapy Intervention Process Model (OTIPM) (Fisher, 1998), the AOTA Framework Occupational Therapy Process (AOTA Commission on Practice, 2008), Model for Planning and Implementing Client-centred OT Services (Baum & Law, 1997), Occupational Performance Process Model (Fearing, Law, & Clark, 1997) and Canadian Practice Process Framework (Davis et al., 2007). These are sum- marised in Table 2.3 in terms of the various stages of the occupational therapy process each espouses. For the purposes of this book, a cyclical process of occupation-centred service delivery for children is proposed and illustrated in Figure 2.1.

First, occupation-centred approaches for children are characterised by an information-gathering process that focuses on the child's occupational and social roles, occupations and the environmental context for performance, goal setting that emphasises occupational performance and participation, and assessment that identifies aspects of the child, occupation and envi- ronment that both facilitate and impede performance. Second, as described earlier, the interventions focus on child- and/or family-chosen goals that emphasise skill acquisition, and modification to occupations/tasks and/or environments to enhance the child's performance of meaningful and pur- poseful occupations. The ultimate objective is to enhance the child's partici- pation in relevant life situations. Hence, using the International Classification of Functioning, Disability and Health (ICF) schema (WHO, 2001) described in Chapter 1, the focus is on intervening at the activities and participation levels and with altering environmental factors to enhance both occupational per- formance and participation. The focus is not on remediating impairments at the body structures or functions level.

Third, evaluation of intervention outcomes focuses on the use of out- come measures that consider occupational performance, roles, habits, val- ues and participation, as well as the child's and family's satisfaction with the process. Hence, the focus of outcome measurement is at the activities and participation levels of the ICF (WHO, 2001). This is a critical difference to 'bottom-up' approaches that evaluate outcomes at the body structures/ functions level. In addition, consideration of child's and family's satisfaction with the service delivery process, outcomes and their perspectives on goal achievement is pivotal to working within an occupation- and client-centred framework.

Table 2.3 Comparison of five occupational therapy process models

Model for Planning and Implementing Client-Centred OT Services (Baum & Law, 1997)	The OT Intervention Process Model (Fisher, 1998)	Occupational Performance Process Model (Fearing & Clark, 2000; Fearing et al., 1997)	OT Practice Framework domain and process summary (AOTA Commission on Practice, 2008)	Canadian Practice Process Framework (CPPF) (Davis et al., 2007)[1]
Name, validate and prioritise client's occupational performance issues	Establish a client-centred performance context	Identifying occupational performance issues (OPIs)	Evaluation – occupational profile	Enter/initiate
Identify potential intervention model(s)	Identify strengths and problems of occupational performance	Selecting a theoretical approach	Evaluation – analysis of occupational performance	Set the stage
Identify occupational performance components and environmental conditions	Implement performance analysis	Identifying performance components and environmental conditions contributing to OPIs	Intervention – intervention plan	Assess/evaluate
Identify strengths and resources	Define actions of performance the person cannot effectively perform	Naming strengths and resources of the client and therapist	Intervention implementation	Agree on objectives/plan
Negotiate targeted outcomes, develop action plans	Clarify or interpret cause	Collaborating on targeted outcomes and making action plans	Intervention review	Implement plan
Implement plans through occupation	Select compensatory or remedial model	Connecting clients with their future through occupation	Outcomes – supporting health and participation in life through engagement in occupation	Monitor/modify
Evaluate occupational performance outcomes	Plan and implement occupational intervention	Evaluating client performance related to targeted outcomes		Evaluate outcome
	Re-evaluate for enhanced occupational performance			Conclude/exit

[1]Occurs within societal and practice context and with use of frame/s of reference.

Client-Centred Practice Framework

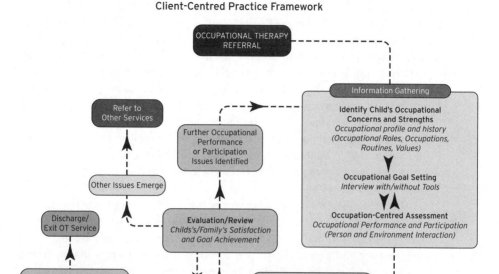

Figure 2.1 Occupation-centred service delivery process for children and families

Information gathering focuses on roles, occupations, occupational performance and environment

Coster (1998) was one of the first authors to apply an occupation-centred or top-down assessment process (first developed for adults) (Fisher & Short-DeGraff, 1993; Trombly, 1993) to occupational therapy practice with children and to explicate the difficulties in doing so. Molineux (2004) described the need to 'start where you mean to finish' (p. 9), encapsulating the need to get the focus of assessment right from the outset, as this will inevitably guide the subsequent stages of the process. Three stages of information gathering are proposed in Figure 2.1. The first involves informal discussions with the child's parent/s and the child (depending on age, developmental level and cognitive capacity). It focuses on the child's pattern of occupational engagement in a particular context, the child's occupational strengths, needs, problems and concerns related to the things he/she needs or wants to do in relevant contexts. This assists the therapist to appreciate the child as an occupational being. Central to this is the profession's belief that access to and participation in meaningful occupations (and associated activities or tasks) is critical to performance of life roles and pivotal to health and well-being (AOTA Commission on Practice, 2008; Molineux, 2004). The Occupational Therapy Practice Framework (AOTA Commission on Practice, 2008) refers to this stage as developing an 'occupational profile', reflecting the client's occupational history and experiences, patterns of daily living, interests, values and needs.

In the Canadian Process Practice Framework (CPPF) (Davis et al., 2007), this refers to the action points of 'enter/initiate' and 'setting the stage'. This appreciation reveals insights into the child's occupational roles (e.g. school student, player, self-carer and soccer player) as well as social roles (e.g. brother, son, friend and team member). Understanding of these roles provides insights into the occupations that are central to these roles (e.g. schoolwork, play and self-care) and the associated activities that are relevant (e.g. academics – writing, reading and mathematics; non-academic – playground games and physical education; extracurricular – football and gymnastics). The therapist is also interested in identifying the child's and family's strengths, resources and support networks (formal and informal), as part of information gathering.

Having developed a perspective on the child's occupational roles and his/her engagement in relevant contexts, the therapist engages in the second stage of information gathering, that is *occupational goal setting* (using appropriate children's goal-setting tools) in discussion with the child and parent/s and/or teacher. Occupational goal setting and a range of tools for children and parents will be addressed in detail in Chapter 6. Based on a discussion about the child's and parent's concerns and goals, the therapist is able to undertake a more detailed third stage of information gathering, that is, *assessment of the child's occupational performance and participation* relevant to the priority goals. The major focus of such assessment is to identify the key tasks/activities that comprise the child's roles and what performance difficulties the child has with these tasks. This is similar to Rogers' (2004) concept of occupational diagnosis of the child's difficulties in occupational performance. Then, the child's skills and abilities specific to the identified occupational performance issues (personal characteristics), identification of performance breakdown (task constraints) and assessment of environmental factors, and his/her participation in life situations can be addressed (Fisher, 1998). This is consistent with the CPPF action point of assess/evaluate (Davis et al., 2007).

When using an occupation-centred approach, the focus is on the occupational performance issues (Rogers, 2004), tasks and environment rather than on underlying performance components, as would be the case when a 'bottom-up' approach is used. Assessment of these components may be required as these may contribute to the child's limitations. They may inform us about *how* to intervene rather than about establishing the *goals* for intervention (Coster, 1998). Identifying performance breakdown requires use of an observational framework of performance analysis such as the Assessment of Motor and Process Skills (AMPS) (Fisher, 1997), Dynamic Performance Analysis (DPA) (Polatajko, Mandich, & Martini, 2000), or use of the Perceive, Recall, Plan and Perform (PRPP) system (Chapparo & Ranka, 1997b). These assessment tools will be described in further detail in Chapters 7–9. Understanding the cultural, physical, personal, social, virtual and temporal environment or context of occupational performance is crucial (AOTA Commission on Practice, 2008). This third stage will lead to consolidation and refinement of the intervention goals in consultation with the child and his/her parents, consistent with the CPPF stage of 'agree on objectives and plan' (Davis et al., 2007). It is recognised that this stage of information gathering is not linear (although it appears that way in Figure 2.1), but rather iterative with some degree of moving back and forwards between stages as more information comes to light. Re-checking the goals with the child and his/her parents before commencing intervention is critical, as these may shift and need clarification during this phase.

Intervention focuses on roles, occupations, occupational performance and environment

Having established the goals for intervention, the therapist selects an *occupation-centred intervention approach* based on his/her clinical experience, professional knowledge and reasoning. In the CPPF, this is known as 'implement the plan' (Davis et al., 2007). The professional reasoning needed involves: (1) the therapist's knowledge of the evidence-base for various interventions with specific diagnostic groups (scientific reasoning); (2) the selection of a frame of reference; (3) the development of a systematic process for information gathering, hypothesis generation and testing throughout the process of therapy (procedural reasoning); (4) knowledge of the child's and family's situation and preferences (narrative reasoning); and (5) considerations about the setting, time and resources available (pragmatic reasoning) (Mattingly & Fleming, 1994; Rogers & Holm, 1991; Schell & Cervero, 1993). In being occupation-centred, the focus is on enabling the child's occupational engagement so as to enhance his/her participation in appropriate and relevant life situations or contexts. Clinical reasoning supports and underpins client-related thinking and decision making. A detailed discussion of how therapists blend their lived clinical experience, the research evidence and their reasoning processes and how these influence their decision making can be found in Chapter 15.

Means versus ends

Various authors have classified occupational therapy interventions in different ways (AOTA Commission on Practice, 2008; Davis et al., 2007; Fisher, 1998) and have also discussed the use of activity and occupations as *means versus ends* (McLaughlin Gray, 1998). A comparison between three different classifications by Fisher (1998), AOTA Commission on Practice (2008) and CPPF (Davis et al., 2007) can be found in Table 2.4. For example, Fisher (1998) described three categories of occupation as *means* (i.e. exercise, contrived occupation and therapeutic occupation) and compensatory occupation as focusing on occupational outcomes or ends. The latter involves using assistive devices, teaching alternative or compensatory strategies and modifying physical or social environments. The AOTA Commission on Practice (2008) classification of *intervention approaches* as either health promotion, compensation or adaptation or disability prevention focuses on occupation as *ends* mostly through occupation-based activity. In contrast, remediation or restoration focuses on *means* through the use of preparatory methods and purposeful or goal-directed activities. Maintenance of client performance abilities, without which abilities would be lost, could equally refer to the use of activity and occupation as *means* as well as *ends*. The point is that occupation-centred practice emphasises the use of activity and occupation as *ends* with the focus being on child- and family-centred and -directed, goal-focused naturalistic interventions which aim to improve occupational performance and participation.

By and large, the compensatory approaches focus on planning and implementing adaptive actions to compensate for ineffective actions and use of adaptive strategies such as providing adapted equipment or assistive technology, teaching alternative or compensatory techniques and/or modifying the task or environment and are *ends* oriented. By contrast, remedial interventions focus on planning and implementing therapeutic occupations to remediate impairments (Fisher, 1998) and are *means* focused. Chapter 14 focuses on the use of assistive technology to enable children's occupational engagement and broader participation. Usually the remedial interventions draw from 'bottom-up' frames of reference (e.g. biomechanical or sensory integration) and apply specific techniques in isolation or out of an occupational context.

The adaptive, compensatory and acquisitional interventions tend to be more consistent with 'top-down' approaches or frames of reference (e.g. skill acquisition and four-quadrant model of facilitated learning) (Greber, Ziviani, & Rodger, 2007) that emphasise occupational performance and participation as the outcomes. The latter are sometimes referred to as performance-focused approaches (Polatajko, Rodger, Dhillon, & Hirji, 2004). These focus on the child's skill acquisition, the role of learning and task or environmental modification to enable motor-based performance (Polatajko et al., 2004). They emphasise adaptive learning, performance outcomes and skill development and acquisition. Some of these approaches include cognitive approaches (e.g. Cognitive Orientation for daily Occupational Performance (CO-OP)) (Polatajko & Mandich, 2004), conductive education (Todd, 1990), PRPP (Chapparo & Ranka, 1997a) and compensatory approaches (e.g. adaptive or specialised equipment). The compensatory approaches described by Polatajko et al. (2004) overlap with those described by Fisher (1998) above. Within the performance-focused approaches, motor problems are viewed as difficulties in learning, with the aim being to enhance the developmental motor process and skill acquisition through facilitating learning (Polatajko et al., 2004).

Cognitive or meta-cognitive approaches (Missiuna et al., 1997) aim to enhance the child's capacity to acquire and use information (i.e. learning) in order to adapt to environmental demands. These approaches are 'top-down' as the emphasis is on organising and integrating the child's motor experiences with greater cognitive awareness while engaged in relevant occupations or

Table 2.4 Classifications of occupational therapy interventions and description in terms of occupation as means versus ends

Occupation as means versus ends	OT Intervention Process Model (Fisher, 1998)	OT Practice Framework domain and process (AOTA Commission on Practice, 2008)	CMOP-E (Townsend & Polatajko, 2007)
Means	*Exercise:* client engaged in rote exercise or practice (purpose originates with therapist, not client), exercise has little/no meaning to client (e.g. theraband or theraputty exercises)	*Remediation/restoration:* change client variables to establish skill/ ability not yet developed or restore these (if impaired) using preparatory methods (exercise, orthotics, modalities) or purposeful activity (goal-directed activities that lead to occupation/s)	*Impairment reduction:* therapeutic use of activities (e.g. acquisitional, biomechanical, cognitive perceptual, sensorimotor approaches)
Means	*Contrived occupation:* exercise with added purpose but purpose originates with practitioner and focus is on remediation of impairments (e.g. throwing bean bags into a hoop/basket)	*Maintain:* interventions that aim to maintain client performance abilities, without which abilities would be lost using preparatory methods (exercise, orthotics, modalities) or purposeful activity (goal-directed activities that lead to occupation/s)	
Means	*Therapeutic occupation:* client actively participates in activities that client identifies as purposeful and meaningful, performance is naturalistic and contextual. Focus remains on remediation of impairments (e.g. addressing attentional issues while playing cards)		

(Continued)

Table 2.4 (Continued)

Occupation as means versus ends	OT Intervention Process Model (Fisher, 1998)	OT Practice Framework domain and process (AOTA Commission on Practice, 2008)	CMOP-E (Townsend & Polatajko, 2007)
Ends	*Adaptive/compensatory occupation:* occupations chosen by client and actively engaged in, activities are purposeful and meaningful and performance is naturalistic and contextual but focus is on improved occupational performance. Involves use of assistive devices, teaching alternative or compensatory strategies, modifying physical or social environments. Emphasis also on grading and adaptation of activity for successful performance	*Compensation/adaptation:* to support performance in naturalistic setting using occupation-based activity (actual occupations part of clients' own context and own goals)	*Adaptation:* adjusting or tailoring occupations based on occupational analysis of the physical, mental, cognitive, social, economic and other environmental demands and requirements of an occupation (p. 117); breaking down tasks for just right challenges *Enable skill acquisition* for individuals, families, groups *Occupational enablement:* Client-centred enablement of client-specific goals/challenges with focus on occupational challenges, using asset-based solutions, client-centred perspective, multidisciplinary knowledge base and professional reasoning (p. 214). Enabling person to change, enabling change in occupation, environment or in combination
Ends		*Disability prevention:* prevent barriers to performance in context *Health promotion:* enrich experiences that will enhance performance for individuals/communities, when disability not necessarily present	

related activities. Cognitive approaches focus on how strategies are taught (Missiuna et al., 1997) and generally use a problem-solving process: (1) define and analyse the task, (2) anticipate the child's performance difficulties, (3) provide a supportive environment to allow exploration of strategies, (4) apply the strategy to the task, and (5) evaluate the utility of the strategy and modify as needed.

Transfer and generalisation of strategies is emphasised. This will be further discussed in Chapter 8 which specifically addresses CO-OP intervention. Two other approaches, PRPP (Chapparo & Ranka, 1997b) and Occupational Performance Coaching (OPC) (Graham, Rodger, & Ziviani, 2009), will be described in Chapters 9 and 10, respectively.

Interventions are whole or finite

McLaughlin Gray (1998) described occupational interventions as being 'whole or finite' or as having an inherent beginning, middle and end. The aspects can be observed both within individual session plans and for the intervention as a whole over a number of sessions. Most therapists as part of their practice context will have to specify to parents, health insurers or employers an approximate number of sessions that might be required to achieve the particular client goals. This may be over an 8-10-week school term or a negotiated block of private therapy. These parameters are discussed with the child's parents in terms of their capacity to bring the child to therapy sessions or agreement for the child to be seen at school, etc. Hence, therapists usually work within a finite time frame (for managing specific goals) even if the child's progress will be reviewed at a later date and more contact is negotiated if required to address other goals, etc.

Individual sessions start with a connecting time with the child and parents and rapport is re-established (e.g. *How has the week been? What progress has been made? What changes have been noticed? What has worked/not worked?*). The middle part of intervention sessions tends to focus on the 'work' of therapy with specific goal/s being addressed and practiced, and activities/occupations or specific techniques used. The final part often focuses on summarising what has been achieved, feedback to parent/s if they were not present during the session and the consideration of tasks to undertake at home to promote generalisation and transfer of outcomes.

Occupation-centred evaluation of intervention outcomes

Intervention outcomes are evaluated from the perspectives of the child's occupational performance gains, his/her goal achievement as well as satisfaction with the intervention process. Both child and parent satisfaction should be addressed. The resulting evaluation may lead to exiting from occupational therapy services if occupational engagement and participation have been enhanced to a level that both parents and the child are satisfied with. Alternately, referral to other services may occur should remaining issues be beyond the domain of concern of occupational therapy (Mosey, 1981). Re-engagement in the occupational therapy process may occur if further occupational performance or participation issues are identified. Tools such as the Canadian Occupational Performance Measure (COPM) (Law et al., 1998) and goal attainment scaling (Kiresuk, Smith, & Cardillo, 1994) can be used to measure changes in goal achievement and performance/satisfaction over the course of intervention. Additionally, therapists utilise tools that measure parent satisfaction with the intervention services provided such as how family-centred they have found them to be (e.g. Measure of Processes of Care (MPOC)) (King, Rosenbaum, & King, 1997). Tools suitable for occupation-centred assessment and evaluation of outcomes will be discussed in Chapter 3 (family-centred practice and satisfaction tools), Chapter 6 (goal-setting tools) and Chapter 7 (occupation-centred assessment tools).

Conclusion

This chapter has highlighted the need to choose an appropriate model of occupational performance (the *what*), and a frame of reference that provides ways to engage the child in his/her roles and occupations, and optimise his/her participation in relevant life contexts (the *how*). Additionally, the differences between 'top-down' and 'bottom-up' approaches have been discussed in relation to the relative importance of each when using an occupation-centred approach. Eleven key characteristics of occupation-centred practice for children have been proposed. Finally, an occupation-centred occupational therapy service delivery process that therapists can use to guide their engagement with children and their families has been described, and will be expanded upon in subsequent chapters.

References

AOTA Commission on Practice. (2008). Occupational therapy practice framework: Domain and process. Second edition. *American Journal of Occupational Therapy, 62*(6), 625–683.

Ayres, J. (1972). *Sensory integration and the child*. Los Angeles, CA: Western Psychological Services.

Barthel, K. A. (2009). A frame of reference for neurodevelopmental treatment. In P. Kramer, & J. Hinojosa (Eds.), *Frames of reference for pediatric occupational therapy* (3rd ed., pp. 187–233). Philadelphia, PA: Walters Kluwer, Lippincott Williams & Wilkins.

Baum, C., & Law, M. (1997). Occupational therapy practice: Focusing on occupational performance. *American Journal of Occupational Therapy, 51*, 277–288.

Berry, J., & Ryan, S. (2002). Frames of reference: Their use in paediatric occupational therapy. *British Journal of Occupational Therapy, 65*(9), 420–426.

Blanche, E. I., & Blanche Kiefer, D. (2007). Sensory integration and neurodevelopmental treatment as frames of reference in the context of occupational science. In S. Dunbar (Ed.), *Occupational therapy models for intervention with children and families* (pp. 11-26). Thorofare, NJ: SLACK Inc.

Brown, G. T., Rodger, S., Brown, A., & Roever, C. (2007). A profile of Canadian paediatric occupational therapy practice. *Occupational Therapy in Health Care, 21*(4), 39-69.

Chapparo, C., & Ranka, J. (1997a). Towards a model of occupational perform-ance: Model development. In C. Chapparo, & J. Ranka (Eds.), *Occupational Performance Model (Australia): Monograph 1* (pp. 24-45). Sydney: Total Print Control (retrieved 10 March 2009 from http://www.occupationalperformance. com index.php).

Chapparo, C., & Ranka, J. (1997b). *The perceive, recall, plan and perform system (PRPP).* Sydney: Total Print Control (retrieved 10 March 2009 from http://www. occupationalperformance.com index.php, originally published in Chapparro, C., & Ranka, J. (1997). *Occupational Performance Model (Australia): Monograph 1* (pp. 199-204)).

Christiansen, C., Baum, C., & Bass-Haugen, J. (Eds.). (2005). *Occupational therapy: Performance, participation and well-being* (3rd ed.). Thorofare, NJ: SLACK Inc.

Colangelo, C. A., & Shea, M. (2009). A biomechanical frame of reference for posi-tioning children for functioning. In P. Kramer, & J. Hinojosa (Eds.), *Frames of ref-erence for pediatric occupational therapy* (3rd ed., pp. 489-567). Philadelphia, PA: Walters Kluwer, Lippincott Williams & Wilkins.

Copley, J., Turpin, M., & Bennett, S. (in press). Decision making in occupational therapy practice with children. In S. Rodger (Ed.), *Occupation centred practice for children: A practical guide for occupational therapists.* Oxford, UK: Wiley Blackwell.

Coster, W. (1998). Occupation-centred assessment of children. *American Journal of Occupational Therapy, 52,* 227-344.

Davis, J., Craik, J., & Polatajko, H. (2007). Using the Canadian Process Practice Framework: Amplifying the process. In E. Townsend & H. Polatajko (Eds.), *Enabling occupation II: Advancing an occupational therapy vision for health, well-being and justice through occupation* (pp. 247-272). Ottawa: CAOT Publications.

Dunbar, S. B. (2007). Theory, frame of reference and model: A differentiation for practice considerations. In S. Dunbar (Ed.), *Occupational therapy models for intervention with children and families* (pp. 1-10). Thorofare, NJ: SLACK Inc.

Dunn, W. (2007). Ecology of human performance model. In S. Dunbar (Ed.), *Occupational therapy models for intervention with children and families* (pp. 127-156). Thorofare, NJ: SLACK Inc.

Fearing, V. G., & Clark, J. (2000). *Individuals in context: A practical guide to client-centred practice.* Thorofare, NJ: SLACK Inc.

Fearing, V. G., Law, M., & Clark, J. (1997). An occupational performance process model: Fostering client and therapist alliances. *Canadian Journal of Occupational Therapy, 64,* 7-15.

Fisher, A. G. (1997). *Assessment of motor and process skills* (2nd ed.). Fort Collins, CO: Three Star Press.

Fisher, A. G. (1998). Uniting practice and theory in an occupational framework. *American Journal of Occupational Therapy, 52,* 509-521.

Fisher, A. G., & Short-DeGraff, M. (1993). Nationally speaking - Improving func-tional assessment in occupational therapy: Recommendations and philosophy for change. *American Journal of Occupational Therapy, 47,* 199-200.

Graham, F., Rodger, S., & Ziviani, J. (2009). Coaching parents to enable children's participation: An approach to working with parents and their children. *Australian Occupational Therapy Journal, 56*(1), 16-23.

Greber, C., Ziviani, J., & Rodger, S. (2007). The four quadrant model of facilitated learning (part 1): Using teaching-learning approaches in occupational therapy. *Australian Occupational Therapy Journal, 54*, S31-S39.

Hinojosa, J., & Kramer, P. (2009). Frames of reference for the real world. In P. Kramer, & J. Hinojosa (Eds.), *Frames of reference for pediatric occupational therapy* (3rd ed., pp. 571-581). Philadelphia, PA: Walters Kluwer, Lippincott Williams & Wilkins.

Iwama, M. (2006). *The Kawa Model.* Toronto, Ontario: Churchill Livingston, Elsevier.

Kaplan, M. T., & Bedell, G. (1999). Motor skill acquisition frame of reference. In P. Kramer, & J. Hinojosa (Eds.), *Frames of reference for pediatric occupational therapy* (2nd ed., pp. 410-430). Philadelphia, PA: Lippincott Williams & Wilkins.

Kielhofner, G. (2007). *The model of human occupation: Theory and application* (4th ed.). Baltimore, MD: Lippincott Williams & Wilkins.

Kimball, J. G. (1999a). Sensory integration frame of reference: Theoretical base, function/dysfunction continua, and guide to evaluation. In P. Kramer, & J. Hinojosa (Eds.), *Frames of reference for pediatric occupational therapy* (2nd ed., pp. 119-168). Philadelphia, PA: Lippincott Williams & Wilkins.

Kimball, J. G. (1999b). Sensory integration frame of reference: Postulates regarding change and application to practice In P. Kramer, & J. Hinojosa (Eds.), *Frames of reference for pediatric occupational therapy* (2nd ed., pp. 129-204). Philadelphia, PA: Lippincott Williams & Wilkins.

King, G. A., Rosenbaum, P. L., & King, S. M. (1997). Evaluating family-centred service using a measure of parents' perceptions. *Child: Care, Health and Development, 23*(1), 47-62.

Kiresuk, T. J., Smith, A., & Cardillo, J. E. (1994). *Goal attainment scaling: Applications, theory and measurement.* Hillsdale, NJ: Lawrence Erlbaum Associates.

Kramer, J. M., & Bowyer, P. (2007). Application of the model of human occupation to children and family interventions. In S. Dunbar (Ed.), *Occupational therapy models for intervention with children and families* (pp. 51-90). Thorofare, NJ: SLACK Inc.

Kramer, P., & Hinojosa, J. (1999). *Frames of reference for pediatric occupational therapy* (2nd ed.). Philadelphia, PA: Lippincott Williams & Wilkins.

Kramer, P., & Hinojosa, J. (2009). *Frames of reference for pediatric occupational therapy* (3rd ed.). Philadelphia, PA: Walters Kluwer, Lippincott Williams & Wilkins.

Law, M. (1998). *Client-centred occupational therapy.* Thorofare, NJ: SLACK Inc.

Law, M., Baptiste, S., Carswell, A., McColl, M., Polatajko, H., & Pollock, N. (1998). *Canadian Occupational Performance Measure manual* (3rd ed.). Ottawa, Ontario: Canadian Association of Occupational Therapists.

Law, M., Baum, C. M., & Baptiste, S. (2002). *Occupation-based practice: Fostering performance and participation.* Thorofare, NJ: SLACK Inc.

Law, M., & Dunbar, S. B. (2007). Person-environment-occupation model. In S. Dunbar (Ed.), *Occupational therapy models for intervention with children and families* (pp. 27-50). Thorofare, NJ: SLACK Inc.

Luebben, A. J., & Brasic Royeen, C. (2009). An acquisitional frame of reference. In P. Kramer, & J. Hinojosa (Eds.), *Frames of reference for pediatric occupational therapy* (3rd ed., pp. 461-488). Philadelphia, PA: Walters Kluwer, Lippincott Williams & Wilkins.

Marr, D. (1999). Bridging a top-down approach in pediatrics. *American Journal of Occupational Therapy, 53*, 114-115.

Mattingly, C., & Fleming, M.H. (1994). *Clinical reasoning: Forms of inquiry in therapeutic practice*. Philadelphia: F.A. Davis.

McLaughlin Gray, J. (1998). Putting occupation into practice: Occupation as ends, occupations as means. *American Journal of Occupational Therapy, 52*, 354-364.

Missiuna, C., Malloy-Miller, T., & Mandich, A. D. (1997). *Cognitive or 'top down' approaches to intervention*. Hamilton, Canada: CanChild Centre for Childhood Disability Research. Retrieved 10 March 2009 from http://www.canchild.ca/default.aspx?tabid=118 (Keeping Current #97-1).

Molineux, M. (2004). Occupation in occupational therapy: A labour in vain? In M. Molineux (Ed.), *Occupation for occupational therapists* (pp. 17-31). Oxford, UK: Blackwell Science.

Mosey, A. C. (1981). *Occupational therapy: Configuration of a profession*. New York: Raven.

Nelson, A., Copley, J., Flanigan, K., & Underwood, K. (2009). Occupational therapists prefer combining multiple intervention approaches for children with learning difficulties. *Australian Occupational Therapy Journal, 56*(1), 51-62.

Olson, L. J. (2009). A frame of reference to enhance social participation. In P. Kramer, & J. Hinojosa (Eds.), *Frames of reference for pediatric occupational therapy* (2nd ed., pp. 306-348). Philadelphia, PA: Lippincott Williams & Wilkins.

Parham, C., & Mailloux, Z. (1998). Sensory integration. In J. Case-Smith, A. Allen, & P. N. Pratt (Eds.), *Occupational therapy for children* (pp. 307-352). Toronto, Ontario: Mosby.

Polatajko, H. J., & Mandich, A. D. (2004). *Enabling occupation in children: The cognitive orientation to daily occupational performance (CO-OP) approach*. Ottawa, Ontario: CAOT Publications ACE.

Polatajko, H. J., Mandich, A. D., & Martini, R. (2000). Dynamic performance analysis: A framework for understanding occupational performance. *American Journal of Occupational Therapy, 54*(1), 65-72.

Polatajko, H., Rodger, S., Dhillon, A., & Hirji, F. (2004). Approaches to the management of children with motor problems. In D. Dewey & D. E. Tupper (Eds.), *Developmental motor disorders: A neuropsychological perspective – The science and practice of neuropsychology series* (pp. 461-486). New York, NY: Guilford Press.

Rodger, S., Brown, G. T., & Brown, A. (2005). Profile of paediatric occupational therapy practice in Australia. *Australian Occupational Therapy Journal, 52*(4), 311-325.

Rogers, J. C. (2004). Occupational diagnosis. In M. Molineux (Ed.), *Occupation for occupational therapists* (pp. 17-31). Oxford, UK: Blackwell Science.

Rogers, J. C., & Holm, M. B. (1991). Occupational therapy diagnostic reasoning: A component of clinical reasoning. *American Journal of Occupational Therapy, 45*(11), 1045-1053.

Royeen, C. B., & Duncan, M. (1999). Acquisition frame of reference. In P. Kramer, & J. Hinojosa (Eds.), *Frames of reference for pediatric occupational therapy* (2nd ed., pp. 377-429). Philadelphia, PA: Lippincott Williams & Wilkins.

Schaaf, R. C., Schoen, S. A., Smith Roley, S., Lane, S. J., Koomar, J., & May-Benson, T. A. (2009). A frame of reference for sensory integration. In P. Kramer, & J. Hinojosa (Eds.), *Frames of reference for pediatric occupational therapy* (3rd ed., pp. 99-186). Philadelphia, PA: Walters Kluwer, Lippincott Williams & Wilkins.

Schell, B. R., & Cervero, R. M. (1993). Clinical reasoning of occupational therapy: An integrative review. *American Journal of Occupational Therapy, 47*, 605-610.

Schoen, S. A., & Anderson, J. (1999). NeuroDevelopmental treatment frame of reference. In P. Kramer, & J. Hinojosa (Eds.), *Frames of reference for pediatric occupational therapy* (2nd ed., pp. 83-118). Philadelphia, PA: Lippincott Williams & Wilkins.

Schneck, C. M. (2009). A frame of reference for visual perception. In P. Kramer, & J. Hinojosa (Eds.), *Frames of reference for pediatric occupational therapy* (3rd ed., pp. 349-389). Philadelphia, PA: Walters Kluwer, Lippincott Williams & Wilkins.

Schön, D. A. (1987). *Educating the reflective practitioner: Toward a new design for teaching and learning in the professions.* San Francisco, CA: Jossey-Bass.

Stanton, M. (1997). *Cerebral palsy handbook: A practical guide for parents and carers.* London, UK: Vermillion.

Sumsion, T. (1996). Implementation issues. In T. Sumsion (Ed.), *Client-centred practice in occupational therapy: A guide to implementation* (pp. 27-37). London, UK: Churchill Livingstone.

Todd, J. (1990). Conductive education: The continuing challenge observations drawn from a recent period of study at the Peto Institute, Budapest. *Physiotherapy, 76,* 13-16.

Todd, V. R (1999). Visual information analysis frame of reference for visual perception. In P. Kramer, & J. Hinojosa (Eds.), *Frames of reference for pediatric occupational therapy* (2nd ed., pp. 205-255). Philadelphia: Lippincott Williams & Wilkins.

Townsend, E., & Polatajko, H. (Eds.). (2007). *Enabling occupation II: Advancing an occupational therapy vision for health, well-being and justice through occupation.* Ottawa, Ontario: CAOT Publications.

Trombly, C. (1993). Anticipating the future: Assessment of occupational function. *American Journal of Occupational Therapy, 47*(3), 253-257.

Turpin, M. (2004). *Clinical reasoning and reflective practice: Postgraduate practicums.* Brisbane, Queensland: Division of Occupational Therapy, University of Queensland.

Weinstock-Zlotnick, G., & Hinojosa, J. (2004). Bottom-up or top-down evaluation: Is one better than the other? *American Journal of Occupational Therapy, 58,* 594-599.

Weston, J., Kinley, E., Hughes, B., & Fishwick, S. (1998). Physical (motor and functional) difficulties. In R. Appleton, & T. Baldwin (Eds.), *Management of brain-injured children* (pp. 71-105). Oxford, UK: Oxford University Press.

World Health Organisation (WHO). (2001). *International Classification of Functioning, Disability and Health (ICF).* Geneva, Switzerland: WHO.

Chapter 3

Child- and Family-centred Service Provision

Sylvia Rodger and Deb Keen

Learning objectives

The objectives of this chapter are to:

- Briefly describe the origins of client-centred practice in psychology and its roots in occupational therapy in the later half of the 20th century.
- Define client-, child- and family-centred practice and services in terms of the existing literature and discuss complexities arising from being both child- and family-centred.
- Identify the personal characteristics of practitioners which enhance child- and family-centred practice.
- Provide guidelines for developing family-centred services at systems/organisation, therapist and client levels.
- Consider how practitioners might engage extended family and community members.

Introduction

This chapter provides an overview of client-centred practice (CCP) as it is operationalised when working with children and their families. Whilst family composition has changed significantly over the past two decades (Darlington & Rodger, 2006), within the family unit there are various family members –children, parent/s, siblings and possibly extended family members. The presence of more than one client makes for a complex context for service delivery. Occupational therapists and other team members must be cognisant of the needs of both the child and the family members. In this chapter, we address how services are provided to children and families from an occupation-centred perspective and about the characteristics of 'best practice' family-centred service (FCS) provision.

Defining the client: who and how many?

A broad definition of occupational therapy clients refers to: '... individuals, families, groups, communities, organizations, or populations who participate in occupational therapy services' (Townsend et al., 2007, p. 96). Whilst 'client' is a term used in business, the term was used by Canadian occupational therapists in the early 1980s (Canadian Association of Occupational Therapists, 1983, 1991) and then by occupational therapists internationally (e.g. Baum & Law, 1997; Sumsion, 1999). This term was chosen because whilst diverse in nature, occupational therapy clients are usually active participants in therapy and their lives (Townsend et al., 2007).

This diversity of practice raises questions regarding who is the client. The individual of concern is not always the purchaser of the service. For example, it is usual that parent/s or carer/s consult with professionals about concerns related to their child's performance, functioning or participation in home, school or community contexts. Hence, from the outset there are potentially at least two clients, the parent/carer and the child him/herself. In school settings, this situation can become more complex with referrals from teachers, so the therapist works with the duality of teacher as client (assisting him/her to work more effectively with the child in the classroom) and the child whose skill acquisition or performance is challenging. In this case, the parent may not be directly involved in therapy which occurs in the school context. As a result, the need for consultation and generalisation of outcomes across both home and school contexts becomes more complicated. Occupational therapy in school settings is addressed further in Chapter 11.

Client-centred practice

The term 'client-centred' was first coined by humanist psychologist Carl Rogers (1946) and further developed (Rogers, 1951) in relation to 'client-centred therapy' which was a revolutionary, non-directive approach to psychotherapy. Considered by some to be heretical, this approach contradicted the more directive behavioural and psychodynamic therapies practiced at the time. Rogers sought to create an accepting and understanding climate for therapy and believed that people move towards growth and healing (self-actualisation) and have a natural capacity to find their own answers. Rogerian therapists listen and aim to understand the client's perspective, check their understanding with the client, treat the client with the utmost respect and regard, and are transparent about their own self-awareness and self-acceptance (Rogers, 1946).

The term 'client-centred' was first adopted by the Canadian Association of Occupational Therapists in 1983, with the initial emphasis on collaboration during assessment and intervention rather than 'doing things to or for' people. An early definition of CCP (Law, Baptiste, & Mills, 1995) focused on:

> an approach to service which embraces a philosophy of respect for, and partnership with, people receiving services. Client-centred practice recognizes the autonomy of individuals, the need for client choice in making decisions about occupational needs, the strengths clients bring to the therapy encounter, the benefits of the client–therapist partnership and the need to ensure that services are accessible and fit the context in which the client lives. (p. 253)

Key concepts common to various definitions of client-centred practice include:

- Clients, their families and their choices are respected.
- Information, physical comfort, emotional support and person-centred communication are provided.
- Clients are facilitated to participate fully in occupational therapy services.
- Clients and families have the ultimate responsibility for decisions about daily occupations and services.
- Occupational therapy service delivery is flexible and individualised.
- Clients are enabled to solve their own occupational performance issues.
- The relationship between person-environment-occupation is the focus of intervention (Sumsion, 2000; Sumsion & Law, 2006).

Client-centred practice: inherent challenges

Whilst occupational therapists appear to universally espouse CCP principles, its effective implementation remains elusive. As is frequently the case, the gap between theory (and its rhetoric) and clinical practice continues to be significant (Mortensen & Dyck, 2006; Sumsion & Law, 2006; Wilkins, Pollock, Rochon, & Law, 2001). Recent qualitative studies have investigated adult clients' perspectives (e.g. Rebeiro, 2000) from their experiences with occupational therapy services and therapists' perspectives of barriers to CCP (e.g. Mortensen & Dyck, 2006; Sumsion & Smyth, 2000). These studies have shed light on the potential challenges of engaging in CCP. Whilst conducted with adults, some common themes are worthy of reflection: (1) issues with goal setting, conflict regarding goals resulting from different values and beliefs, and relinquishing therapist control regarding intervention goals; (2) a focus on impairment rather than wellness (Rebeiro, 2000; Sumsion & Smyth, 2000); and (3) institutional issues such as diagnostic clinical protocols, as well as conflict when therapists' views of safety and unreasonable risk-taking conflict with clients' preferences (Mortensen & Dyck, 2006).

Unequal power in relationships

The issue of power has emerged as a critical factor in better understanding the implementation of CCP (Mortensen & Dyck, 2006; Sumsion, 1996; Sumsion & Law, 2006). Sumsion (1996) described 'power over' as well as 'power to' within CCP. Power 'over' influences behaviour and decisions in relation to conformity, authority and control. Rather than exerting power 'over' clients, therapists should attempt to give 'power to' clients, focusing on effectiveness, goal setting and achieving objectives. Clients can be disempowered by institutional culture such that they may not be able to fully participate in their health care and choice making. Whilst this can be challenging, CCP operates to shift the power from dependence to interdependence and towards partnership between therapist and client. Access to information in a way that is understood by clients is critical and leads to more involvement in decision making regarding treatment options, prognosis and improved client satisfaction (Hall, Roter, & Katz, 1988). Through CCP power is no longer held by the therapist, rather it is shared equally with the client (Sumsion, 1996).

Recognising expertise and goal setting

Another issue can be that of recognising the expertise that clients bring to the partnership. Clients bring knowledge about themselves (and their family members), their occupations and life situations/contexts. This is possible providing that they have insight into their own needs, which may be compromised for individuals with some mental health conditions and cognitive impairments. Ideally, they are actively involved in goal setting and determining outcomes and choosing the occupations important to them that will become the focus of intervention. Rosenbaum, King, Law, King, and Evans (1998) highlighted the importance of developing collaborative therapeutic alliances between parents and therapists by acknowledging therapists as technical experts with knowledge and skills about the condition, the child's developmental status and life stage, the range of appropriate interventions and their evidence base, and provision of information about these (Sumsion & Law, 2006; Tickle-Degnen, 2002). Health professionals are increasingly expected to tailor interventions within the context of the family and to support the child and family members within the community where they live, work and play (Law, 2002).

Effective partnerships also require parents to actively participate in goal selection and collaboration with health professionals. This can be challenging for therapists who may develop their own treatment goals based on the child's development, health condition and their knowledge of the child's context. Shifting between these in favour of listening to parents' concerns takes time and effort on the part of the therapist who may feel that he/she knows best. The therapist's role is to listen and then to facilitate an informed and balanced discussion about goal selection. In this discussion, whilst being cognisant of parents' goals, therapists bring their expert knowledge to the interaction. They need to integrate their developmental knowledge about the child and his/her condition and its likely trajectory with parents' perspectives and wishes.

This becomes obvious when designing home programmes based on parents' goals (Novak & Cusick, 2006). For example, a child may present as happy and quiet whilst watching TV and a parent may prioritise this over correct positioning of the child whilst engaged in this activity. A therapist may be concerned that too much time spent in a poor position engaging in a passive type of activity may have long-term consequences on muscle balance, joint alignment, posture as well as pain/comfort, effective performance and reducing play occupations. In this case, the child's cognitive limitation makes him unable to voice an opinion, and the parents may not share the therapists' priority of addressing a meaningful play occupation (self-amusement), cognisant of positions that support postural alignment and maximise successful performance. The therapist is not obligated to accept the parents' view but rather to provide meaningful information (with clinical and research evidence where possible) about the potential impact of this long-term positioning and degree of passivity. This is consistent with our ethical code of doing no harm (non-maleficence). Over time, not intervening may well cause harm. Parents may (with time, discussion and provision of appropriate information) be prepared to revisit this issue. This raises concerns about the 'timeliness' of intervention. In long-term contact with a client and family, there is an opportunity to revisit such issues at a later stage, particularly when the parent is ready or able to hear these perspectives and able to implement changes as required. However, in many situations the opportunity for ongoing contact is not possible. In these cases, therapists are most challenged by the consequences of not addressing the issue and may impose their views/goals because there is not an opportunity to delay intervention until the family is ready.

Sometimes following a balanced presentation of the issue, parents choose not to address it at that time, that is their prerogative. However, it is the therapist's responsibility to document the discussion with the parents, so that in future therapists and others are aware that the issue had been raised and that the parents chose to pursue other goals at that time. If there is no change in child status, therapists should continue to raise their concerns with parents over time when goals are renegotiated.

Child-centred practice

Rarely is *child*-centred practice defined separately to *client*-centred practice. In recognising the child as the focus, the therapist's practice is consistent with all aspects of CCP already discussed (e.g. mutual respect, provision of choice, engagement with goal setting and decision making). The therapist also needs to be cognisant of the child's developmental level, likes/dislikes, strengths and challenges, family context, roles, occupations and performance demands. Child-centred practice involves listening to and respecting what children have to say, focusing on their needs, seeing their perspective and seeing children as individuals as well as members of a group (e.g. family or school class).

Many therapists, who consider they are child-centred, are actually 'child-friendly', that is, they work in an environment (waiting room and clinic) that has children's toys, games, furniture and equipment, and they utilise age-appropriate activities. However, they work on therapist goals developed from their assessment, perhaps in consultation with teachers and parents. However, if they do not utilise children's goal-setting tools or at the very least have a conversation with the child about his/her concerns and what he/she wishes to address (where the child is cognitively able to participate) and then use these concerns as the focus of assessment and intervention, they are not being child-centred. Given the important role of family members, particularly parents, there is a need for high levels of communication with parents and the child requiring listening, negotiation and perhaps at times conflict resolution.

There may be times when neither the parent nor the child feels comfortable with what appears 'to be giving the child the control' and the therapist needs to negotiate a way forward, bringing his/her expertise into the equation. In situations where the child is developmentally or cognitively unable to determine the focus of intervention, the therapist is necessarily reliant on parents, and/or the child's teacher, to assist with developing goals. However, the therapist still provides the child with some developmentally appropriate choices and tries to understand his/her perspective.

Another important consideration is that meaningful occupations are not always enjoyable. For example, the child needs to get ready for school in the morning and for many this routine is not enjoyable but a necessary occupation. When we refer to meaningful occupation, some therapists frame this by asking the child 'what do you want to work on?' This is particularly important in school environments where the child is required to comply with a number of expectations and requirements. The child, who does not want to write, remain in his/her seat or restrain from interrupting, is still required to do so. It would be rare for a child to identify these goals, unless the motivator is simply 'to get the teacher off my back'. Parents, too, sometimes lack an awareness of the way classrooms operate. The challenge for therapists in this situation is to help children and families to understand the centrality of some mundane occupations.

Family-centred practice and service provision

This section focuses on family-centred practice and service provision. First, the role of the family is discussed, followed by family-centred care (FCC) models, the critical component of collaboration and then definitions of family-centred practice, services and care. Finally features of FCS and their outcomes are addressed.

The family unit

When working with children, the family unit is pivotal. Family members will provide the child with life-long support; they have expert knowledge about the child through their daily lived experiences with him/her, and have an understanding of his/her likes/dislikes, roles, occupations and the environmental contexts in which these occur. Finally, in most cases family members will continue to be the child's best advocates in the health, education and welfare systems that they will engage with throughout the lifespan. Family members are not only contextually important for the child with occupational performance issues, but they are also individuals who have needs of their own and may experience their own occupational performance issues. Additionally, the family as a whole engages in occupations that are characteristic of that family and they need to be able to participate meaningfully in everyday family life (Werner DeGrace, 2004).

Werner DeGrace (2004) challenged practitioners to learn how families collectively construct their meanings of family (i.e. how family members interact, share time, space and life experiences). She argued that families are defined not just by what they 'do' (the tasks they engaged in and roles fulfilled), but also by who they 'are' (i.e. family 'being') and encouraged therapists to understand families' 'doing' occupations and how they are meaningfully occupied as a family unit. This requires families to establish a sense of connection and inner satisfaction in their daily patterns of 'doing'. She proposed that we need to focus not only on the child with special needs/occupational performance issues in the context of his/her family, but also on family routines and rituals. It is argued that rituals (such as birthday celebrations, family gatherings, bedtime stories and meal times) preserve a sense of family meaning, identity and cohesion because they make special time out of ordinary time, linking people through shared meanings. Through rituals, family relationships are built. Some research has demonstrated that families of children with developmental disabilities such as autism are over-routinised and revolve around the needs of the child with autism (Werner DeGrace, 2004), leaving limited time for engagement in meaningful family occupations and the development of cohesive rituals that support family well-being. Werner DeGrace (2004) proposed that FCS provision needs to extend beyond helping children not only to meet their developmental needs within their home/family environment, but also to facilitate families' engagement in rituals and meaningful family occupations (such as family outings or eating a meal together) (Evans & Rodger, 2008) which strengthen their identity as a family unit and the well-being of family members.

FCC models which advocate collaboration and mutual respect for clients and family members began to emerge in the late 1980s with increasing attention to the potential influences of therapy on parent–child interactions, home programmes and family life (Lawlor & Mattingly, 1998). The concept of working with families is not new, but the way occupational therapists work with family members has changed. Historically, occupational therapy intervention was provided with a child-centred focus, whereby therapists set goals that focused on the child and these were usually separate from other family members (Bazyk, 1989). Parents typically saw professionals as the experts and were expected to be passive recipients of therapy rather than acknowledged experts themselves (Brown, 2003). In the last decade, there has been a growing recognition of parents' own needs and the importance of considering the parents and other family members when planning and executing therapy goals (Law, 2002; Lawlor & Mattingly, 1998; Rodger, 2006; Rodger, Braithwaite, & Keen, 2004).

Family-centred practice, family-centred services and family-centred care

Different terms are used by different professions such as FCC by nurses in hospitals (e.g. Franck & Callery, 2004; MacKean, Thurston, & Scott, 2005; Shields, Pratt, Davis, & Hunter, 2007; Shields, Pratt, & Hunter, 2006), and FCP and FCS in early intervention (Carpenter, 2007; Edwards, Millard, Praskac, & Wisniewski, 2003) and disability and rehabilitation contexts (King, Rosenbaum, & King, 1997; Law et al., 2003). A consensus definition (Allen & Petr, 1996) is:

> FCS delivery, across disciplines and settings, views the family as the unit of attention. This model organises assistance in a collaborative fashion in accordance with each individual family's wishes, strengths, and needs. (p. 64)

FCS recognises the central role of the family as the primary unit for promoting the development of a child and that both the family and the health or education professional bring different knowledge and skills to their working relationships in order to effectively provide care and therapy to the family (Hanna & Rodger, 2002). The needs and priorities of the family determine how and when services are provided, with the emphasis on the strength and resources of the whole family and not individual family members. Goals and desired outcomes are mutually defined by the family and the health and/or education professional.

Rosenbaum et al. (1998) identified some guiding principles of FCS:

- Parents have ultimate responsibility for the care of their children.
- Family members are treated with respect as individuals.
- The needs of all family members are considered.
- Parents' expertise about the child's and family's status and needs is recognised.
- Families have an opportunity to decide on the level of involvement they wish in decision making for their child.
- The involvement of all family members is encouraged.

FCP and FCS are both underscored by the premise that collaboration and partnership is a central means that therapists, service providers and families use to work together towards common goals and combine efforts to achieve mutually agreed-upon outcomes which benefit not only the child, but also the family (Case-Smith, 1999).

FCC refers to the professional support of the hospitalised child and family through involvement, participation and partnership, underpinned by empowerment and negotiation (Smith, Coleman, & Bradshaw, 2002). This definition also recognises parents' choice about how they participate in their child's care during hospitalisation.

The terms FCC, FCP and FCS are sometimes used interchangeably in the literature across children's health care and early educational intervention. They share concepts of parental participation, partnership and collaboration between professionals and parents in decision making, family-friendly environments that normalise family those of functioning and care/support of family members and their needs, as well as children (Franck & Callery, 2004). The next section will address some of the practicalities about how to become a more child- and family-centred practitioner.

Becoming a child- and/or family-centred practitioner

The importance of working in partnership with clients was highlighted earlier in this chapter and is pivotal to being client- and family-centred. Characteristics of effective partnerships have been identified in the literature and include: mutual respect, trust and honesty; mutually agreed-upon goals; and shared planning and decision making. In this section, we will examine these characteristics in order to define practitioner skills and behaviours that are important when adopting a family-centred approach.

Relationship development

Identifying practitioner skills and behaviours that facilitate the development of effective partnerships is important because the development of a trusting and respectful relationship is unlikely to occur automatically or easily (Dunlap, Fox, Vaughn, Bucy, & Clarke, 1997; Dunst, Trivette, Davis, & Cornwell, 1994; Summers et al., 2005). Dunst, Trivette, and Johanson (1994) conducted a survey of parents and professionals to ascertain their perceptions of what makes a good partnership. The highest ranked characteristic was 'trust', followed by mutual respect, open communication and honesty. As practitioners are often required to work with a diverse range of families with complex and differing needs, it can be challenging to successfully build a strong and respectful relationship with every family (Rodger, Keen, Braithwaite, & Cook, 2008). A practitioner may have success in developing rapport with one family but not another, as was found in a study conducted by Rodger et al. (2008) with families who had a recently diagnosed child with autism. In this case, practitioners conducted home visits to a number of families involved in the study, helping them to identify and work towards intervention goals for their child. Feedback from assessments and interviews with families and practitioners highlighted how individual characteristics of the family may alter the rapport-building process.

As this research showed, to some degree, compatibility between practitioner and family appears to reflect a 'goodness-of-fit'. Understanding the ecology of a family and ensuring a good fit between that ecology and the intervention has been found to influence intervention outcomes (Fox, Vaughn, Dunlap, & Bucy, 1997; Lucyshyn, Albin, & Nixon, 1997; Moes & Frea, 2000; Vaughn, Dunlap, Fox, Clarke, & Bucy, 1997). There are a number of ways in which practitioners may gain an understanding of family ecology and use this information to establish rapport and guide goal setting and intervention such that it is compatible with family goals and priorities. One technique is to gather information about family rituals and routines which help to define the family and how time is spent by family members individually and as a family unit. Alternatively, there are several tools that can help to focus on relevant aspects. Research using the *Enabling Practices Scale* (EPS) (Dempsey, 1995), for example, has shown parents felt more able to obtain supports and resources they needed when they also had a choice about which staff worked with them (Dunst & Dempsey, 2007). Whilst it may not always be practicable to provide clients with this choice, on some occasions it may be possible to re-allocate the family to another practitioner in instances of incompatibility. Another tool that can be used is the *Helpgiving Practices Scale* (HPS) (Dunst, Trivette, & Hamby, 1996) which has been helpful in showing the importance parents place on being able to obtain needed resources, supports and services. These scales can be used as a self-assessment technique and can assist practitioners to identify key practices that are associated with a family-centred approach (see Table 3.1).

Goal identification and setting

The importance of mutually agreed-upon goals has been emphasised in much of the partnership literature (Dunst et al., 1994). The actual process of goal identification has received some attention in the clinical and research literature (Dempsey & Carruthers, 1997; Lucyshyn, Dunlap, & Albin, 2002; Rodger et al., 2004; Sperry, Whaley, Shaw, & Brame, 1999). Individualised planning using an individual education plan (IEP) or individualised family service plan (IFSP) has been one mechanism commonly used for goal iden-tification. Parent and client participation in these planning processes is encouraged and, in some countries, mandated. In the USA, for example, the Individuals with Disabilities Education Act (IDEA) amendments of 1997 and 2004 (Commission on Education and the Workforce, 2004) mandated the inclusion of parents as members of the IEP team and in the development of the IFSP associated with provision of early intervention services.

Table 3.1 Family-centred practice assessment scales

Assessment Scale	Enabling Practices Scale (EPS) (Dempsey, 1995)	Helpgiving Practices Scale (HPS) (Dunst et al., 1996)	Family-Centredness Scale (FCS) (Thompson et al., 1997)	Family-Focused Intervention Scale (FFIS) (Mahoney, O'Sullivan, & Dennebaum, 1990)
Description	The EPS is a 24-item scale which assesses parents' perceptions of the nature of support provided to them and their child with a disability by service providers. The items were designed to address 12 enabling practices identified by Dunst et al. (1988) as important in family-centred practice	The HPS is a 25-item scale that measures a variety of help-giving behaviours and practices. Each item includes five responses from which the respondent selects a behaviour that best describes a particular help-giving practice that they have received	The FCS is a 14-item rating scale which measures the family-centred nature of all services received by the family. Items in this scale ask for the degree to which service providers work in partnership, meet the needs of the entire family, help plan for the future, deliver services in a timely manner, are courteous and facilitate networking with other families	The FFIS is a 40-item rating scale which assesses the degree to which respondents receive a range of intervention services from their provider and the perceived benefits of these services. There are five subscales including systems engagement, child information, family instructional activities, personal-family assistance and resource assistance.
Properties	The scale has three factors that show high internal consistency: comfort with relationship, collaboration and parental autonomy.	The scale has high internal consistency and criterion related validity	The scale has high internal consistency and satisfactory concurrent validity	The scale has acceptable internal consistency and validity. Administration time is approximately 15–20 min
Availability	Available free of charge from authors	Contact HPS authors	Contact FCS authors	Contact FFIS authors

The actual involvement of parents in IEP or IFSP processes, however, can vary widely (Ashman & Elkins, 2002; Dabkowski, 2004) and parents are not always partners in the decision-making process (Harry, Allen, & McLaughlin, 1995; Salembier & Furney, 1997). To agree on intervention goals, there must be a shared understanding of those goals which can best be achieved by defining the goals in quite specific ways so that parents and practitioners interpret the goals in a similar way (Murray, 2000). Broadly defined goals are open to differing interpretations that can then lead to misunderstandings. In an effort to work in partnership with parents to identify parental priorities and establish shared early intervention goals (Rodger et al., 2004), the *Canadian Occupational Performance Measure* (COPM; Law et al., 1998) has been used. The COPM was developed by Law et al. (1998) from a CCP framework and has been used to document occupational performance and satisfaction. In their study, Rodger et al. used the COPM to discuss with parents of young children with autism their child's performance in areas of self-help, play, behaviour and communication (instead of productivity/work). Parents identified priorities for intervention by rating their child's performance and satisfaction with that level of performance for each area. Parents can often feel overwhelmed with the many skills they feel their child needs to acquire and areas in which they would like to see their child develop. Assisting parents to work out which of these areas are most important is not only advantageous to goal setting, but also provides a starting point for establishing mutual respect and trust.

Shared decision making

Whilst genuine sharing of decision making between families and professionals has been identified as a critical element to parent's sense of lifestyle control (Knox, Parmenter, Atkinson, & Yazbeck, 2000), parents in this study found that professionals were unwilling to share control. As a consequence, parents felt they had to fight for control by being pushy and assertive. True partnerships require professionals to view parents as key decision makers rather than simply consumers or clients of a service (Brown, Nolan, & Davies, 2001; Knox et al., 2000; Murray, 2000). The techniques outlined in this section can assist practitioners to take account of family ecology and to build positive and meaningful partnerships.

Developing family-centred services

This section focuses on the service/s in which the practitioner works, rather than the practitioner him/herself. Occupational therapists comprise one of the many professional groups who are part of inter-professional teams working with children and their families. Hence, there is a need for effective team work if the vision of coordinated and effective FCS delivery is to be achieved. In this section, we will address a number of considerations for making services more family-centred, and discuss ways of appreciating a continuum of parental/family involvement and ways of evaluating FCS from the families' and service providers' perspectives.

Considerations for family-centred service delivery

There is preliminary research evidence to demonstrate that FCS constitutes a 'best practice' approach to meeting the needs of children with disabilities and their families (King et al., 2002; Law et al., 2003). The next section will address how to operationalise FCS at multiple levels.

Client-, therapist- and systems-level issues

Operationalisation of the philosophy of FCP in an actual service requires integration and alignment of practice at the level of organisational systems and processes, as well as the level of therapist or practitioner and client (Wilkins et al., 2001). This is similar to Restall, Ripat, and Stern (2003) who also identified a framework focusing on five categories of strategies for family-centred practice – personal reflection, client-centred processes (both at the therapist level), practice settings, community organisation, and coalition advocacy and political action (at the organisational systems/processes level). Wilkins and colleagues documented strategies necessary for the effective implementation of client- and family-centred practice based on secondary analysis of transcripts from interviews with service providers who participated in three published studies by Chiu and Blumberger (1997), Rosenbaum et al. (1998) and Wilkins and Mitra (1994) cited in Wilkins et al. (2001). Examples of operational strategies for each level are summarised in Table 3.2.

Systems/organisational-level considerations

First and foremost evidence of the existence and operationalisation of a service mission and philosophy (that is grounded in values such as human worth and dignity, the right to be with a nurturing family, to participate optimally in desired life situations, to achieve one's human potential and to make informed decisions about services) is critical. These values and principles shape the organisational culture which promotes partnerships which are at the core of CCP (Lawlor & Mattingly, 1998). Organisational culture refers to norms, values, basic assumptions and shared meanings that guide the work of an organisation and are taught to new members. This culture plays a key role in determining health care provided by organisations (Hemmelgarn, Glisson, & Dukes, 2001). Figure 3.1 illustrates a vision and mission statement, values and principles of a service based in Brisbane, Australia, providing in-home therapy and respite services for children with high support needs and their families. This information is available to all families on their website and also includes information about families' rights and responsibilities. This philosophical stance is foundational to this organisation, and is referred to, discussed and reflected upon at staff retreats and

Table 3.2 Strategies for implementation of child- and family-centred services

Systems/organisation-level strategies	Practitioner/therapist-level strategies	Client-level strategies
Commitment to principles and values of CCP[1] and FCS[2] as part of organisational culture	Assistance with translating principles into practice	Clarify from outset who is the client (e.g. referring person, family, teacher, child). Is there a single client or multiple stakeholders? Is there any conflict between stakeholders/multiple clients?
Open communication	Sharing ideas and practical strategies regarding what works/does not work	Consider how therapists introduce occupational therapy in initial interactions, description of role and that of client. Ask client what they think you can do for them
Commitment to ongoing support and education for service providers and clients	Mentoring staff by asking challenging questions about practice/encouraging reflection	Consider how information is provided to clients. Are clients informed sufficiently so that they can make choices?
Responsibility with individual or group to move organisation forward to become more client-centred	Education to develop skills in negotiation, consultation, conflict resolution and client education	Re-examine client information materials (e.g. clarity, literacy levels, translations to other languages)
Seek input of clients and families through opportunities for feedback and active participation in change processes	Soliciting feedback from individual clients formally or informally	Ask clients how they prefer to work. What type of partnership works best for them?
Participatory management style to engage staff in new directions	Discussing creative solutions for engaging client who is more challenging (e.g. cultural or language barriers, issues with insight/cognition)	Find out client's priority issues using range of strategies (e.g. interview, goal-setting tools, pictures of occupations)
Rewarding effort in embracing client-centred practices	Opportunities to reflect on therapists' own practice style, relationship formation, modus operandi Personal reflection exploring own knowledge, values and beliefs about personal and professional experiences/tasks	Provide clients with information needed to participate equally in partnerships and to make choices

		Outline continuum of involvement enabling clients to make choices about level of involvement
		Engage clients in evaluation of their performance (e.g. COPM,[3] GAS[4]) and their satisfaction with services (e.g. MPOC[5])
Regular review of institutional policies and procedures and possible barriers to CCP	Recognise individual differences in how clients wish to relate to service providers (continuum of involvement/client-centred interactions)	
Environmental scan of documentation (mission statement, staff appraisal tools, programme evaluations, job descriptions, client documentation) to ensure principles of CCP are embedded	Be aware of power differentials in relationships with clients	
Modelling and coaching of staff to increase confidence in CCP	Be aware of and use evidence regarding this approach to intervention	
Formation and use of parent advisory groups/committees	Develop skills in community development, planning, leadership capacity, community needs and capacity assessment	
Engagement in coalition advocacy and political action to bring together diverse individuals and groups to advocate for system changes through policy change, resource development and ecological change. Targets can be local or national		

Based on Mortensen and Dyck (2006), Restall et al. (2003), Sumsion (2005) and Wilkins et al. (2001).

[1]CCP: client-centred practice.

[2]FCS: family-centred services.

[3]COPM: Canadian Occupational Performance Measure.

[4]GAS: goal attainment scaling.

[5]MPOC: Measure of Processes of Care.

Xavier Children's Support Network

Vision Statement

To provide excellence in service provision through innovation and empowerment of families.

Mission Statement

To provide a network of services which supports and enables families of children with high support needs to maintain an appropriate quality of life for their children in a family and community environment.

Values

- That each child with a disability is treated with dignity and as a valued member of their community
- That children with a disability have a right to and are best placed within a nurturing family environment
- That each child with a disability has a right to reach their individual potential and an appropriate level of independence
- That children with a disability have the right to participate in inclusive community activities available to all children
- That each child with a disability and their family has the right and is empowered to make decisions concerning the services they receive

Principles

- Family centred support practice
- Inclusion in family and community is promoted
- Natural family supports are valued
- A flexible and individual support response is ensured
- Family integrity is protected
- Family empowerment and responsibility must be strengthened

Figure 3.1 Example of family-centred philosophy embedded in a service mission, values and principles (Xavier Children's Support Network, n.d.). Reproduced with permission

implemented by staff, executive officers and directors providing organisational governance. The policies, procedures and practices that emanate from the organisation's mission, values and principles need to be addressed regularly to ensure that they are continuing to facilitate FCS. Feedback from clients and service providers regarding this is critical. Seeking this input is a crucial aspect of quality assurance processes and acting on this leads to continuous improvement. The engagement of both service providers (i.e. staff at all levels within the organisation) and clients who are consumers of the

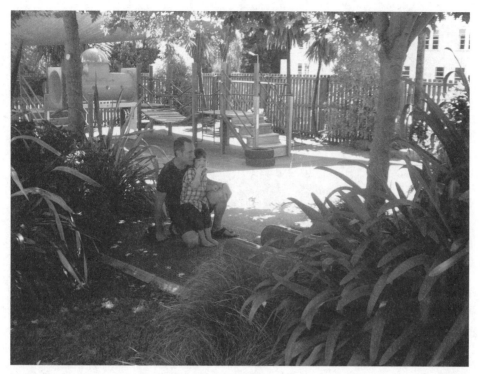

Figure 3.2 Family-friendly playground at an early intervention centre. Reproduced with permission

service supports change management through active participation (Wilkins et al., 2001).

Provision of *welcoming child- and family-friendly environments, procedures and practices* is congruent with FCP principles and attainable with due consideration to features such as: (1) attractive spaces for children and family members' waiting rooms with play areas, tea/coffee facilities and resources for parents, children and siblings (e.g. Garwick, Kohrman, Wolman, & Blum, 1998); (2) well-trained sensitive and empathic reception/front of office staff, and (3) professional staff who are cognisant of child and family needs and able to provide emotional support to family members (Hemmelgarn et al., 2001). See Figures 3.2 and 3.3 which illustrate some child- and family-friendly environments.

Family-friendly procedures and practices might include scheduling of appointments considering parent work commitments (e.g. weekends or after hours), service documentation requirements such as standards for reports and written documentation for families that consider literacy levels, cultural appropriateness and use of family-friendly diagrams and summaries. Hence, therapists need to develop skills in report writing that can transcend three levels of writing (e.g. family, organisation and medico-legal requirements) and be able to move effectively between the three styles as required.

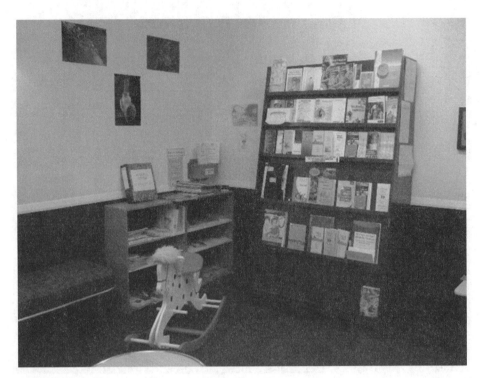

Figure 3.3 Parent and family waiting room at an early intervention centre. Reproduced with permission

Child-specific and individualised information in reports and details such as use of lay explanations, functional implications of assessment findings, specific recommendations and plans for further intervention, and implications of findings were found to be positively regarded by parents (Donaldson, McDermott, Hollands, Copley, & Davidson, 2004). Families also need information about FCS, what this means and what they can expect from the organisation and individual service providers.

Some organisations also embed a *strengths focus* that is competency enhancing rather than deficit focused into their FCP philosophy (Cooley & McAllister, 1999; MacKean et al., 2005; Viscardis, 1998). Strengths-focused practices aim to assist families and carers of young children with disabilities to identify family strengths and hold an empowered view of their child's and their family's future (Brun & Rapp, 2001; McCashen, 2005; Rapp, 1998).

Another organisational practice that is congruent with FCP is the *facilitation of family-to-family support and informal and formal networking*. This recognises the expert knowledge families have to share with one another, their capacity to empathise through shared but individual lived experiences and the importance of facilitating both formal and informal community networks. It is recognised that families with the least formal (e.g. friends, relatives and neighbours) supports require more assistance from professionals to engage with other families who might be able to provide mutual support through more formal networking (e.g. support group meetings and coffee mornings organised by parents or professionals) (Darlington & Rodger, 2006). Hanna and Rodger (2002) also highlighted the need to incorporate practices that strengthen family systems and encourage a wider use of community resources. In the final section of this chapter, an example of building the capacity of families' extended family and informal networks will be provided.

Practitioner- or therapist-level considerations

Attitudinal considerations at the practitioner or therapist level require attention to factors such as whether the individual professional's philosophical stance is congruent with that of the organisation in terms of: (1) values/ beliefs (e.g. respect and dignity), attitudes towards team work, cooperation and willingness to work with staff and family team members to reach satisfactory solutions for individual families; and (2) the practitioner's knowledge and skills in communication and collaboration leading to development of effective partnerships (i.e. mutual trusting relationships with parents, child and other family and team members). At a personal level, practitioners need a high degree of personal and professional adaptability to respond to the multiple issues influencing how families with children, particularly those with special needs, manage on a daily level. Therapists need to recognise that there will always be tension between what seems to be a natural human tendency to judge and the need to be open to a family's cultural and contextual practices in order to enable goal attainment. Minimising the tension is sometimes the very best we can do.

Availability of mentors for staff working to implement FCS and encouragement of reflection and sharing of ideas and brainstorming solutions among staff for improving FCS provision is recommended particularly when issues of language and cultural diversity and power differentials add to the complexity of practice with families (Wilkins et al., 2001). Development of high-level communication skills (e.g. negotiation, consultation and conflict resolution) to aid in the development of collaborative partnerships with parents is also critical. Provision of information/client education taking into consideration educational levels, literacy, cultural and language issues, adult learning principles and learning style preferences also needs to be well developed in family-centred practitioners (Rodger, 2006).

Continuum of parental involvement: respecting families' choices

There is a continuum of possible family involvement within FCS provision (Brown, 2003; Hutchfield, 1999). Just as all families are individual, so are their choices in terms of how they engage with service providers, their level of involvement and confidence. In modern families with a pattern of life that often involves before-school, after-school and vacation care, some families actually remain somewhat uninformed about the child's performance in many occupations that are central to childhood but which occur predominantly during periods outside of family time. Homework is sometimes completed at after-school care when parents are absent and this can lead to a lack of knowledge about the child's school-based therapy programmes.

Hutchfield (1999) described a continuum of FCC in hospitals from *parental involvement* (where the parent is advocate and emotional supporter of child, recipient and provider of information), through *parental participation* (where parents participate in care giving and nursing care if desired, share knowledge and collaborate with nurses) and *parental partnerships* (in which parent and nursing roles are negotiated, support needs are identified, parents are empowered to give care and equal status of parents as caregivers and experts on child is acknowledged) to *fully immersed FCC* (in which the parent leads the child's care, is expert in all aspects of care, is recognised as an expert on child's illness and treatment and is mutually respected and engaged at the policy level). Corlett and Twycross (2006) found that the need for professionals to have effective negotiation and communication skills in working with families and children was paramount. Equally parents need to be able to negotiate the nature or their roles and participation with the care of their hospitalised child, as well as to be involved in decision making. Hence, professionals need to create relationships with parents in which they feel empowered to do this.

Similarly, Brown (2003) described a continuum of participation with respect to delivery of therapy services in which the role of the family is either one of: (1) informant, (2) assistant, (3) co-worker, (4) partner, (5) collaborative team partner/member, or (6) service director.

Outcomes of FCP and FCS and their measurements

A final method of ensuring that services are family-centred is gaining feedback from parents/families and service providers themselves. This can be undertaken using valid and reliable evaluation methods and then utilising this information for service improvement. Two extensively researched evaluation tools are the Measure of Processes of Care (MPOC) (King et al., 1997) and the Measure of Processes of Care-Service Providers (MPOC-SP) (Woodside, Rosenbaum, King, & King, 2001). These tools and their uses and psychometric properties are summarised in Table 3.3. Practitioners must also keep abreast of the research evidence about the effectiveness of their interventions and practice philosophies such as FCP (see Chapter 15).

FCC and FCS claim to improve child and family outcomes and satisfaction, build on family strengths, increase service provider satisfaction and lead to more effective use of resources (Franck & Callery, 2004). However, high-level empirical evidence for the impact of FCC on children and family members is lacking (Shields et al., 2006). A Cochrane review (Shields et al., 2007) about FCC for hospitalised children revealed a dearth of high-quality quantitative research about FCC outcomes. However, there have been a number of qualitative studies about FCC demonstrating that negotiation between staff and families, perceptions of parents and staff roles, and costs (both financial and emotional) influenced the delivery of FCC.

Table 3.3 Summary of MPOC and MPOC-SP tools

Properties of evaluations	MPOC-56 (King, King, King, & Rosenbaum, 2004; King, Rosenbaum, & King, 1995, 1996; King et al., 1997)	MPOC-SP (Woodside, Rosenbaum, King, & King, 1998; Woodside et al., 2001)
Who should complete it?	The Measure of Process Care (MPOC) is a self-report tool for parents that measures the extent to which they perceive a service to be family-centred. It takes 15–20 min to complete	The MPOC-SP is a self-assessment tool for paediatric service providers that measures the extent to which the services they provide are family-centred. It takes 10–15 min to complete
Scales and items	MPOC contains 56 items which have five-factor analytically determined scales: • Enabling and partnership • Providing general information • Providing specific information about the child • Coordinated and comprehensive care for the child and family • Respectful and supportive care For each item parents respond to a common question: 'To what extent do the people who work with your child ...'. A 7-point response scale is used, with three of the options being: 7, 'to a great extent'; 4, 'sometimes'; and 1, 'never'. There is also a 'not applicable' category A respondent's data yield five scores, one for each of the factors or scales. A scale score is obtained by computing the average of the items' ratings. Instructions for scoring are included in the manual	This outcome measure is based on the MPOC and comprises 4 scales and 27 items. For each item, service providers respond to a common question: 'In the past year, to what extent did you ...'. A 7-point response scale is used, with the following response options available: '7' indicates that the service provider engaged in this behaviour to a very great extent, '6' to a great extent, '5' to a fairly great extent, '4' to a moderate extent, '3' to a small extent, '2' to a very small extent and '1' not at all. A score of '0' indicates that the item is 'not applicable' A respondent's data yield five scores, one for each of the factors or scales. There is no total score. Each scale score is obtained by computing the average of the relevant items' ratings
Purposes	The Measure of Processes of Care is a well-validated and reliable self-report measure of parents' perceptions of the extent to which the health services they and their child(ren) receive is family-centred. The original version of MPOC is a 56-item questionnaire; as of 1999 there is a shorter, 20-item version The purpose of the MPOC is to assess parents' perceptions of the care they and their children receive from children's rehabilitation treatment centres. It is a means to assess family-centred behaviours of health care providers Validated on samples of parents whose children range in age from 0 to >17 years and who had a variety of neuron developmental disabilities or maxillofacial disorders	Useful for purposes of professional development, educational and research initiatives in clinical settings The MPOC-SP provides one element of a comprehensive programme evaluation initiative. It provides the perspectives of service providers regarding how well they perceive that they provide services that fulfil FCP principles.

(Continued)

Table 3.3 (Continued)

Properties of evaluations	MPOC-56 (King, King, & Rosenbaum, 2004; King, Rosenbaum, & King, 1995, 1996; King et al., 1997)	MPOC-SP (Woodside, Rosenbaum, King, & King, 1998; Woodside et al., 2001)
Psychometric properties	Various studies of MPOC-56's reliability and validity have been conducted. These demonstrated good internal consistency (Cronbach's alpha ranging from .63 to .96){and test-retest reliability (intra-class correlation coefficients ranging from .78 to .88). Validity has been shown with: (a) positive correlations between MPOC scale scores and a measure of satisfaction, and (b) negative correlations between MPOC scale scores and a measure of the stress experienced by parents when dealing with their child's treatment centre. Also, responses to MPOC indicate that various components of service provision are experienced differently by parents, with data showing variations across scale scores by both individuals and groups of parent respondents	Various studies of MPOC-SP's reliability and validity as a discriminative measure have been conducted. These analyses demonstrated good internal consistency (Cronbach's alpha ranging from .76 to .88), test-retest reliability (intra-class correlation coefficients ranging from .79 to .99) and validity (i.e. including cross-disciplinary scale score comparisons and real-ideal comparison testing)
Innovation and uses	MPOC measures parents' perceptions of important aspects of care on a specific behavioural level, and is a very useful tool for programme evaluation. It is a theoretically sound measure of family-centred service. The scales fit well with the key constructs about care giving found in the literature that are fundamental to family-centredness and are associated with client outcomes MPOC has wide applicability. Over 1600 parents from across the province of Ontario have been involved in its development. Both mothers and fathers have participated, and their children were receiving a variety of services and were not limited to any specific diagnostic categories. Parents have found MPOC to be user-friendly with simple instructions and lay language. As a self-administered questionnaire, it is very suitable for mailed surveys and use in clinic settings, without the need of an interviewer	Includes service providers in the programme evaluation process. The MPOC-SP measures the perceptions of service providers – this is an important aspect of health service delivery effectiveness. Wide applicability – the MPOC-SP is useful across long-term paediatric settings. It is not limited in applicability to any specific diagnostic category or form of health care User-friendly and short Self-administered – This feature of the MPOC-SP makes it suitable for mailed surveys and in-clinic settings, without the need for an interviewer
Ordering	The MPOC manual can be downloaded free of charge: http://www.canchild.ca/Default.aspx?tabid=200	To order the MPOC-SP: send an email to canchild@mcmaster.ca. Include the title of the measure (i.e. the MPOC-SP) in your message

Based on information from the CanChild website (www.canchild.ca/), retrieved 16 February 2009.

With regards to FCS, there is an increasing number of both qualitative and quantitative studies that have addressed various aspects of FCS provision from the perspectives of parents and service providers both in Canada and elsewhere (e.g. Dyke, Buttigieg, Blackmore, & Ghose, 2006; Law et al., 2003; Raghavendra, Murchland, Bentley, Wake-Dyster, & Lyons, 2007). However, there is a need for more research addressing the outcomes of FCP/FCS philosophy from child's, parent's and service provider's perspectives and satisfaction with these.

The extended family and community

We know that there can be many different 'family' configurations sharing a variety of different living arrangements (Darlington & Rodger, 2006). Relatives may be close or more distant and differ in the way they participate in the life of the child. The family network generally extends beyond relatives to include friends, neighbours, paid carers and other members of the community with whom the family has regular contact (e.g. a swimming teacher, sports coach or church member).

The family's network of relatives, friends and community members has the potential to be an important source of support to the child and family but their capacity to be supportive is related to their acceptance of the child with a disability or occupational performance difficulties and their ability to acknowledge the many challenges faced by parents in raising a child with a disability (Cuskelly & Hayes, 2004). This acceptance and acknowledgement may not happen easily or automatically as previous research has shown. For example, grandparents have been found to fall into one of two categories: those who do and those who do not provide support to parents. In most cases, grandparents who are less supportive and involved seem to have difficulties accepting their grandchild's disability (Mirfin-Veitch & Bray, 1997).

When extended family and friends are unable or unwilling to provide support, families may need more formal supports and may also find that they increasingly associate with others in their communities who have a child with a disability (Begun, 1996). This can limit the range and type of experiences the family has and the informal supports available to the family in the longer term. By recognising the importance of support from within the family's own networks and the potential need for intervention to enable this support to occur, practitioners may be well placed to provide assistance in this area. To illustrate, we shall describe a component of an early intervention programme that was developed for families with a child diagnosed with autism. The Stronger Families program provided education and support to parents of children newly diagnosed with autism (Keen, Rodger, Doussin, & Braithwaite, 2007; Rodger et al., 2004). Parents participated in a 2-day workshop followed by 10 home visits conducted by a home facilitator. During this time, they received information about autism, play, social communication, behaviour and a range of strategies to use in the home that would facilitate the child's communication and social interaction skills. Home facilitators assisted parents to identify intervention goals and strategies that could be used in the home and within daily routines to achieve those goals.

Parents were also offered a 'Community Session' to which they could invite any number of people from their personal networks. The session was held in the evening to facilitate attendance. In most instances, participants in the program invited extended family members (the child's aunts, uncles and grandparents), paid carers (e.g. child care staff), early childhood educators and play group leaders. The session lasted for approximately 90 min during which time information was given about autism and parenting strategies that were encouraged through the Stronger Families program. The final 15 min was dedicated to answering questions for those who attended.

Written feedback gathered from Community Session participants highlighted the success of the session in facilitating a better understanding and possible acceptance of the child's disability and the challenges associated with parenting a child with autism. Some examples include:

> I was not very sure about the disorder but after tonight I now have a better understanding. Very informative session. (Grandmother)

> I guess you can never really understand what it is like to be a parent of a child with ASD unless you are one. The child with ASD will benefit greatly from this workshop and helping others to understand. (Family friend)

> The evening was fantastic full of relevant, useful and practical information which was shared in a way that was user friendly and achievable for staff in a childcare group setting who are caring for children with ASD. (Childcare staff member)

> Presented in a manner which was easy to understand and extremely useful. Certainly put my mind to how frustrated the child would feel trying to communicate. (Aunty)

Conclusion

This chapter has addressed issues that might be faced by practitioners in implementing child-centred services and FCS. Whilst there is rhetoric about the benefits of CCP research in this area is still emerging. Incorporating the principles of CCP and FCP into everyday practice with children and families is not easy and requires support at all levels (therapist, team and institution) as these philosophies must permeate the organisational culture as well as individual practitioners' activities if they are to be successfully implemented. This chapter has provided information about how this may be achieved, the characteristics of family-centred practitioners and how FCS might be broadened to meet the needs of extended family and members of the families' informal support networks.

References

Allen, R., & Petr, C. G. (1996). Toward developing standards and measurements for family centred practice in family support programs. In G. Singer, L. Powers, & A. Olson (Eds.), *Redefining family support: Innovations in public private partnerships* (pp. 57-86). Baltimore, MD: Paul H. Brookes.

Ashman, A., & Elkins, J. (2002). Rights and learning opportunities. In A. Ashman, & J. Elkins (Eds.), *Educating children with diverse abilities* (pp. 41-72). Frenchs Forest, NSW: Pearson Education Australia.

Baum, C. M., & Law, M. (1997). Occupational therapy practice: Focusing on occupational performance. *American Journal of Occupational Therapy, 51*(4), 277-288.

Bazyk, S. (1989). Changes in attitudes and beliefs regarding parent participation and home programs: An update. *American Journal of Occupational Therapy, 43*, 723-728.

Begun, A. (1996). Family systems and family-centered care. In P. Rosin, A. Whitehead, L. Tuchman, G. Jesien, A. Begun, & L. Irwin (Eds.), *Partnerships in family-centered care: A guide to collaborative early intervention* (pp. 33-63). Baltimore, MD: Paul H. Brookes.

Brown, G. (2003). Family centred care, mothers' occupations of care giving and home therapy programs. In S. A. Esdaile, & J. A. Olson (Eds.), *Mothering occupations: Challenge, agency and participation* (pp. 346-371). Philadelphia, PA: FA Davis Company.

Brown, J., Nolan, M., & Davies, S. (2001). Who's the expert? Redefining lay and professional relationships. In M. Nolan, S. Davies, & G. Grant (Eds.), *Working with older people and their families* (pp. 19-32). Buckingham, UK: Open University Press.

Brun, C., & Rapp, R. C. (2001). Strengths-based case management: Individuals' perspectives on strengths and case manager relationship. *Social Work, 46*(3), 278-288.

Canadian Association of Occupational Therapists. (1983). *Guidelines for the client-centred practice of occupational therapy*. Ottawa, ON: CAOT Publications ACE.

Canadian Association of Occupational Therapists (CAOT). (1991). *Occupational therapy guidelines for client centred practice*. Toronto, ON: CAOT Publications ACE.

Carpenter, B. (2007). The impetus for family-centred early childhood intervention. *Child: Care, Health & Development, 33*(6), 664-669.

Case-Smith, J. (1999). The family perspective. In W. Dunn (Ed.), *Pediatric occupational therapy: Facilitating effective service provision* (pp. 319-331). Thorofare, NJ: SLACK Incorporated.

Commission on Education and the Workforce. (2004). *Individuals with Disabilities Education Act*. Retrieved 17 March 2009 from http://frwebgate.access.gpo.gov/cgi-bin/getdoc.cgi?dbname=108_cong_public_laws&docid=f:publ446.108.

Cooley, W. C., & McAllister, J. W. (1999). Putting family-centred care into practice: A response to the adaptive practice model. *Journal of Developmental and Behavioural Pediatrics, 20*, 120-122.

Corlett, J., & Twycross, A. (2006). Negotiation of parental roles within family-centred care: A review of the research. *Journal of Clinical Nursing, 15*, 1308-1316.

Cuskelly, M., & Hayes, A. (2004). Characteristics, contexts and consequences. In J. M. Bowes (Ed.), *Children, families and communities: Contexts and consequences* (2nd ed., pp. 29-51). South Melbourne, Vic.: Oxford University Press.

Dabkowski, D. M. (2004). Encouraging active parent participation in IEP team meetings. *Teaching Exceptional Children, 36*(3), 34-39.

Darlington, Y., & Rodger, S. (2006). Families and children's occupational performance. In S. Rodger, & J. Ziviani (Eds.), *Occupational therapy for children: Understanding children's occupations and enabling participation* (pp. 22-40). Oxford, UK: Blackwell Science.

Dempsey, I. (1995). The Enabling Practices Scale: The development of an assessment instrument for disability services. *Australia and New Zealand Journal of Developmental Disabilities, 20,* 67-73.

Dempsey, I., & Carruthers, A.(1997). How family-centered are early intervention services: Staff and parent perceptions. *Journal of Australian Research in Early Childhood Education, 1,* 105-114.

Donaldson, N., McDermott, A., Hollands, K., Copley, J., & Davidson, B. (2004). Clinical reporting by occupational therapists and speech pathologists: Therapists' intentions and parental satisfaction. *Advances in Speech Language Pathology, 6*(1), 23-38.

Dunlap, G., Fox, L., Vaughn, B., Bucy, M., & Clarke, S. (1997). In quest of meaningful perspectives and outcomes: A response to five commentaries. *Journal of the Association for Persons with Severe Handicaps, 22,* 221-223.

Dunst, C., & Dempsey, I. (2007). Family/professional partnerships and parenting competence, confidence and enjoyment. *International Journal of Disability, Development and Education, 54,* 305-318.

Dunst, C., Trivette, C., Davis, M., & Cornwell, J. (1994). Characteristics of effective help giving practices. In C. J. Dunst, C. M. Trivette, & A. G. Deal (Eds.), *Supporting and strengthening families: Methods, strategies and practices* (Vol. 1, pp. 171-186). Cambridge, MA: Brookline Books.

Dunst, C., Trivette, C., & Deal, A. (1988). *Enabling and empowering families: Principles and guidelines for practice.* Cambridge, MA: Brookline Books.

Dunst, C., Trivette, C. M., & Hamby, D. W. (1996). Measuring the helpgiving practices of human services program practitioners. *Human Relations, 49,* 815-835.

Dunst, C., Trivette, C., & Johanson, C. (1994). Parent-professional collaboration and partnerships. In C. Dunst, C. M. Trivette, & A. G. Deal (Eds.), *Supporting and strengthening families: Methods, strategies and practices* (Vol. 1, pp. 197-211). Cambridge, MA: Brookline Books.

Dyke, P., Buttigieg, P., Blackmore, A. M., & Ghose, A. (2006). Use of the Measure of Process of Care for families (MPOC-56) and service providers (MPOC-SP) to evaluate family-centred services in a paediatric disability setting. *Child: Care, Health and Development, 32*(2), 167-176.

Edwards, M., Millard, P., Praskac, L. A., & Wisniewski, P. A. (2003). Occupational therapy and early intervention: A family-centred approach. *Occupational Therapy International, 10*(4), 239-252.

Evans, J., & Rodger, S. (2008). Mealtimes and bedtimes: Windows to family routines and rituals. *Journal of Occupational Science, 15*(2), 98-104.

Fox, L., Vaughn, B., Dunlap, G., & Bucy, M. (1997). Parent-professional partnership in behavioral support: A qualitative analysis of one family's experience. *Journal of the Association for Persons with Severe Handicaps, 22,* 198-207.

Franck, L. S., & Callery, P. (2004). Re-thinking family-centred care across the continuum of children's healthcare. *Child: Care, Health & Development, 30*(3), 265-277.

Garwick, A. W., Kohrman, C., Wolman, C., & Blum, W. (1998). Families' recommendations for improving services for children with chronic conditions. *Archives of Pediatric and Adolescent Medicine, 152*(5), 440-448.

Hall, J. A., Roter, D. L., & Katz, N. R. (1988). Meta-analysis of correlates of provider behaviour in medical encounters. *Medical Care, 26,* 657–675.

Hanna, K., & Rodger, S. (2002). Towards family centred practice in paediatric occupational therapy: A review of the literature on parent–therapist collaboration. *Australian Occupational Therapy Journal, 49,* 14–24.

Harry, B., Allen, N. A., & McLaughlin, M. (1995). Communication versus compliance: African-American parents' involvement in special education. *Exceptional Children, 61,* 364–377.

Hemmelgarn, A. L., Glisson, C., & Dukes, D. (2001). Emergency room culture and the emotional support component of family-centered care. *Children's Health Care, 30*(2), 93–110.

Hutchfield, K. (1999). Family-centred care: A concept analysis. *Journal of Advanced Nursing, 29*(5), 1178–1187.

Keen, D., Rodger, S., Doussin, K., & Braithwaite, M. (2007). A pilot study of the effects of a social-pragmatic intervention on the communication and symbolic play of children with autism. *Autism: The International Journal of Research and Practice, 11,* 7–15.

King, G., King, S., Law, M., Kertoy, M., Rosenbaum, P., & Hurley, P. (2002). *Family centred service in Ontario: A 'best practice' approach for children with disabilities and their families.* Ontario, Canada: CanChild Centre for Childhood Disability Research, McMaster University.

King, S., King, G., & Rosenbaum, P. (2004). Evaluating health service delivery to children with chronic conditions and their families: Development of a refined Measure of Process of Care (MPOC-20). *Children's Health Care, 33,* 35–57.

King, S., Rosenbaum, P., & King, G. (1995). *The Measure of Processes of Care: A means to assess family-centred behaviours of health care providers.* Hamilton, ON: McMaster University, Neurodevelopmental Clinical Research Unit.

King, S., Rosenbaum, P., & King, G. (1996). Parents' perceptions of care-giving: Development and validation of a measure of processes. *Developmental Medicine and Child Neurology, 38,* 757–772.

King, G. A., Rosenbaum, P. L., & King, S. M. (1997). Evaluating family-centred service using a measure of parents' perceptions. *Child: Care, Health and Development, 23*(1), 47–62.

Knox, M., Parmenter, T., Atkinson, N., & Yazbeck, M. (2000). Family control: The views of families who have a child with an intellectual disability. *Journal of Applied Research in Intellectual Disabilities, 13,* 17–28.

Law, M. (2002). Participation in the occupations of everyday life: 2002 Distinguished Scholar Lecture. *American Journal of Occupational Therapy, 56,* 640–649.

Law, M., Baptiste, S., Carswell, A., McColl, M., Polatajko, H., & Pollock, N. (1998). *Canadian Occupational Performance Measure manual* (3rd ed.). Ottawa, ON: Canadian Association of Occupational Therapists.

Law, M., Baptiste, S., & Mills, J. (1995). Client-centred practice: What is it and does it make a difference? *Canadian Journal of Occupational Therapy, 62,* 250–257.

Law, M., Hanna, S., King, G., Hurley, P., King, S., Kertoy, M., et al. (2003). Factors affecting family-centred service delivery for children with disabilities. *Child: Care, Health & Development, 29*(5), 357–366.

Lawlor, M. C., & Mattingly, C. (1998). The complexities embedded in family centred care. *American Journal of Occupational Therapy, 52,* 259–267.

Lucyshyn, J., Albin, R., & Nixon, C. (1997). Embedding comprehensive behavioral support in family ecology: An experimental, single-case analysis. *Journal of Consulting and Clinical Psychology, 65,* 241–251.

Lucyshyn, J., Dunlap, G., & Albin, R. (Eds.). (2002). *Families and positive behavior support*. Baltimore, MD: Paul H. Brookes.

MacKean, G. L., Thurston, W. E., & Scott, C. M. (2005). Bridging the divide between families and health professionals' perspectives on family-centred care. *Health Expectations, 8*(1), 74-85.

Mahoney, G., O'Sullivan, P., & Dennebaum, J. (1990). Maternal perceptions of early intervention services: A scale for assessing family-focused intervention. *Topics in Early Childhood Special Education, 10*, 1-15.

McCashen, W. (2005). *The strengths approach*. Bendigo, Vic.: St Luke's Innovative Resources.

Mirfin-Veitch, B., & Bray, A. (1997). Grandparents: Part of the family. In B. Carpenter (Ed.), *Families in context: Emerging trends in family support and early intervention* (pp. 76-88). London, UK: David Fulton Publishers.

Moes, D., & Frea, W. (2000). Using family context to inform intervention planning for the treatment of a child with autism. *Journal of Positive Behavior Interventions, 2*, 40-46.

Mortensen, W. B., & Dyck, I. (2006). Power and client-centred practice: An insider exploration of occupational therapists' experiences. *Canadian Journal of Occupational Therapy, 73*(5), 261-271.

Murray, P. (2000). Disabled children, parents and professionals: Partnership on whose terms? *Disability and Society, 15*, 683-698.

Novak, I., & Cusick, A. (2006). Home programmes in paediatric occupational therapy for children with cerebral palsy: Where to start? *Australian Occupational Therapy Journal, 53*, 251-264.

Raghavendra, P., Murchland, S., Bentley, M., Wake-Dyster, W., & Lyons, T. (2007). Parents' and service providers' perceptions of family-centred practice in a community-based, paediatric disability service in Australia. *Child: Care, Health & Development, 33*(5), 586-592.

Rapp, R. C. (1998). *The strengths model*. New York, NY: Oxford University Press.

Rebeiro, K. L. (2000). Client perspectives on occupational therapy practice: Are we truly client-centred? *Canadian Journal of Occupational Therapy, 67*(1), 7-14.

Restall, G., Ripat, J., & Stern, M. (2003). A framework of strategies for client-centred practice. *The Canadian Journal of Occupational Therapy, 70*(2), 103-112.

Rodger, S. (2006). Children and families: Partners in education. In K. M. Kenna, & L. Tooth (Eds.), *Client education: A partnership approach for health practitioners* (pp. 88-111). Sydney, NSW: University of NSW Press.

Rodger, S., Braithwaite, M., & Keen, D. (2004). Early intervention for children with autism: Parental priorities. *Australian Journal of Early Childhood, 29*, 34-41.

Rodger, S., Keen, D., Braithwaite, M., & Cook, S. (2008). Mothers' satisfaction with a home based early intervention program for children with ASD. *Journal of Applied Research in Intellectual Disabilities, 21*, 174-182.

Rogers, C. R. (1946). Significant aspects of client-centered therapy. *American Psychologist, 1*, 415-422.

Rogers, C. R. (1951). *Client-centred therapy: Its current practice, implications and theory*. Boston, MA: Houghton Mifflin.

Rosenbaum, P., King, S., Law, M., King, G., & Evans, J. (1998). Family-centred service: A conceptual framework and research review. *Physical & Occupational Therapy in Pediatrics, 18*(1), 1-20.

Salembier, G., & Furney, K. S. (1997). Facilitating participation: Parents' perceptions of their involvement in the IEP/transition planning process. *Career Development for Exceptional Individuals, 20*(1), 29-42.

Shields, L., Pratt, J., Davis, L., & Hunter, J. (2007). Family-centred care for children in hospital. *Cochrane Database of Systematic Reviews* 2007, Issue 1. Art. No.: CD004811. DOI: 10.1002/14651858.CD004811.pub2 http://www.cochrane.org/reviews/en/ab004811.html.

Shields, L., Pratt, J., & Hunter, J. (2006). Family centred care: A review of qualitative studies. *Journal of Clinical Nursing, 15*(10), 1317–1323.

Smith, L., Coleman, V., & Bradshaw, M. (Eds.). (2002). *Family-centred care: Concept theory and practice*. Basingstoke, UK: Palgrave MacMillan.

Sperry, L., Whaley, K., Shaw, E., & Brame, K. (1999). Services for young children with autism spectrum disorder: Voices of parents and providers. *Infants and Young Children, 11*(4), 17–33.

Summers, J. A., Hoffman, L., Marquis, J., Turnbull, A., Poston, D., & Nelson, L. L. (2005). Measuring the quality of family–professional partnerships in special education services. *Exceptional Children, 72,* 65–81.

Sumsion, T. (1996). Implementation issues. In T. Sumsion (Ed.), *Client-centred practice in occupational therapy: A guide to implementation* (1st ed., pp. 27–37). London, UK: Churchill Livingstone.

Sumsion, T. (1999). A study to determine a British occupational therapy definition of client-centred practice. *British Journal of Occupational Therapy, 62,* 52–58.

Sumsion, T. (2000). A revised occupational therapy definition of client-centred practice. *British Journal of Occupational Therapy, 62,* 52–58.

Sumsion, T. (2005). Facilitating client-centred practice: Insights from clients. *Canadian Journal of Occupational Therapy, 72*(1), 13–20.

Sumsion, T., & Law, M. (2006). A review of evidence on the conceptual elements informing client-centred practice. *Canadian Journal of Occupational Therapy, 73*(3), 153–162.

Sumsion, T., & Smyth, G. (2000). Barriers to client-centeredness and their resolution. *Canadian Journal of Occupational Therapy, 67,* 15–21.

Thompson, L., Lobb, C., Elling, S., Herman, S., Jurkiewicz, T., & Hulleza, C. (1997). Pathways to family empowerment: Effects of family-centered delivery of early intervention services. *Exceptional Children, 64,* 99–113.

Tickle-Degnen, L. (2002). Client-centered practice, therapeutic relationship, and the use of research evidence. *American Journal of Occupational Therapy, 56*(4), 470–474.

Townsend, E., Beagan, B., Kumas-Tan, Z., Versnel, J., Iwama, M., Landry, J., et al. (2007). Enabling: Occupational therapy's core competency. In E. Townsend, & H. Polatajko (Eds.), *Enabling occupation II: Advancing an occupational therapy vision for health, well-being, and justice through occupation* (pp. 87–133). Ottawa, ON: CAOT Publications.

Vaughn, B., Dunlap, G., Fox, L., Clarke, S., & Bucy, M. (1997). Parent–professional partnership in behavioral support: A case study of community-based intervention. *Journal of the Association for Persons with Severe Handicaps, 22,* 186–197.

Viscardis, L. (1998). The family-centred approach to providing services: A parent perspective. *Physical & Occupational Therapy in Pediatrics, 18*(1), 41–53.

Werner DeGrace, B. (2004). The everyday occupations of families with children with autism. *American Journal of Occupational Therapy, 58,* 543–550.

Wilkins, S., Pollock, N., Rochon, S., & Law, M. (2001). Implementing client-centred practice: Why is it so difficult to do so? *Canadian Journal of Occupational Therapy, 68*(2), 70–79.

Woodside, J., Rosenbaum, P., King, S., & King, G. (1998). *The Measure of Processes of Care for Service Providers (MPOC-SP)*©. CanChild Centre for Childhood Disability Research, McMaster University.

Woodside, J., Rosenbaum, P., King, S., & King, G. (2001). Family-centred service: Developing and validating a self-assessment tool for pediatric service providers. *Children's Health Care, 30*(3), 237–252.

Xavier Children's Support Network. (n.d.). *Our mission*. Retrieved 10 April 2009 from http://www.xcsn.org/content.mission.asp.

Chapter 4

Cultural Influences and Occupation-centred Practice with Children and Families

Alison Nelson and Michael Iwama

Learning objectives

In aim of this chapter is to:

- Extend the readers' views of how culture might be viewed within occupational therapy practice.
- Explore some of the implications this view of culture has on occupational therapy practice with children and their families.
- Present some examples of use of the Kawa Model with children to illustrate how the river metaphor may be used to understand the child's perspectives on their life flow.

Introduction

Culture is a fundamental facet of how we ascribe meaning to and make sense of occupations. Occupation as a culturally bound construct has received much attention in the occupational therapy literature recently (e.g. Hocking & Whiteford, 1995; Iwama, 2005, 2006; Kondo, 2004). These authors have pointed out that 'cultural bias is inadvertently embedded in occupational therapy' (Kondo, 2004, p. 174). In Western countries, culture is commonly defined along positivist/objectivist and universalistic lines and culture is inferred to be more an individual embodiment rather than a contextual concern. In other words, we have usually described culture as relating to an individual's association with a particular 'cultural group' (e.g. being Indian, Aboriginal or Japanese) rather than a more complex examination of *all* of the cultural contexts an individual may be influenced by (e.g. childhood, urban living, gender and socio-economic status).

Throughout this chapter, we will use examples of working with Indigenous children as a way of trying to highlight the taken-for-granted assumptions we make about not just Indigenous children but *all* children in our everyday practice. It is hoped that using one 'other' cultural group (Indigenous Australians) will highlight the issues and possibilities surrounding our work with all 'other' cultural groups, including that of children.

Culture and the occupations of the child

In practice, traditional occupational therapy for identified groups of people, including children, has followed a familiar pattern borrowed or transplanted from rehabilitation of adults. This pattern is based on the 'able-ist' social norm of autonomy, independence, instrumental function and competency (or the ability to compete). The general expectation extending from these norms for children is that they are able to perform the roles consistent with child-hood such as those of son/daughter, student, self-carer, etc. As occupational therapists working with children and families, we therefore bring our own enculturated view of children, childhood and childhood occupations to our interactions and interventions.

Our theoretical models and frameworks have also followed this familiar pattern, and many are merely extensions of a particular worldview that favours or privileges an adult, autonomous, individual-centric 'occupational' being which is the 'norm' within the culture of contemporary occupational therapy. The authors of these models have, after all, developed their models from the very social and cultural contexts in which they abide and have experienced the realities that they are trying to describe and explain. These models are often predicated on the experience of normal (Western) adulthood and being.

It should come as little surprise then that established approaches to occu-pational therapy for children have also reflected the features that adults who hold this view would consider normal or ideal. In the Western world, this is often observed in the values inherent in occupational therapy practice with children including independence, autonomy, rational choice and future (goal-setting) orientation. This bias is not always easy to see for those of us who represent the dominant Western culture because we often come from a sub-conscious position that 'our' beliefs and practices are 'the norm' (Awaad, 2003; Iwama, 2006; MacNaughton & Davis, 2001).

In order to practice in a truly occupation-centred way with children, we need to recognise that we are *all* culturally situated (Bonder, Martin, & Miracle, 2004), that is, we have all been influenced by the cultures, families, beliefs and values that we were brought up in, taught or learnt as we devel-oped into adults. When we become more aware of our own position, our own values and beliefs, we are less likely to project our own view of what is 'normal' onto clients. This is a starting point in enabling us to fit our therapy with the meanings and realities of the children and families who are our clients (Iwama, 2006; Nelson, 2007).

We advocate a broader definition of culture by expanding its location and interpretation outside of the individual, into the social realm of shared experience and collective meanings of shared phenomena and objects in the world. By doing this, we recognise that the culture of the child is not necessarily racially or ethnically bound. The forms, functions and meanings (Yerxa et al., 1989) of occupation can be comprehended through the cultural experiences of the child rather than on assumptions that are stereotypically attributed to the child by authorities or dominant groups representing an 'other' *sphere of shared experiences* (culture). In other words, the cultural features of children as a defined cultural entity or group may, in many complex ways, differ markedly from the cultural views of reality held by adults, which in contemporary occupational therapy still commands the standard: authority in analysis, interpretation, categorisation and explanation of a child's occupational performance, intervention and outcome measurement. To illustrate this point, consider, for example, engaging in a sporting activity such as soccer. To the adult (and particularly the occupational therapist), the shared meanings we ascribe to soccer may include the development of gross motor skills, opportunities for socialisation and gaining physical fitness through a form of exercise. Some adults may have also constructed meanings of soccer based on seeing elite sportsman, exposure to the World Cup, their own competence and belonging to a club. For children, the sphere of shared experiences in playing soccer may mean having fun with friends, winning or losing, or eating hot chips afterwards.

Just as in instances when explanations and interpretations of human acts of an 'other' cultural group are performed by another dominant group, occupational therapists may have engaged in a similar process of interpreting or making assumptions about the form, function and meaning of children's occupations (Yerxa et al., 1989). As Burgman and King (2005) stated, 'we need to be mindful of how our ways of thinking about childhood affect the ways we make our own meanings and communicate these to the children we are serving' (p. 154). From the vantage of many adults, children are seen to be unable to articulate their thoughts and feelings, 'adequately'. They appear to lack the insight in a way that adults can comprehend. This is even more dramatically demonstrated when the child has an illness, injury or disability which further hinders his/her ability to communicate or express his/herself. Thus, tuning in to the occupational world of the child-client represents a profound undertaking. This is not only because the child is considered to lack the necessary (adult) skills of cognition and insight, but perhaps also because we unwittingly insist that the child's experience be comprehended and valued through Western-centric, rational, autonomous standards of the adult health professional/ occupational therapist.

The privilege of occupational therapy

We as occupational therapists carry a great privilege of being well-educated and having knowledge about health and education systems (another culture or shared sphere of experience and meaning) that many of our clients may not have experienced or comprehended (consider, e.g., how 'foreign' it felt the first time you entered a large hospital institution as a therapist or student). For some of us, we also have the privilege of growing up as the cultural 'norm' against which all 'others' are measured (Moreton-Robinson, 2000). This privilege carries a potential danger if left unchecked, that in a well-intentioned desire to 'help' we come from a subliminal position of superiority as the 'expert' where the child is positioned as lesser and powerless and we see only the 'needs' and fail to see the assets, capabilities and gifts that they offer (Townsend, 2003).

Occupational therapy has at its core a value of being non-judgemental. However, this is very difficult to do. We are products of our environments, each with a set of values that causes us to see the world and our place in it in a particular way. We cannot help but be influenced by the attitudes of family, friends and the media. In Australia, for instance, we have grown up with media portrayals of Indigenous people as fantastic athletes, noble savages or drunk, unemployed and neglectful of their children. Whilst we may disagree with these portrayals, these images and stories are part of our collective psyche and unless we actively seek to critique them, we may operate under their influence. We need to seek therefore not so much to be non-judgemental as to be critical of the unconscious judgements we will unwittingly make. This is essential if we are to be both child- and occupation-centred. The ability to do this requires making our own assumptions visible and examining the 'unsaid' power relationships behind those assumptions. Some of these power relationships were also discussed in Chapter 3. For example, if we take the portrayals of Indigenous people given above we might ask, who benefits from portraying Indigenous people in these ways? How do these portrayals give power to or disempower Indigenous people? What is the role of non-Indigenous people in creating these circumstances? Once we begin asking these questions, we can also practice empathy by trying to think about the circumstances of 'the other' from their vantage (e.g. taking away my land, removing me from my home and taking my children away from me might well result in my life being one of poverty, depression and substance abuse). This can help us to challenge our assumptions about what is 'normal' when faced with a shared sphere of experience which is different from our own.

Cultural safety in occupational therapy

This recognition of power differentials in our interactions with clients is a core tenet of cultural safety (Gray & McPherson, 2005). Cultural safety recognises the effect of past and present political actions on the current health status of many (often colonised) peoples. We must acknowledge that these health conditions will not change 'without a significant redistribution of power, authority and control of resources' (Jungerson, 2002, p. 5). Culturally safe practice also requires the therapist to critically examine his/her own values and attitudes and how these have been influenced by a socio-political context. For example, as a mother in a Western society, I (Alison) hold certain assumptions about my role of being 'the teacher' and the one who 'knows best' for my child. Whilst as an occupational therapist I may also adhere to the principals of client-centred practice, I still unwittingly bring my 'Western mothering lens' to my encounters with clients. I cannot separate this from my practice but I do need to question these attitudes as a therapist (uncomfortable as that may be) if I am to see the ways these attitudes may potentially disempower my child-clients to express their needs. We propose the metaphorical notion of side-to-side processes (rather than expert-driven) connoting a lateral structure of the patient–therapist dynamic, mirroring a more balanced client–environment relationship. As Watson (2006) has stated, the 'doing' of occupational therapy will flow out of the partnership we establish where we can 'make the most of what each has to offer' (p. 156). This partnership is reflective of Indigenous cultures and often requires a conscious effort for therapists from White Western culture which values busyness, activity and time efficiency, as building a partnership of this nature will necessarily take time.

We recognise, however, that to a large extent, our views of children and their occupations, and our Western centredness *will* influence our practice as occupational therapists. In grappling with how to practice in a way that values the child's cultural context, we are painfully aware that it is always a flawed process. However, we have adopted an approach of self-reflection and caution where we attempt to be sensitive to the possibilities of danger in our assumptions and seek to move beyond these to a new realm of shared spheres of experience in occupational therapy.

For example, when working as non-Indigenous people with Indigenous families, we may be well aware that Indigenous people often face poverty, disease and lack of access to appropriate education and health services. However, there is a danger that in our Western 'ways of knowing' which value statistics, epidemiological data and causal relationships, we then (perhaps subconsciously) assume that Indigenous children are 'lacking' in nearly every facet of life. Bond (2005) reported that as an Aboriginal woman, researcher and health worker, she resisted the notion that her Aboriginality was a risk factor for high rates of ill-health and disease. For her, being Aboriginal carried many other (positive and wonderful) meanings, yet when working in health, it was reduced to health status and 'risk'. In addition, even those Indigenous Australians who *do* deal with poverty and ill-health on a daily basis may display great resilience and have much to teach us as health professionals and fellow human beings, about dealing with complex social and health issues and how these can be overcome or lived with. The pathologising of Indigenous people further disempowers us as health professionals from seeing Indigenous people as possessing valuable resources which can assist the therapeutic process. When we choose to work in partnership with Indigenous Australians and to take an attitude of humility and being a 'learner', not a 'teller', we are far more likely to be enabling practitioners. This example highlights the ways in which we can inadvertently hold a view (of an Aboriginal child or of *any* child) which disempowers when ideally our aim is to enable and indeed learn from the children and families we see.

Meeting the individual needs and learning from the individual experiences of Indigenous Australians requires that we do not take an essentialist view of who Indigenous people are. That is, we recognise that just as all children have a unique personality and set of needs and abilities, there are innumerable experiences of being Indigenous (Paradies, 2006). In reality, our identities are complex and multi-faceted and it is important that we do not assume that because a client is Indigenous or even because a client is a child, they will fit a particular 'profile' that has usually been ascribed to them by someone else (Paradies, 2006).

How should we proceed, then, to gain a better, more equitable approach to the occupational life and context of the child? Whilst we contemplate and innovate better ways, we may need to first acknowledge the inadequacies and the cultural boundaries of our current forms, functions and meanings of practice (Yerxa et al., 1989). We may need to appreciate the cultural biases embedded in our tools and models and even acknowledge when a specific model or procedure is wrong, disadvantageous and therefore 'unsafe' for the client.

There is support for a critical re-evaluation of our theory and practices in occupational therapy for children, to move away from an individual-centred focus where the determination of problems and needs is predicated on pathologies embodied in the child, towards encompassing the physical and social environmental factors, and viewing the child's family as an integrated unit of concern known as the 'client'. See Chapter 3 for further details. Environment has long been acknowledged as an important factor in shaping, enabling and also limiting and constraining the individual client, but when doing so, the client is still viewed and comprehended to be a separate and distinct entity from the environment. Contrast this popular worldview with another one shared by Eastern societies and Aboriginal groups of the world, who hold to the view that there is no such thing as a (rational) separation between self and the environment/context and that all aspects of nature are inseparably inter-related. These distinctly differing worldviews can be demonstrated by explaining that 'the child is in the environment' and 'the environment is in the child as much as the child is in the environment'.

If we can re-conceptualise culture to mean shared spheres of experience and the ascription of meaning to objects and phenomena in the world, then not only can we consider the world of shared experience of childhood as a cultural entity, but we can also recognise that the structure and mechanisms for how these meanings are expressed, comprehended/measured and transmitted (in occupational therapy) are also culturally determined. In an extreme sense, such models, instruments and frameworks, through which we filter children's responses, might also be deemed culturally 'unsafe'. So in order to better comprehend the occupational world of the child, and to appreciate it closer to the way to which that child might comprehend it, we may need alternative approaches that afford a better view.

The Kawa Model: a tool for culturally safe practice

One recent development in occupational therapy theory that may offer an alternative way for occupational therapists to comprehend the child in a familiar context is the Kawa (Japanese for 'river') Model. The model uses a familiar metaphor of the river as a narrative or explanation of the life course to gain a broader and more comprehensive view of the client in the context of his/her daily realities – from the client's vantage. Life, as described in the Kawa Model, is like a river; its starting point may be up in the distant hills, and may meander down an eventful course, towards a distant sea which symbolically represents end of life. At any point along one's life course, one's river can be appreciated as a configuration of contextual factors. Water in this metaphor symbolises life flow, and life energy. In some cultural contexts, the water has also been conceptualised to symbolise and explain 'occupation'. As long as there is water in the river course, there is life or potential for greater life flow. River walls which give shape and volume to the flow of water may symbolise factors such as the social and physical environment. Rocks, of different shape, size and number, can appear in the river course affecting the quality of water flow at that location. Rocks symbolise difficulties and challenges. These rocks might have been there since birth or may have, like an acquired illness or accident, suddenly appeared. Driftwood, which has a serendipitous character, may flow by inconsequently, push structures like rocks and walls aside to create greater flow or become caught up between rocks, resulting in compounding impediment or a slowing down of water (life) flow at that particular point in the life course. By using these four simple elements that depict a river, the occupational therapist is transformed into becoming a facilitator of each client's life flow (Table 4.1).

Enabling or facilitating a person's life flow

Occupational therapists using the *kawa* metaphor are able to conceptualise or imagine the child's life journey in the fullness of the child's daily life context. When the child/client is unable to exploit the *kawa* metaphor by him/herself, members of the family, surrogates and others who hold the client's interests at heart are invited to participate in filling out the metaphorical representation of the child's life flow and circumstances. Depictions of the river flow characteristics can be compared with other views of the client's life flow retrospectively as well as prospectively. Occupational therapy's mandate is to enhance and even maximise the child's life flow.

Until now, we have proceeded with an approach of 'adults know best'. We are not used to anything else, especially those of us who have grown up in shared spheres of experience of being a part of a dominant group in which our ideas have eluded critical reflection, and adjustment. This situation is not unlike that of dominant nations during the colonial era where the subjugation of other groups of people was justified by a need to 'cultivate' the other to meet the dominant group's standard of 'normal'.

Table 4.1 Using the Kawa framework with an urban Indigenous family to direct intervention and approaches in context: examples of *culturally safer* practices in action[1]

Kawa/context location	Approach and intervention options	Contextual considerations/ideas to support and enable culturally safer approaches
Environmental factors – river walls	Develop a relationship	• Understand key people in child's life (may not be mum and dad but aunts/ uncles, etc.) • Have a long-term therapist and take time to build trust. Share something of your own life • Use an Indigenous liaison person • Be aware of differences in communication style, for example, lack of eye contact, non-verbal communication • Be a 'learner not a teller'
Environmental factors – river walls	Assessment processes	• Understand the client's environment including socio-economic status, family make-up and social factors such as employment, the level of literacy of parents and the presence of social supports, violence or alcohol abuse
All four components of Kawa Model (river walls, rocks, driftwood and water)	Assessment tools	• Use Kawa Model as a way of understanding the child in his/her context • Tools such as the Person–Environment– Occupation (PEO) model have assisted therapists in identifying areas of occupational performance concern
Problems – rocks Environmental factors – river walls	Intervention tools that value culture	• Use colours of the Aboriginal flag • Use Indigenous art on worksheets (with permission) • Use photos and pictures to show therapeutic techniques (values the child and helps parents with reduced literacy levels)
Environmental factors – river walls, water, life flow	Intervention processes	• See children in small groups (this helps reduce a sense of shame at being singled out from others) • Remain occupation-centred by adapting group to meet individual needs of each child within the session
Environmental factors – river walls	Organisational- level considerations	• Plan services so that logistical issues such as attendance, location and timing of the service are more appropriate for Indigenous clients

Table 4.1 (Continued)

Kawa/context location	Approach and intervention options	Contextual considerations/ideas to support and enable culturally safer approaches
		• Seeing children in local settings such as their schools where they do not need to organise additional transport to minimise the impact of socio-economic barriers • Seeing children in natural setting also helps therapist understand context
Environmental factors – river walls; personal assets and liabilities – driftwood	Develop community links	• Attend special 'cultural' days of celebration (e.g. concerts, sporting events) to meet community members and gain a deeper understanding of the world of your client • Enables the therapist to see the 'assets' (driftwood) of clients and families in their context
Environmental factors – river walls	Be self-reflective	• As with all occupational therapy practice, these strategies have been developed within a particular cultural and social context. They have emerged in an urban setting and as such may be different from what is required in more remote Indigenous communities. Our intention therefore is not to prescribe a particular way of practising but rather to provide stimulus for thought about how one might adapt practice for a particular context or situation

[1] This information is provided by Alison, a White woman who has grown up in Australia as one of the privileged representatives of the dominant Western culture. Whilst this does not prescribe my views or values about many issues (indeed I resist and abhor many of the views about Indigenous Australians portrayed in popular media), I am nevertheless a product of this environment.

We propose that two guiding principals may be useful: first, allowing children, if they can, to express their occupational views through their own words and through media that are not limited to the sophisticated world of (adult) literacy. Children will often use symbols and non-language-based expression of their thoughts and experiences (Burgman & King, 2005). Second, when the child-client is not capable of expressing his or her needs and circumstances, we need to trust the insights of loved ones who hold the child's best interests at heart, to contribute to a comprehensive appreciation of the child's occupational performance and needs. This may take the form of a conference around the child's needs, in which a number of voices are speaking to the child's river (i.e. life flow and circumstances).

Case study: the broader context

The following section of this chapter provides an example of occupation-centred practice with Indigenous Australian children. Whilst this book will also be read by those living outside Australia, it is anticipated that many of the principles outlined will have some relevance in other cultural contexts. In fact, the authors believe that there are profound lessons that occupational therapists can learn about meeting the challenges of diversity, difference and client-centred practice from such cases featuring Indigenous people. We are not presenting this as a *cultural* case per se. To present this case as 'Aboriginal' would suggest that culture and difference is located in the child as embodiment, rather than a set of features that emerges from an integration of self and context, of shared spheres of experience. Every person is unique and represents a unique constellation of internal (self) and external (context) factors. We could easily take the identifying label, aborigine, and leave it off. The case would still show the child's situation in context, and lead to a more meaningful and relevant occupational therapy response that is uniquely tailored to each child's unique situation, regardless of race and ethnicity. The use of identifiers such as 'Aboriginal' is to broaden the reader's comprehension of the broader context of the case, which brings important factors such as history and polity that have an ultimate bearing on the form, functions and meanings of occupation (Yerxa et al., 1989).

Kerrey is a 13-year-old girl living in an urban setting. She was asked to draw 'her river' and show what made it easier or more difficult to be active and healthy (see Figure 4.1). The focus of this exercise was around the occupations of leisure and play. When talking with Kerrey, not only was I (Alison) interested in her perceptions of her life and health, but I also drew upon my own observations. This is consistent with the notion of using objective and subjective assessment and demonstrates the ways in which the Kawa Model can be used both as a direct tool with clients and as an organising framework for the therapist's assessment processes.

Therapists' observations and knowledge of environmental context

The river walls and river bed

Indigenous Australians have, as the original inhabitants of Australia, a unique history and culture that are in many ways different from the experiences and history of those from diverse cultures who have come to make Australia their home following European invasion.

Australia is a colonised nation. Since European settlement, Indigenous Australians have experienced dispossession of land, active destruction of culture and language and disruption to family, culminating with a government

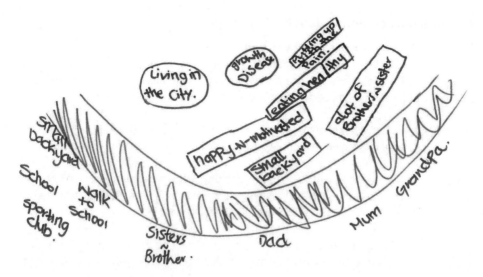

Figure 4.1 Kerrey's river. Reproduced with permission

policy of the removal of Indigenous children from their families for several decades of the last century. This has resulted in a health status which is now well below that of other Australians, with Indigenous Australians expecting to live an average 17 fewer years than their non-Indigenous peers, be 2-4 times more likely to experience infant mortality, be 17 times more likely to develop diabetes and be at greater risk for a range of lifestyle diseases (National Aboriginal Community Controlled Health Organisation (NACCHO), 2001; Thomson et al., 2008). The health needs of Indigenous Australians appear to be similar in many ways across urban, rural and remote areas (NACCHO, 2001). On a global scale, the gap in life expectancy is significantly greater than that of Indigenous peoples living in other Westernised nations such as the Maori in New Zealand or the Indigenous nations of North America (Ring & Brown, 2003). Whilst many would argue we are now living in a post-colonial age, for many Indigenous Australians, colonisation continues in many, perhaps less obvious, forms.

For occupational therapists working with children, we need to be aware of the ways in which the knowledge and practices of Indigenous families continue to be viewed negatively, or at least as inferior, when compared to the knowledge and practices of White Western medicine and education. In addition, the history of colonisation and the resultant governmental policies have left not only a legacy of physical, emotional and social ill-health for Aboriginal families, but also a legacy of often unspoken and unacknowledged attitudes within non-Indigenous Australians towards Indigenous families that disempower and disadvantage. Not surprisingly then, Indigenous families are often suspicious of what they call 'mainstream' services. This context is the one in which occupational therapists will be seen in while and trying to support Indigenous families.

Kerrey's observations about her environment

The river walls and river bed

Kerrey identified that in her social environment, her family members enabled her to be active and healthy by driving her to sporting commitments, cooking healthy meals and playing with her.

> ... like I've got a big family and it makes it easier to kind of exercise 'cos you can never be alone. You won't be alone by yourself if some go.

Kerrey also identified that in her physical environment, her ability to be active was limited by a small backyard and living in the city but facilitated by living close enough to school that she could walk.

> 'Cos we grew up back [in the country] real sporty and that. And moving here [the city] there's nowhere to run. You can't ride your bike or anything.

The school environment also enabled her to be active through sporting activities.

Interestingly, Kerrey did not mention any broader political aspects to her river walls and river bed. This perhaps reflects the difference between an adult view and that of a child. In other conversations with Kerrey, it was apparent that she was acutely aware of issues of 'race' and the impact on her as an Aboriginal person in a colonised country but in her day-to-day life, she did not recognise this political environment as directly affecting her health or daily leisure pursuits. It may also reflect the differences between shared spheres of experience as a White woman and that of a young Aboriginal woman.

Therapist's observations/knowledge about problems (rocks) and assets and liabilities (driftwood)

Kerrey appeared to be active and healthy. She was observed running around at school and her parents reported that she engaged in soccer and athletics on a regular basis. However, Kerrey's mother sustained an injury which meant she was no longer able to drive Kerrey to her sporting activities. This was identified by the therapist as a problem in terms of Kerrey's ability to pursue these leisure activities.

Kerrey's interpretation of her rocks and driftwood

Kerrey identified rocks in her river that made it harder to be active and healthy. A small backyard and living in the city again featured as problems. Kerrey also described having a 'growth disease' as a problem as it caused her pain to run. However, she immediately added a log (driftwood) which she identified as an asset of putting up with the pain and another which she described as being a happy and motivated person.

> And our doctor said we had to either put up with the pain or stop running and we put up with the pain because we want to keep running.

This demonstrated her resilience and ability to see 'a way through' her pain at this point in time. Kerrey also identified that she was happy and motivated and that this was an asset to her health and activity.

Using the river metaphor with Kerrey provided an opportunity for her to express her view of her world. Reflecting on Kerrey's river also gave the therapist an opportunity to critically examine her own assumptions about the 'lived reality' of a young Indigenous Australian woman.

Intervention planning possibilities

An initial assessment of Kerrey's situation may well identify her knee pain as a major barrier to her leisure pursuits. However, after using the Kawa Model as a framework for understanding Kerrey's context, it became apparent that the biggest issues for her accessing physically active leisure were transportation and her immediate physical environment. Thus, intervention may be aimed more at addressing these needs in the first instance.

Additional observations of using the Kawa Model with young Indigenous Australians

In trialling the Kawa Model with a number of Indigenous young people (aged 11–14 years), results have been varied in terms of how well they engaged with the metaphor of the river but in all cases, additional information was provided through the use of the Kawa Model that was not otherwise recorded through a direct interview process. At times, the young people needed a lot of examples of what could go in the river (e.g. a rock might be an injury) and this was a limiting factor in its use. Generally girls engaged with the river drawing more than boys and appeared to relate more to the use of metaphor. This may have been because it involved drawing, with some boys feeling the need to pre-empt their drawings with an explanation that ... I'm not a good drawer (Willy).

The young man who drew the river depicted in Figure 4.2 chose to use a more Indigenous style of drawing rather than following the therapist's example of a more 'traditional western river'. However, his interpretation of the metaphor was more concrete. He tended not to assign metaphorical meaning to the objects in his river. Nevertheless, it gave him an opportunity to express how he 'sees' a river and provides an insight into how even our idea of how a river 'looks' is culturally bound.

Using the Kawa Model also provided opportunities for Indigenous young people to exert their power in the relationship. Rather than answering the therapists' questions, they were able to exert their authority as the author/ s of their rivers, challenging my assumptions about what they had drawn or what 'should' be a problem. For example, one participant when asked if being on crutches was a problem as a barrier to his participation in physical activity responded:

> ... but see when I broke my toes I was on crutches and I had to walk around everywhere with them and we always go places and I had to always walk around and I'd always go to the footy club. I'd go all the way down to the footy club on crutches, to support my team and then walk back up home. (Willy)

So clearly he did not see his injury as a rock and using the river metaphor helped me see where I may have jumped to the conclusion that an injury was a barrier to physical activity participation.

Culturally appropriate goal setting

Client-centred practice necessitates that therapists and clients collaborate to meet goals that are meaningful for the client (Canadian Association of Occupational Therapists, 1997). Goal-setting with children in an

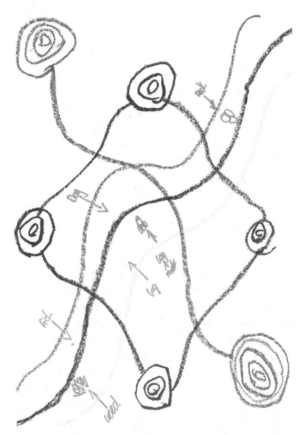

Figure 4.2   Patrick's river. Reproduced with permission

occupation-centred way is still developing in practice. However, like much occupational therapy theory, many of the current goal-setting tools used in occupational therapy practice are embedded in White Western ways of knowing about the world and indeed about occupation. The Kawa Model was used in these cases to help the therapist and the Indigenous young person gain a shared understanding of the young person's occupational needs and context. The Kawa Model provided a visual way for the children to create their current life situation through the illustration of their own 'river'. This can lead to discussions between therapist and child about his/her priorities and perspectives regarding aspects of his/her life that can be changed, and the influence of the environment (river bed), problems (boulders/rocks) as well as assets and liabilities (driftwood) on the flow of the 'river'.

The crux of using the Kawa Model is to explicate and illuminate context. Context is what explains the form, function and meaning (Yerxa et al., 1989) of occupations. The cases described above illuminate the importance of appreciating the deeper, unique contextual factors, in concert with the more emergent and readily apparent contexts of meanings that combine to limit and enable flow of a person's life and occupations.

Making the invisible visible

Nature or the ecological environs is infinitely complex and still forms the media through which we navigate our occupational lives. Rationally oriented people, with a quest to make things and processes more efficient (and in a way which privileges humans), have attempted to simplify their comprehension of nature and have positioned the 'self' above it. Our models in occupational therapy have reflected this particular worldview by treating the self and environs in a rational dualism where the 'self' is a separate entity from his/her environment. Unwittingly, our models have also privileged the 'adult' and able skills of insight, language and literacy, using adult-made structures and frameworks as the media through which occupational narratives are filtered and processed. 'Occupation', for example, is often justified by the need to conjoin this artificially separated dichotomy.

In this chapter, two cases involving (Aboriginal) young people were utilised to illuminate the cultural influences on the performance and meaning of their occupations. The Kawa Model was used as a framework to appreciate the unique features of children's occupations and their perspectives of factors impacting these occupations. For occupational therapists to practice in a way which can truly be enabling for all clients, we must learn to think and act critically about the value patterns and assumptions embedded in both our theories and our broader contexts (Kronenberg, Algado, & Pollard, 2005). This necessitates learning to reflect at both a macro and a micro level. Not only do we need to reflect on aspects of our day-to-day practice (e.g. Did the child meet the goals we had for this session? Did I use myself therapeutically?), but we also need to make time to reflect on the ways in which our attitudes and values have been shaped. We can do this formally through activities like writing down our personal values and how these might impact on our practice. However, we also need to reflect informally on a regular basis as a tool for making visible what is often invisible to us when we are embedded in our own seemingly 'normal' context. The cases outlined above have illustrated the ways in which the Kawa Model is one tool which can help to make these assumptions more visible.

To be a reflective practitioner requires us to ask 'why' when we are confronted by difference. We then need to ask 'what can I do to change?' For example, when working with Indigenous Australian families, we might be confronted by different views of time. If an Indigenous client has a 9 a.m. appointment but typically arrives 20 min late (or not at all), we might be tempted to assume they do not value the service we provide or they are disrespectful of our time. What we need to do in order to be enabling practitioners is to examine these assumptions and ask 'why might they be coming late or not arriving?' (e.g. they are relying on public transport, they do not have money for transport, they got lost in the hospital grounds, they had another family commitment that needed attending to, they thought of 9 a.m. as being any time after 9 a.m., etc.; the list could go on). We then need to ask 'what can I do to change?' (e.g., make a visit to them, liaise with an Aboriginal community group to arrange transport, have a drop-in time for appointments in the mornings and call the day before the appointment to check if they can make it). These strategies may assist Indigenous people in accessing services without rigid timeframes, for example, having a time before lunch on a Tuesday when families may drop in and have a drink, a chat and some therapy. All of these options will take time and effort and possibly financial investment but they are necessary if we want to 'avoid contributing to the oppression of the very people we intend to help' (Kronenberg et al., 2005, p. xvi). Here, we also emphasise that these strategies are but an example of the ways in which we need to approach practice with *all* children from their vantage and context and then modify our practice (and often our attitudes) to suit.

Relationship: the art of occupational therapy

Gray and McPherson (2005) have argued that the development of a culturally safe relationship necessitates the examination of power relationships between the therapist and client in order for open communication of needs to occur. Being reflective in practice is an important first step in developing meaningful relationships with Indigenous (and indeed *all*) families (Nelson, Allison, & Copley, 2006). Having an effective relationship with children is the cornerstone of occupation-centred practice. It is from this relationship that the importance of different occupational roles can be understood and meaningful goals established. A well-developed relationship also enables the therapist to gather accurate information about the child's abilities and difficulties as well as providing effective interventions (Nelson & Allison, 2007). Taking time to do this is not always easy in the current therapy environment of increased efficiency and prioritisation. However, working with children and their families will require several changes in approach and priorities if services are to be appropriate, effective and truly occupation-centred.

There are times when occupation-centred practice with families involves working with more than just the individual child and his or her parent(s). Building an effective relationship enables the occupational therapist to gain a better understanding of the key people within each child's life and the ways in which these people impact on his/her occupations. This relationship helps us to develop a shared understanding of what is meaningful to the child and his/her family. Many of our future and present clients will hold quite different meanings of the word 'family' from a White Western interpretation. For example, for many Indigenous Australians, 'family' means not just the inclusion of extended family as an integral part of daily life, but also as those who may carry certain responsibilities for care of a child, other than the biological mother or father. These family members are no less important than mum and dad and need to be considered with great respect. For example, it may be that the child's grandmother has responsibility for caring for a child with a disability within the home whilst the older brother or sister or cousin may be responsible for care at school. Occupational therapists therefore would need to consider all these people in any intervention plan.

These issues of providing culturally safe services present many challenges when working with children in an occupation-centred way. What are the meaningful occupations of this child, within his/her cultural and familial context? How are these occupations enacted within this child's context, for example, are they performed individually or collectively? And how can occupational therapy best meet the occupational needs of this child within his/her context? For some families, the answers to these questions may not be terribly far removed from the values underpinning conventional occupational therapy practice with children. For others, it may be that their occupational needs cannot and should not be addressed through traditional occupational therapy practices but through advocacy and the provision of resources that enables families to move from being 'in need' (Whiteford, 2007). For other families, it may be that an approach embracing both these ways of practicing is required. Consider, for example, those living in poverty in remote Indigenous communities with limited access to appropriate or adequate health care. For these people, the occupational needs are issues of access and equity which are beyond individual-level needs. As Mbambo (2005) stated, 'poverty is an impairment because it makes people unable to reach their full potential at times' (quoted in Watson, 2006, p. 157).

Ultimately, using a family-centred approach in its broadest sense will help to explore the occupational needs of our clients (Whiteford & Wright St-Clair, 2002). If we approach each client and his/her family and community on a case-by-case basis, we can establish whether the occupational needs of each client are best met in an individual-, family- or community-centred manner,

Indeed, it may be that the family or community become our 'client' rather than the individual.

Assumptions of normal function imposed from the spheres of experience around adult competency, like independence, autonomy, self-determinism, etc., are often unwittingly imposed upon children in occupational therapy practice. This creates difficulties on one hand because many of the children that we are trying to help either have not developed that standard of competency (such as in neonates, and children with severe disabilities) or are just in the early stages of developing that context. Added to this are the dilemmas around other cultural assumptions (such as an Aboriginal child being evaluated according to cultural norms of occupation by a non-Aboriginal adult).

Conclusion

This chapter has sought to demonstrate the ways in which occupation-centred practice with children must start with a critical examination of those assumptions embedded in our own personal and professional views of children and childhood occupations. It is only when we understand the meanings of occupations from the perspectives of our child-clients and families within their cultural contexts that we can begin to practice in a truly occupation-based way. The *kawa* metaphor is one way of enabling children who represent diverse and infinitely complex spheres of experience to share their view of their occupational lives with us.

References

Awaad, T. (2003). Culture, cultural competency and occupational therapy: A review of the literature. *British Journal of Occupational Therapy, 66*(8), 356-362.

Bond, C. (2005). A culture of ill-health: Public health or Aboriginality? *Medical Journal of Australia, 183*(1), 39-41.

Bonder, B., Martin, L., & Miracle, A. (2004). Culture emergent in occupation. *American Journal of Occupational Therapy, 58*(2), 159-168.

Burgman, I., & King, A. (2005). The presence of child spirituality. Surviving in a marginalized world. In F. Kronenberg, S. S. Algado, & N. Pollard (Eds.), *Occupational therapy without borders. Learning from the spirit of survivors* (pp. 152-165). London, UK: Elsevier.

Canadian Association of Occupational Therapists. (1997). *Enabling occupation: An occupational therapy perspective*. Ottawa, ON: CAOT Publications ACE.

Gray, M., & McPherson, K. (2005). Cultural safety and professional practice in occupational therapy: A New Zealand perspective. *Australian Occupational Therapy Journal, 52*, 34-42.

Hocking, C., & Whiteford, G. (1995). Multiculturalism in occupational therapy: A time for reflection on core values. *Australian Occupational Therapy Journal, 42*, 172-175.

Iwama, M. (2005). Situated meaning. An issue of culture, inclusion, and occupational therapy. In F. Kronenberg, S. S. Algado, & N. Pollard (Eds.), *Occupational therapy without borders. Learning from the spirit of survivors* (pp. 127-139). London, UK: Elsevier.

Iwama, M. (2006). *The kawa model: Culturally relevant occupational therapy.* Toronto, ON: Elsevier.

Jungerson, K. (2002). Cultural safety: Kawa Whakaruruhau – An occupational therapy perspective. *New Zealand Journal of Occupational Therapy, 49*(1), 4-9.

Kondo, T. (2004). Cultural tensions in occupational therapy practice: Considerations from a Japanese vantage point. *American Journal of Occupational Therapy, 58*(2), 174-184.

Kronenberg, F., Algado, S. S., & Pollard, N. (2005). *Occupational therapy without borders. Learning from the spirit of survivors.* London, UK: Elsevier.

MacNaughton, G., & Davis, K. (2001). Beyond 'othering': Rethinking approaches to teaching young Anglo-Australian children about Indigenous Australians. *Contemporary Issues in Early Childhood, 2*(1), 83-93.

Moreton-Robinson, A. (2000). *Talkin' up to the white woman. Aboriginal women and feminism.* Brisbane, Qld: University of Queensland Press.

National Aboriginal Community Controlled Health Organisation (NACCHO). (2001). *Submission to the Commonwealth Parliamentary Inquiry into the needs of urban dwelling Aboriginal and Torres Strait Islander Peoples.* Retrieved 14 March 2009 from http://www.naccho.org.au/Files/Documents/Urbaninquirysubmission.pdf.

Nelson, A. (2007). Seeing white: A critical exploration of occupational therapy with Indigenous Australian people. *Occupational Therapy International, 14*(4), 237-255.

Nelson, A., & Allison, H. (2007). Relationships: The key to effective occupational therapy practice with urban Australian Indigenous children. *Occupational Therapy International, 14*(1), 57-70.

Nelson, A., Allison, H., & Copley, J. (2006). Understanding where we come from: Occupational therapy with urban Indigenous Australians. *Australian Occupational Therapy Journal, 53*, 1-12.

Paradies, Y. (2006). Beyond black and white: Essentialism, hybridity and indigeneity. *Journal of Sociology, 42*(4), 355-367.

Ring, I., & Brown, N. (2003). Indigenous by definition, experience or world view. *British Medical Journal, 327*, 404-405.

Thomson, N., Burns, J., Burrow, S., Hardy, A., Krom, I., Stumpers, S., et al. (2008). *Overview of Australian Indigenous health.* Perth, WA: Australian Indigenous HealthInfoNet. Retrieved 14 March 2009 from http://www.healthinfonet.ecu.edu.au/health-facts/overviews.

Townsend, E. (2003). Reflections on power and justice in enabling occupation. *Canadian Journal of Occupational Therapy, 70*(2), 74-87.

Watson, R. (2006). Being before doing: The cultural identity (essence) of occupational therapy. *Australian Occupational Therapy Journal, 53*(3), 151-158.

Whiteford, G. (2007). The Koru unfurls: The emergence of diversity in occupational therapy thought and action. *New Zealand Journal of Occupational Therapy, 54*(1), 21-25.

Whiteford, G., & Wright St-Clair, V. (2002). Being prepared for diversity in practice: Occupational therapy students' perceptions of valuable intercultural learning experiences. *British Journal of Occupational Therapy, 65*(3), 129-137.

Yerxa, E., Clark, F., Frank, G., Jackson, J., Parham, D., Pierce, D., et al. (1989). An introduction to occupational science, a foundation for occupational therapy in the 21st century. *Occupational Therapy in Healthcare, 6*(4), 1-17.

Chapter 5

Enabling Children's Spirituality in Occupational Therapy Practice

Imelda Burgman

Learning objectives

The objectives of this chapter are to:

- Appreciate the contribution of spirituality to children's self-esteem, agency and resilience.
- Understand the importance of enabling spirituality in children's everyday lives.
- Develop an understanding of the ways in which children may express their spirituality.
- Identify ways of supporting children's expression of their spirituality in daily occupational therapy practice.

Introduction

Why is spirituality important to children's occupational performance? Let me begin by telling you a story about two little boys. On a cold autumn day in the Bronx, New York, at a preschool for children with special needs, surrounded by razor wire and nestled among the tenements, I met Jacob. He had severe cerebellar ataxia and was unable to speak, but his joy of being alive shone from his eyes and radiated from his smile. Jacob gave life everything he had. He was filled with determination, to be included, to be seen as capable and intelligent and to be loved. He fell and picked himself up again, literally and figuratively. He would not use any adaptive device he viewed as making him different and was fierce in his suspicion and refusal of them. He built friendships with the children in his class, cared for them and looked after their interests. He was adamant in his desire to experience everything life had to offer him, finding the courage, hope and trust he needed to survive in a world that was often harsh. Jacob was a child I believed would emotionally survive no matter what life cast his way. He had an inner strength of self. I worked with Jacob for a year and he taught me so much about his way of being in the world.

A few years later, on a hot summer day in an Australian country town, I met Ben. Ben was the same age as Jacob, had a severe developmental delay and, like Jacob, he was unable to speak. Ben screamed for the hour of my visit. He found the world terrifying; screaming was his way of keeping the world away, to be left alone. He was scared of new places, people (whether adults or children), toys, sounds, foods and textures. His only joy was being held by his mother or at home with his family, where he felt safe. His life was very restricted. I spent the next 2 years, helping Ben to deal with his fears and to find pleasure in life outside his confined world.

With children like Jacob, what enables them to sustain their resilience, continuing their engagement in occupational roles? For children like Ben, what helps to reduce their vulnerability and enable their occupational engagement? This chapter will aim to answer this question, at least in part.

The primary focus of occupational therapy intervention for children with disabilities is to assist them in the development of their occupational roles and performance, and optimise their participation (Case-Smith, 2005; Rodger & Ziviani, 2006). The outcome of this focus is the enhancement of children's abilities to adapt, grow and change in harmony with their physical/sensory (Gilfoyle, Grady, & Moore, 1990), cognitive (Piaget, 1955) and emotional development (Erikson, 1963). However, the occupational performance of children with disabilities is affected not only by their impairment(s), but also by their response to the social construction of their 'disability'.

Children's beliefs and values about themselves and the world in which they live shape their responses to the world and hence their experiences (Merleau-Ponty, 1964). Bronfenbrenner (1979) and others (e.g. Morris, 1991; Shakespeare, 1996) strongly argued that these beliefs are shaped by children's close relationships with and responses from others. However, children also influence their world (Bronfenbrenner & Morris, 1998; James, Jenks, & Prout, 1998). How children define their sense of agency and purpose and sustain their resilience through their relations with others are important questions to consider in our therapeutic relationships with them.

Occupational therapy's traditional focus on medical and psychological understandings of children does not fully reflect children's abilities to be actively engaged in the world. Prescriptive understandings of children often position them within restrictive models of intervention, where their desires are secondary to professional goals of developmental achievement. These understandings are not sufficient to engage respectfully and effectively with children like Jacob and Ben. With both of these children, I needed to re-evaluate my professional direction if I wanted to facilitate their engagement in all aspects of their lives. I needed to consider other ways of understanding them, such as appreciating their spiritual selves beyond that of their clinical diagnosis or developmental achievements.

Spirituality and children

How spirituality supports adults to experience purpose and seek engagement in their lives have been important questions for the occupational therapy profession over the past decade (e.g. Collins, 2007; Hasselkus, 2002; Peloquin, 1997). Current understandings of spirituality in occupational therapy practice provide a general thread to follow in exploring its potential significance in the lives of children like Jacob and Ben. The importance of spirituality to general physical and emotional well-being has also been explored in the fields of medicine, psychiatry and psychology (e.g. White, 2006; Wright & Sayre Adams, 2000). The spiritual care of children with life-threatening or chronic illnesses (Hufton, 2006) and the spiritual needs of those who are dying (Kübler-Ross, 1969, 1975, 1981) have been explored in the fields of nursing and psychiatry. Exploring the needs and care of children from these perspectives has highlighted the common themes of spirituality experienced by children with diverse life experiences. Spirituality may be a primary enabler for successful adaptation to the challenges in children's lives. Their ability to utilise spiritual qualities including belonging, hope and trust may impact on their ability to maximise their potential in all aspects of their lives.

Children's ways of understanding and drawing on the spiritual dimension, as distinct from the religious expression of spirituality, have implications for occupational therapy theory and practice. In order to facilitate change in the lives of children, we need to remain aware of the impact of children's spirituality in relation to their ability to achieve in a way that is meaningful for them (Coles, 1990; Moustakas, 1959).

Ideas about children's spirituality are known largely through the writings of religious and moral thinkers that place children's understandings and expressions within developmental models. However, from those who have listened to children, other understandings of children have arisen. In this chapter, the concept of spirituality will be clarified by identifying the nature of spiritual qualities. Within the understandings of qualities such as belonging, hope and trust, there lies a commonality of meaning and expression. Although the expression of spirituality is bound by culture, meanings transcend religious and cultural boundaries, and the expressions are at once common and unique to each person. The lived expression of spiritual qualities is embedded in the daily rituals, rhythms and challenges of life for children, as is the case for adults. How we reflect upon and appreciate these expressions contributes to our understanding of children's spirituality, and its importance in the therapeutic context.

The importance of the relationship between occupational therapists and children is in our ability to support therapeutic change in children's lives (Mosey, 1986). Through this relationship, occupational therapists facilitate children's use of their physical, cognitive, emotional and spiritual resources to enhance their occupational performance and to optimise their participation (Townsend & Polatajko, 2007). Our understanding, and therefore application, of this relationship with children needs to include a focus on children's needs and resources (Mandich & Rodger, 2006; Rodger & Ziviani, 2006).

Why does spirituality matter in occupational therapy practice?

Meaning also brings life to occupation. Occupational therapy's focus on meaning through engagement opens a door to a consideration of spirituality. Purpose embodied through meaning gives children the motivation to keep trying, to endure life's difficulties and to feel they are making a difference to themselves and others (Clinton, 2008; Coles, 1990). Constructive discourses within the profession have led to the development of theoretical models that include spirituality or spiritual dimensions of being. The Canadian Model of Occupational Performance and Engagement (CMOP-E) (Townsend & Polatajko, 2007) and the Occupational Performance Model (Australia) (OPM Aust.) (Chapparo & Ranka, 1996) present the influence of spirituality in different ways, but both clearly discuss its importance in the experiences of all human beings. There are also occupational therapy models that incorporate the importance of spiritual values and beliefs which support meaning in people's lives (e.g. Iwama, 2006; Kielhofner, 2008).

Developmental understanding

The most extensive work to date in relation to children and spirituality has been from the focus of Christian faith development (Fortosis, 1992; Fowler, 1974; Helminiak, 1996). Religious understandings of children foreground the development of cognitive abilities as a pre-requisite to the 'correct' understanding of religious concepts. These theorists have assumed children must achieve a certain level of cognitive maturity before adults accept that children have a knowledge of themselves and their spirituality. Often this is based on children's verbal responses and ability to explain abstract thought. However, the ability to value children's spiritual knowing is constrained within the arbitrary boundaries of psychological and sociological developmental research that seeks to measure and objectify a highly subjective area of experience.

Exploring the individual meaning of spirituality in everyday experiences provides a way of understanding its place in children's lives. Children's use of language, embedded with personal meaning, is an example of the expression of spirituality. However, the expression of spirituality occurs through all aspects of children's participation in the world (Adams, Hyde, & Woolley, 2008). Spirituality is reflected in children's relationships, play, work and learning. The narratives documented in *The Spiritual Life of Children* (Coles, 1990) demonstrate the diversity of children's spiritual experiences. Common spiritual underpinnings weave their way through each child's story. Children from diverse religious backgrounds spoke of the central importance of connection with family and community, and caring for others. Children living in segregated societies as well as those for whom religious beliefs could not be separated from their connection with nature expressed their views of love and compassion for others and the world. The importance of a relationship with a divinity (or divinities) was evident in their religious understandings, as was the impact this relationship had on their actions. Central themes included the role of God (or another divinity) in their lives and what children needed to do in order to live in harmony with their divinity's teachings. These children questioned the meaning of life and significant life experiences, and connected their personal philosophies with their everyday lives. All of the children pondered, discussed and wrestled with spiritual issues, blending these into discussions of who they would become when they grew up, the way the world was and the way they wished it could be. Their philosophies wove their way into conversations about their relationships with their families, peers and communities, the disagreements, aspirations and challenges to their sense of self-knowing. The questioning and discussions of these children reflected understandings positioned outside of the traditional medical and social constructions of childhood. These understandings challenge the positioning of children's knowledge as lesser than adult knowledge and highlight that adults need to listen to children (Alderson, 2008).

For those children who had not been part of a religious upbringing, the same need for purpose, ethical congruence and connection with others and the world was also evident. Although the expression of these themes was outside religious boundaries, they were still centrally important to the lives of these children. These children also considered the apparent divorce of religious from lived beliefs within the practices of their societies. They preferred to live out their spiritual understandings in ways that were authentic, for example, through caring for their family and establishing ethical relationships with peers (Coles, 1990). The work of Coles (1990) complements that of Robinson (1977) and Hart (2003). Respondents in these works identified a sense of purpose, connection (to others, a divinity and nature) and faith that was part of their inner knowing throughout childhood. Inherent in these childhood narratives is the lesson that spiritual understanding is not tied to religious education, cognitive or emotional development (Adams et al., 2008). Ultimately, children's expressions of spirituality were as varied as their lives.

Considering spirituality

The question of how spirituality is 'considered' forms part of the ongoing discussions about spirituality within the occupational therapy literature. The profession is actively engaged in understanding the spirituality of adults who come within its care, highlighting the importance of spirituality in theoretical frameworks and practice (Kang, 2003; McColl, 2003; Unruh, Versnel, & Kerr, 2002). In these discourses, personal understandings of spirituality are apparent in the worldviews presented, through its perceived nature and expression in life (do Rozario, 1997; McColl, 2003). Adults' experiences have been explored within the therapeutic relationship and within the rhythms, challenges and relationships of their lives (e.g. Egan & DeLaat, 1994, 1997; Frank et al., 1997; Wilding, 2002).

Research by do Rozario (1997) and McColl (2000) highlighted the uniqueness and richness of every person's life story and the influence of each person's spirituality in his or her search for understanding. The embodiment of spiritual qualities can have a significant impact on an adult's life. This has been highlighted in case studies (Clark, 1993; Peloquin, 1995) in which spiritual threads of belonging, purpose and sustaining a sense of self bind each narrative, as does spirituality in everyday occupation. The meaningfulness of everyday occupation interests all occupational therapists regardless of their worldviews on spirituality (Urbanowski, 2003).

Simo Algado and Burgman (2005) explored the role of spirituality in the resilience and emotional recovery of children who have survived traumatic life experiences. The spiritual strength of children experiencing adversity is evident within this work with refugee children in Kosovo, as is their desire to express, make sense of and integrate their experiences.

Everyday spirituality

Current understandings of children's spirituality do not encompass an understanding of the contribution of spirituality to the construction of their identity, agency and resilience. Broadening and deepening occupational therapy understandings will help us to recognise and build upon spiritual qualities with children like Jacob, and enable us to assist children like Ben to use their spiritual qualities to engage with the world. The concept of spirituality is often perceived to be abstract, but it can become more 'concrete' through awareness of its daily expression. We can integrate our awareness of spirituality through our openness towards children's ways of being in the world. Everyday negotiations with family, friends, teachers, peers and neighbours all call upon spiritual qualities. Children draw upon spiritual qualities to meet life's challenges as well as to offer love and friendship to others.

Spiritual qualities are enacted in the relationships that shape children's identities. These qualities are both 'inner' and 'outer' (i.e. more overt or explicit), and are developed and performed through engagement in everyday relationships. They are not separate from children's immediate worlds. Rather, through the self, they are intimately entwined with others and the experience of being in the world. The weaving of spiritual qualities in everyday life speaks of a relational experience of spirituality with the world, an experience that is fluid in its expression and response; thus, spiritual qualities affect identity, and consequently impact on relationships with family, school, community and society (Adams et al., 2008). In Table 5.1, spiritual qualities are presented with everyday examples, which were shared with me by a group of children with disabilities (Burgman, 2005).

The art of occupational therapy practice

Reflective and respectful practice enables the expression of children's spirituality within the formation of their identities in the world, through actions and relationships with others (including therapists) and themselves. In respectful practice, we embrace reflection and wisdom, foregrounding the meaning of children's lives through narrative (Mattingly, 1998). When practice is 'considered' from the perspective of spirituality, we need to extend our knowledge of children's spirituality and how we may enfold their expressions of spirituality within the art of our practice. This can be done through quieting ourselves and listening carefully to children.

Listening to children

Children's knowledge of themselves is not usually foregrounded within client-centred or family-centred practice. Knowledge of children typically comes from others, or is learnt incidentally through children's responses. If we wish to build effective relationships with children, based on trust and respect, then we need to ask children to tell us about themselves (Mattingly, 1998; Peloquin, 2003). Their stories will enable us to hear what holds purpose and joy in their lives. We will discover how they see themselves in relation to the world and the dreams they have for themselves. This knowledge will in turn enable us to engage meaningfully with children. Children may wish to express themselves through: telling, reading, writing or acting out stories; playing at being an animal who is strong or fearless; being a character in a movie, or a computer game (Camilleri, 2007; Sinats et al., 2005). Entering this world of children's metaphor (Lakoff & Johnson, 1980) brings insight into what children see in, and desire for, themselves. Through this avenue of understanding and connection, children can share with us the spiritual qualities they seek to embody in their daily lives, and we can seek to encourage children's spiritual expression. Children express their wisdom as they seek to express their identities within their experience of being in the world. We can engage with children's hopes and their faith in themselves. As they imagine themselves, we need to approach children as having the potential to be more than we have imagined (Alderson, 2008).

The space between

In relationships with children, connecting with their sense of self and learning about what they need from us is paramount. Connecting respectfully,

Table 5.1 Spiritual qualities in everyday life

Spiritual quality	Everyday meaning[1]	Children's examples (Burgman, 2005)
Belonging	Being part of something/someone Connection to family, friends and others, nature, a divinity	Getting a cuddle from mum Playing with my brothers Playing basketball with my friends Praying Going to Sunday school Spending time at the beach Playing with my pets Surfing
Love	Unconditional love; giving without expectations	God's love Loving mum/dad (author's note: even if the parent is abusive or abandons the child) Loving a pet My best friend
Grace	An extension of love Experiencing unexpected support or kindness from a divinity, or person	Helping a stranger Being friendly to a child who is lonely Having your hand held by a nice nurse when you are trying not to be scared about going into surgery
Compassion	Caring for others, understanding the needs of others even if very different from your own. Forgiving yourself, and others	Caring about people who are homeless Caring about war and poverty in other countries Forgiving myself for yelling at someone or being unfair Accepting others who are different from me, who have different needs and wants
Ethics	Considering the needs of others, and the consequences of one's actions on others	Being quiet when someone else is sleeping/sick Not telling lies Being fair when sharing toys and food, or playing games
Purpose	Having direction or meaning in life, or in the activities of life	My mum needs me to help her with the others (siblings) I'm going to be a vet I look after my baby brother I help my friends with their problems
Hope	Believing in life; trusting that life has purpose and therefore meaning	I hope that I won't have my disability anymore I'm going to be a vet when I grow up If I keep trying, one day I'll have a friend (at school) One day I won't be in my wheelchair anymore
Faith	Belief in myself, others or a divinity	In mum and dad's love In friends 'sticking up' for you In God caring about me

(Continued)

Table 5.1 (Continued)

Spiritual quality	Everyday meaning[1]	Children's examples (Burgman, 2005)
Trust	That life has a purpose. Belief in life and people	Mum and dad will keep their promises to you Like faith Your friends will keep secrets
Courage	To continue living, being alive, even when scared or doubtful	Being brave about surgery Being scared, but still being able to call the police Going to school, even though I get bullied in class Wearing my glasses, even though I get called names
Wisdom	Seeing the truth in one's self and in others	Understanding why kids are mean to me Understanding why my mum gets sad Understanding how to take care of myself (emotionally) Knowing how to help my friends with their problems
Awe/wonder	Touching and being touched by the world	Being able to ride my bike without help from dad Surfing the biggest wave I'd ever seen, and being ok
Joy	The self becomes more than and at one with one's spirituality and the world	Complete happiness Being with my baby brother Playing with my baby rabbits
Creativity	The spirit is freed and shines through the self	My drawings Telling stories Finding lots of ways to stop my baby brother from crying Dancing to music in my room Finding ways to keep drawing when my fingers were falling off

[1] References: Ackerman (1999), Burgman (2005), Dalai Lama (1996, 1997), Dalai Lama and Cutler (1998), Frankl (1959), Friesen (2000), Goleman (1997), Hillman (1989), Maslow (1999), McGrath (1999), Moore (1992, 1996, 2002), Moustakas (1967), Pieper (1963), Tillich (1952), Vardey (1995) and Weil (1952).

allowing children to sense safety, not to be overwhelmed or to feel controlled, and to let them lead and set the tone and pace of the interaction will enable the children to sustain their sense of agency (Piper, 1999; Rogers, 1951, 1961). Here, the physical context becomes irrelevant, as a relational space is created in which children can create what they need it to be, enabling their self to emerge in safety. Ultimately, it is a child's self that we wish to see and to connect with meaningfully, not a child's identity as prescribed by the world. When we are in this space, our therapeutic power is quieted and we must be patient (Peloquin, 2003). This is not always easy as our acculturated professional self keeps wanting to resurface and take charge, giving prescriptive choices in the name of empowerment. When we succeed in remaining quiet, the relationship that develops is one of mutual respect and enjoyment. There is a deeper pleasure that comes from being *with*, from a sense that this relationship will be a journey of discovery and sharing. For a little while we are his or her companion, establishing a meaningful relationship with a child within his or her world.

Children's contexts and spirituality

Home

For all children, expressions of selfhood and sameness are lived within home and family, and shaped through love and the challenges of negotiating relationships (Ricoeur, 1992). Children's identities are formed by the repetition of experiences through family relations, rhythms and rituals (Bronfenbrenner & Morris, 1998). Their identities are shaped by their sameness as a child and sibling, subject to family mores, discipline and responsibilities, and by selfhood created through desires for agency, negotiating conflict and caring for the self.

In our relations with families, we need to look for the unique ways in which children interact with their family members. Children's interactions are not only an expression of identity, but also a means of sharing their hearts and spirits. Children seek to give and receive love and belonging, perhaps through creating drawings and paintings, telling stories of their adventures or listening to their parents' stories. Children show compassion to parents who are sad or sick, and show hope when times are difficult. They have faith in their family to survive those difficult times and to continue caring for each other. By creating spaces in which children can express their values and opinions, we enable children's identities to be heard. Our interventions should be designed based on the needs and desires of both parents and children, appreciating the dynamics of these relationships. This will in turn provide a greater understanding of how identity is created and intertwined in these foundational relations between self and other. There may be differences in the way children and family members wish to engage. We should explore with children how they wish to negotiate with others in order to meet their own needs and maintain their sense of identity. Doing so will contribute to the fostering of engagement through respect, contributing to children's resilience.

Inclusion of siblings in the therapeutic partnership may facilitate skills of independence in ways we had not imagined, for example, through the purpose of caring for a younger brother or sister (Brannen, Heptinstall, & Bhopal, 2000; Burgman, 2005). Children with significant disabilities give love and compassion to their siblings. Siblings care for one another and provide a sense of belonging

(Figure 5.1). Sibling relationships are also spaces for developing the qualities of joy, grace and ethical understanding, through engagement in play, sharing chores and negotiating differences/privacy/rules of engagement (Figure 5.2). Enabling children to experience the depth and breadth of sibling relationships and all they have to offer assists them to express their spirituality.

In considering the family, we also need to include pets as members of children's families. Pets need to be considered as more than a source of enjoyment; they can be friends, confidants and playmates, and sources of love, belonging and trust. Children's pets can serve as a very powerful source of comfort and encouragement during difficult times that may include mastering challenges or persisting with painful treatment (Velde, Cipriani, & Fisher, 2005) (Figure 5.3). Pets can help children to be resilient and courageous. We need to ask children about their relationships with their pets and to consider including their pets in therapy interventions.

Children need spaces to replenish their spirits, even within the family. They will establish rituals for themselves, for example, listening to music, drawing, doing craft or shooting basketball hoops, to regain their spiritual balance (Figure 5.4). In our practice, we need to consider how children are caring for themselves through their rituals, choice of activities and their enactment. It is important also to appreciate that children need quiet times for themselves in the busyness of daily family life. The co-constructed spiritual environment of family (Hockey & James, 2003) enables children to build their resilience. Spiritual qualities support the ongoing creation of their identity, one that will be carried into other relational contexts. A focus on these aspects can help

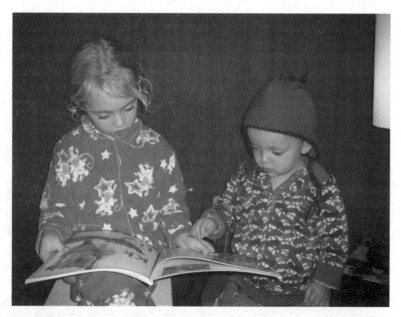

Figure 5.1 Bedtime ritual; caring for a younger brother by reading him a story. Reproduced with permission

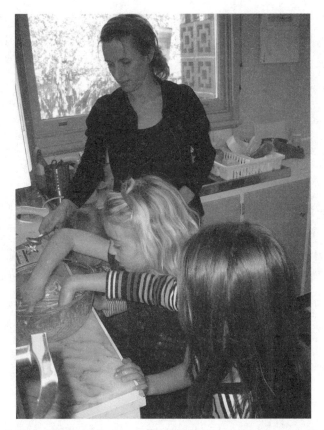

Figure 5.2 Siblings and friends helping in the kitchen. Reproduced with permission

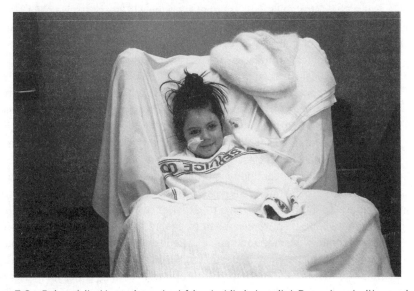

Figure 5.3 Being visited by an important friend while in hospital. Reproduced with permission

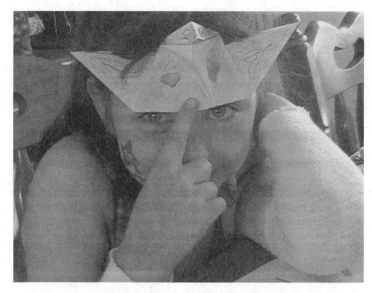

Figure 5.4 Making origami animals. Reproduced with permission

support the reciprocal relationships that contribute to the creation of children's identities as resilient and agentic.

School

As discussed further in Chapter 11, in school contexts we need to build supportive relationships with children based on trust and respect. We need to respect children as capable of creative problem-solving and ask them to share their strategies with us. When working with teachers, we can help them to reframe children's behaviours (Richardson, 2002) as needed, fostering perceptions of children as compassionate and ethical. In this way, we can advocate for children within the classroom, suggesting alternate methods to enable positive relationships in which children can be seen and heard. When working with school support personnel (e.g. aides and volunteers), we need to be aware of the meaning of these relationships for children (Hemmingsson, Borell, & Gustavsson, 2003; Skar & Tamm, 2001). If it is a relationship of mutual trust and respect, it can build the resilience of children in managing challenging classroom and learning experiences (Burgman, 2005). The importance of continuity, mutual liking and respect asks us to advocate for children to maintain relationships with preferred support staff over their primary years. If children are to experience resilience through connection (Hunter, 2001), then we also need to enable them to participate in activities that promote the development of friendships (Law, Petrenchik, Ziviani, & King, 2006; Richardson, 2002; Staub, 1998). Friendship-building activities will engender a sense of belonging with others (Morrison & Burgman, in press), and hope and faith in the self. The development of children's social skills will enable them to gain confidence in approaching and being with other children (Staub, 1998). Being perceived by other children as valuable group members will help children to build a sense of positive identity.

If we wish to support children's resilience within friendships, we need to enable them to develop ways of negotiating disconnection (e.g. disagreements and fights), minimising the threat to their sense of self. Helping children to define their emotional boundaries will help to sustain their identities, through their understanding of their compassion and sense of ethics. Helping them to develop the skills they need to deal with friendship conflicts will also help them to negotiate bullying and isolation experienced within other peer relationships. We can play a vital role in helping children to cope with the challenges of negative stereotyping. We can build children's resilience by enabling them to build their self-esteem. Helping children to be aware of the spiritual qualities they have, and how they already use them in their everyday lives, can reinforce in them that they have internal resources on which they can rely. For example, discussing with children their use of courage, ethics, love, belonging, faith and hope will highlight their ability to use these qualities in challenging situations. Discussing strategies with them to care for themselves emotionally and physically will position them as capable of meeting these needs.

Play (and leisure) occurs in social contexts (Poulsen & Ziviani, 2006; Rigby & Rodger, 2006). When we evaluate children's occupational performance skills, we must also consider the complexities of social interaction. Shared play and leisure at school impacts on children's identities through the interpersonal skills they learn (Law et al., 2006; Morrison & Burgman, in press). We can enable children to build their resilience through pleasurable engagement with their peers (Hunter, 2001) and the creative use of resourcefulness, adaptability and flexibility (Sheldrake, 1989), and develop through the spiritual qualities of love, belonging, trust, purpose and joy.

Children seek to be valued, to be active and creative agents of their learning within the classroom and the playground (Davis & Watson, 2002). How they seek and experience belonging with their teachers and peers tells us of their need to be seen as both unique and the same (Ricoeur, 1992). We need to advocate for the creation of resilient school environments in which there is adult support, engagement in learning, reciprocal friendships and participation with peers.

Community

Children's community spaces include those of their neighbourhood, leisure forums and religious faith communities. These are spaces of active negotiation in which children express themselves and contribute. Children, like adults, see their participation as a valued part of life within the community. Their participation enables the possibility of avenues of agency and belonging. However, community participation can also raise issues of isolation, disrespect and vulnerability. Acknowledging and addressing this diversity of children's emotional experiences is important when enabling them to interact within their communities.

Through sport and recreation, children facilitate their own performance and development rather than these being constructed through therapeutic means (Aitchison, 2003). They are the agents of their own 'learning'. Thus, leisure provides avenues for seeing the self as agentic, sharing skills and giving dedication and support to others. Whether within a neighbourhood or in organised sport, participation in community leisure creates possibilities for the forming of friendships. Children can develop their intrinsic motivation, and experience joy and challenges, through participating in activities that have no goals but pleasure in and through the self (Figure 5.5).

As occupational therapists, we need to enable children to experience 'leisure as "freedom to" engage in activities of choice, in freely chosen spaces, for positive benefit' (Aitchison, 2003, p. 963). Careful consideration needs to be given to leisure activities in the lives of children (King et al., 2003; Specht, King, Brown, & Foris, 2002). Engagement in activities enables belonging, purpose, joy, creativity and transcendence. Through being with others, discovering more about the self and extending the self, children are exploring and shaping their identities. If we wish them to be socially active and engaged, then we must enable children to participate in activities that are meaningful for them. Working in conjunction with recreation specialists can lead to inclusive opportunities beyond the therapeutic interaction (Aitchison, 2003). This is discussed further in Chapter 12.

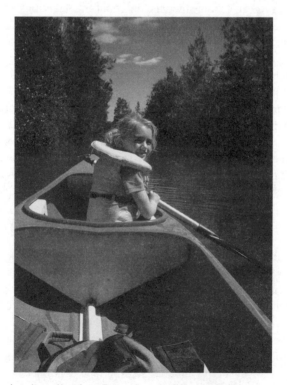

Figure 5.5   Canoeing down the river. Reproduced with permission

For some children, religious faith is an important part of their lives. Their religious faith enables them to cope with pain, sadness and loss, providing emotional strength in difficult times (Coles, 1990). We need to respect the support children may derive from their faith by enabling them to engage in religious practices, such as prayer or Sunday school. The sense of belonging that may occur within a religious community needs to be maintained. Living in the world and meeting its challenges means children call on their spirituality every day. We need to support children through enabling them to replenish their spirit (e.g. through a preferred activity or being in nature). We also need to support children to draw on their spirituality, through supporting them in their engagement in daily occupations.

Conclusion

Spirituality fosters and supports children's self-esteem and sense of agency, and builds resilience in their everyday lives. It supports their ability to engage in occupations, whether at home, school or in the community. Spirituality also supports children to take risks in pursuing their dreams and to continue trying even when life is difficult. By supporting children's connection with their spirituality, we support their engagement with their lives. Children like Jacob, who are engaged and resilient, can tell us much about how to support and encourage children like Ben who have so much difficulty engaging with the world. Jacob's desire and ability to offer love, compassion and trust to others in his life meant that he also received these qualities in return. His ongoing hope and faith in life and in himself enabled him to survive life's challenges and to pursue a path which he found meaningful. Children may express their spirituality in many different ways. They may choose to be determined and vocal, like Jacob, or they may choose to quietly move through the world. We need to be open to how children choose to share their spirituality and how they choose to meet their own needs.

Supporting children's spirituality means supporting the ways they choose to live their lives, and helping them to draw on their spiritual qualities. I have not seen Jacob again, but I still see Ben from time to time. Ben still does not speak or walk. However, he is very loved by his family, and he loves them. He seeks meaningful occupations at school and home, and now is willing to engage in new experiences. He has a strong spirit, one that is nurtured by his large family and his determination to be heard. He is no longer afraid of the world, and that has been his greatest achievement.

References

Ackerman, D. (1999). *Deep play*. New York, NY: Vintage.
Adams, K., Hyde, B., & Woolley, R. (2008). *The spiritual dimension of childhood*. London, UK: Jessica Kingsley.

Aitchison, C. (2003). From leisure and disability to disability leisure: Developing data, definitions and discourses. *Disability & Society, 18*(7), 955-969.

Alderson, P. (2008). *Young children's rights* (2nd ed.). London, UK: Jessica Kingsley.

Brannen, J., Heptinstall, E., & Bhopal, K. (2000). *Connecting children: Care and family life in later childhood*. London, UK: Routledge Falmer.

Bronfenbrenner, U. (1979). *The ecology of human development. Experiments by nature and design*. Cambridge, MA: Harvard University Press.

Bronfenbrenner, U., & Morris, P. A. (1998). The ecology of developmental processes. In W. Damon, & R. M. Lerner (Eds.), *Handbook of child psychology. Theoretical models of human development* (5th ed., Vol. 1, pp. 993-1028). New York, NY: John Wiley & Sons.

Burgman, I. (2005). *Reflections on being: Spirituality within children's narratives of identity and disability*. University of Sydney, Sydney: Unpublished doctoral dissertation.

Camilleri, V. A. (Ed.). (2007). *Healing the inner city child*. London, UK: Jessica Kingsley.

Case-Smith, J. (Ed.). (2005). *Occupational therapy for children* (5th ed.). St. Louis, MO: Elsevier Mosby.

Chapparo, C., & Ranka, J. (1996). *Occupational performance model (Australia). Monograph 1*. Sydney, NSW: Occupational Performance Network.

Clark, F. (1993). Occupation embedded in to real life: Interweaving occupational science and occupational therapy. *American Journal of Occupational Therapy, 47*(12), 1067-1077.

Clinton, J. (2008). Resilience and recovery. *International Journal of Children's Spirituality, 13*(3), 213-222.

Coles, R. (1990). *The spiritual life of children*. Boston, MA: Houghton Mifflin.

Collins, M. (2007). Spiritual emergency and occupational identity: A transpersonal perspective. *British Journal of Occupational Therapy, 70*(12), 504-512.

Dalai Lama. (1996). *The good heart*. Sydney, NSW: Rider.

Dalai Lama. (1997). Medicine and compassion. In D. Goleman (Ed.), *Healing emotions* (pp. 243-250). Boston, MA: Shambhala.

Dalai Lama, & Cutler, H. C. (1998). *The art of happiness: A handbook for living*. Sydney, NSW: Hodder Headline.

Davis, J., & Watson, N. (2002). Countering stereotypes of disability: Disabled children and resistance. In M. Corker, & T. Shakespeare (Eds.), *Disability/postmodernity* (pp. 159-174). London, UK: Continuum.

do Rozario, L. (1997). Spirituality in the lives of people with disability and chronic illness: A creative paradigm of wholeness and reconstitution. *Disability and Rehabilitation, 19*(10), 427-434.

Egan, M., & DeLaat, M. D. (1994). Considering spirituality in occupational therapy practice. *Canadian Journal of Occupational Therapy, 61*(2), 95-101.

Egan, M., & DeLaat, M. D. (1997). The implicit spirituality of occupational therapy practice. *Canadian Journal of Occupational Therapy, 64*(3), 115-121.

Erikson, E. H. (1963). *Childhood and society* (2nd ed.). New York, NY: W.W. Norton.

Fortosis, S. (1992). A developmental model for stages of growth in Christian formation. *Religious Education, 87*(2), 283-298.

Fowler, J. W. (1974). Religious institutions: Toward a developmental perspective on faith. *Religious Education, LXIX*(2), 207-219.

Frank, G., Bernardo, C. S., Tropper, S., Noguchi, F., Lipman, C., Maulhardt, B., et al. (1997). Jewish spirituality through actions in time: Daily occupations of young orthodox Jewish couples in Los Angeles. *American Journal of Occupational Therapy, 51*(3), 199-206.

Frankl, V. E. (1959). *Man's search for meaning*. London, UK: Hodder and Stoughton.

Friesen, M. F. (2000). *Spiritual care for children living in specialized settings. Breathing underwater*. New York, NY: Haworth Press.

Gilfoyle, E. M., Grady, A. P., & Moore, J. C. (1990). *Children adapt* (2nd ed.). Thorofare, NJ: SLACK Inc.

Goleman, D. (1997). Afflictive and nourishing emotions: Impacts on health. In D. Goleman (Ed.), *Healing emotions* (pp. 33–46). Boston, MA: Shambhala.

Hart, T. (2003). *The secret spiritual world of children*. Maui, HI: Inner Ocean.

Hasselkus, B. R. (2002). *The meaning of everyday occupation*. Thorofare, NJ: SLACK Inc.

Helminiak, D. A. (1996). *The human core of spirituality. Mind as psyche and spirit*. Albany, NY: State University of New York Press.

Hemmingsson, H., Borell, L., & Gustavsson, A. (2003). Participation in school: School assistants creating opportunities and obstacles for pupils with disabilities. *Occupational Therapy Journal of Research, 23*(3), 88–98.

Hillman, J. (1989). *A blue fire*. New York, NY: Harper & Row.

Hockey, J., & James, A. (2003). *Social identities across the life course*. Basingstoke, Hampshire: Palgrave Macmillan.

Hufton, E. (2006). Parting gifts: The spiritual needs of children. *Journal of Child Health Care, 10*(3), 240–250.

Hunter, A. J. (2001). A cross-cultural comparison of resilience in adolescents. *Journal of Pediatric Nursing, 16*(3), 172–179.

Iwama, M. (2006). *The Kawa model: Culturally relevant occupational therapy*. New York, NY: Churchill Livingstone.

James, A., Jenks, C., & Prout, A. (1998). *Theorizing childhood*. Cambridge, UK: Polity Press.

Kang, C. (2003). A psychospiritual integration frame of reference for occupational therapy. Part 1: Conceptual foundations. *Australian Occupational Therapy Journal, 50*(2), 92–103.

Kielhofner, G. (2008). *Model of human occupation: Theory and application* (4th ed.). Baltimore, MD: Lippincott Williams & Wilkins.

King, G., Law, M., King, S., Rosenbaum, P., Kertoy, M. K., & Young, N. L. (2003). A conceptual model of the factors affecting the recreation and leisure participation of children with disabilities. *Physical & Occupational Therapy in Pediatrics, 23*(1), 63–90.

Kübler-Ross, E. (1969). *On death and dying*. London, UK: Tavistock.

Kübler-Ross, E. (1975). *Death. The final stage of growth*. Englewood Cliffs, NJ: Prentice-Hall.

Kübler-Ross, E. (1981). *Living with death and dying. How to communicate with the terminally ill*. New York, NY: Touchstone.

Lakoff, G., & Johnson, M. (1980). *Metaphors we live by*. Chicago, IL: University of Chicago Press.

Law, M., Petrenchik, T., Ziviani, J., & King, G. (2006). Participation of children in school and community. In S. Rodger, & J. Ziviani (Eds.), *Occupational therapy with children. Understanding children's occupations and enabling participation* (pp. 67–90). Oxford, UK: Blackwell.

Mandich, A., & Rodger, S. (2006). Doing, being and becoming: Their importance for children. In S. Rodger, & J. Ziviani (Eds.), *Occupational therapy with children. Understanding children's occupations and enabling participation* (pp. 115–135). Oxford, UK: Blackwell.

Maslow, A. (1999). *Toward a psychology of being* (3rd ed.). New York, NY: John Wiley & Sons.

Mattingly, C. (1998). *Healing dramas and clinical plots*. Cambridge, UK: University Press.

McColl, M. A. (2000). Spirit, occupation and disability. *Canadian Journal of Occupational Therapy, 67*(4), 217-228.

McColl, M. A. (Ed.). (2003). *Spirituality and occupational therapy*. Ottawa, ON: Canadian Association of Occupational Therapists.

McGrath, A. E. (1999). *Christian spirituality*. Oxford, UK: Blackwell.

Merleau-Ponty, M. (1964). *Primacy of perception: And other essays on phenomenological psychology, the philosophy of art, history, and politics*. Evanston, IL: Northwestern University Press.

Moore, T. (1992). *Care of the soul*. New York, NY: HarperCollins.

Moore, T. (1996). *The re-enchantment of everyday life*. Rydalmere, NSW: Hodder & Stoughton.

Moore, T. (2002). *The soul's religion*. Sydney, NSW: HarperCollins.

Morris, J. (1991). *Pride against prejudice*. London, UK: Women's Press.

Morrison, R., & Burgman, I. (2009). Friendship experiences among children with disabilities who attend mainstream Australian schools. *Canadian Journal of Occupational Therapy, 76*(3 145-152)

Mosey, A. C. (1986). *Psychosocial components of occupational therapy*. New York, NY: Raven Press.

Moustakas, C. E. (1959). *Psychotherapy with children: The living relationship*. New York, NY: Harper & Row.

Moustakas, C. (1967). *Creativity and conformity*. Princeton, NJ: Van Nostrand.

Peloquin, S. M. (1995). The fullness of empathy: Reflections and illustrations. *American Journal of Occupational Therapy, 49*(1), 24-31.

Peloquin, S. M. (1997). The spiritual depth of occupation: Making worlds and making lives. *American Journal of Occupational Therapy, 51*(3), 167-168.

Peloquin, S. M. (2003). The therapeutic relationship: Manifestations and challenges in occupational therapy. In E. B. Crepeau, E. S. Cohn, & B. A. Boyt Schell (Eds.), *Willard & Spackman's occupational therapy* (10th ed., pp. 157-170). Philadelphia, PA: Lippincott Williams & Wilkins.

Piaget, J. (1955). *The construction of reality in the child* (M. Cook, Trans.). London, UK: Routledge & Kegan Paul.

Pieper, J. (1963). *Leisure. The basis of culture*. Markham, ON: Penguin.

Piper, D. E. (1999). Pleasures, pitfalls and perplexities: The content of counseling and supervision. In P. Milner, & B. Carolin (Eds.), *Time to listen to children* (pp. 29-47). London, UK: Routledge.

Poulsen, A., & Ziviani, J. (2006). Children's participation beyond the school grounds. In S. Rodger, & J. Ziviani (Eds.), *Occupational therapy with children. Understanding children's occupations and enabling participation* (pp. 280-298). Oxford, UK: Blackwell.

Richardson, P. K. (2002). The school as social context: Social interaction patterns of children with physical disabilities. *American Journal of Occupational Therapy, 56*(3), 296-304.

Ricoeur, P. (1992). *Oneself as another* (K. Blamey, Trans.). Chicago, IL: University of Chicago Press.

Rigby, P., & Rodger, S. (2006). Developing as a player. In S. Rodger, & J. Ziviani (Eds.), *Occupational therapy with children. Understanding children's occupations and enabling participation* (pp. 177-199).Oxford, UK: Blackwell.

Robinson, E. (1977). *The original vision*. Oxford, UK: The Religious Experience Research Unit.

Rodger, S., & Ziviani, J. (2006). Children, their environments, roles and occupations in contemporary society. In S. Rodger, & J. Ziviani (Eds.), *Occupational therapy with children. Understanding children's occupations and enabling participation* (pp. 3–21). Oxford, UK: Blackwell.

Rogers, C. R. (1951). *Client-centered therapy. Its current practice, implications, and theory*. Boston, MA: Houghton Mifflin.

Rogers, C. R. (1961). *On becoming a person. A therapist's view of psychotherapy*. London, UK: Constable & Company.

Shakespeare, T. (1996). Disability, identity and difference. In C. Barnes, & G. Mercer (Eds.), *Exploring the divide: Illness and disability* (pp. 94–113). Leeds, UK: Disability Press.

Sheldrake, R. (1989). *The presence of the past*. London, UK: Fontana.

Simo Algado, S., & Burgman, I. (2005). Occupational therapy intervention with children survivors of war. In F. Kronenberg, S. Simo Algado, & N. Pollard (Eds.), *Occupational therapy without borders: Learning from the spirit of survivors* (pp. 253–268). London, UK: Elsevier.

Sinats, P., Scott, D. G., McFerran, S., Hittos, M., Cragg, C., Leblanc, T., et al. (2005). Writing ourselves into being: Writing as spiritual self-care for adolescent girls. Part one. *International Journal of Children's Spirituality, 10*(1), 17–29.

Skar, L., & Tamm, M. (2001). My assistant and I: Disabled children's and adolescents' roles and relationships to their assistants. *Disability & Society, 16*(7), 917–931.

Specht, J., King, G., Brown, E., & Foris, C. (2002). The importance of leisure in the lives of persons with congenital physical disabilities. *American Journal of Occupational Therapy, 56*(4), 436–445.

Staub, D. (1998). *Delicate threads*. Bethesda, MD: Woodbine House.

Tillich, P. (1952). *The courage to be*. New Haven, CT: Yale University Press.

Townsend, E., & Polatajko, H. J. (2007). *Enabling occupation II: Advancing an occupational therapy vision for health, well-being, and justice through occupation*. Ottawa, ON: CAOT Publications ACE.

Unruh, A. M., Versnel, J., & Kerr, N. (2002). Spirituality unplugged: A review of commonalities and contentions, and a resolution. *Canadian Journal of Occupational Therapy, 69*(1), 5–19.

Urbanowski, R. (2003). Spirituality in changed occupational lives. In M. A. McColl (Ed.), *Spirituality and occupational therapy* (pp. 95–114). Ottawa, ON: Canadian Association of Occupational Therapists.

Vardey, L. (1995). *God in all worlds*. Sydney, NSW: Millennium.

Velde, B. P., Cipriani, J., & Fisher, G. (2005). Resident and therapist views of animal-assisted therapy: Implications for occupational therapy practice. *Australian Occupational Therapy Journal, 52*(1), 43–50.

Weil, S. (1952). *Gravity and grace*. London, UK: Routledge & Kegan Paul.

White, G. (2006). *Talking about spirituality in health care practice. A resource for the multi-professional health care team*. London, UK: Jessica Kingsley.

Wilding, C. (2002). Where angels fear to tread: Is spirituality relevant to occupational therapy practice? *Australian Occupational Therapy Journal, 49*(1), 44–47.

Chapter 6

Occupational Goal Setting with Children and Families

Nancy Pollock, Cheryl Missiuna, and Sylvia Rodger

Learning objectives

The objectives of this chapter are to:

- Describe the challenges of involving children in goal setting.
- Discuss the critical connection between goal setting and motivation.
- Review several tools that are available to assist in this process.
- Outline how to embed occupation-based goal setting into a family-centred practice framework.
- Present several case studies to demonstrate goal setting with different children using some of these tools and describe the link to outcome measurement.

Introduction

One of the most important steps in the occupation-centred occupational therapy process (described in Chapter 2) is goal setting. As the therapist and client(s) move from assessment and analysis of the client's occupational strengths and needs to intervention, the desired outcomes of therapy should be clearly articulated. In order to practice using a client- or family-centred approach, the occupational goals must come from the client and family. Goals need to be set *by* the client, not *for* the client.

Giving children a voice

Explicit collaborative goal setting between children, family members and therapists within the occupation-centred occupational therapy process has a number of benefits including:

- Children and family members have the opportunity to clearly state their values and preferences.
- The therapist sends a signal that the children's and family members' voices are being heard and their values are respected within this partnership.
- The therapy is meaningful for children and parents as the connection between the intervention and the goals is made explicit, enhancing achievement motivation.
- Goals are stated in occupation-centred terms.
- The outcomes of therapy are easily measured through goal attainment.

In child- and family-centred practice, the therapist and child, parents and family members work as partners (Law & Mills, 1998; Rosenbaum, King, Law, King, & Evans, 1998). Central to the partnership is the understanding of the client's (child's and parent/s') priorities as these inform the therapy process. Clients need to be able to make their wishes known to the therapist if they are to truly collaborate in therapy (Clark & Bell, 2000). For many clients, goal setting is quite a simple process; the client articulates his or her concerns and priorities through the assessment process and goals are easily identified. While this is the ideal, the reality often differs. Eliciting the client's priorities may not always be a simple process (Wilkins, Pollock, Law, & Rochon, 2001). Clients who are cognitively impaired, who lack insight or who have limited motivation to change may be unable or unwilling to identify their goals. Young children also pose a significant challenge in collaborative goal setting. The ability to self-assess and determine one's goals requires a level of abstract reasoning that most children do not attain until 8 or 9 years of age. As a result, therapy goals are often set by the adults involved: parents, teachers or the therapists themselves. While it is important to involve the family in setting goals within a family-centred practice framework, it is also important for children to be able to articulate their own goals.

It is often assumed that young children are not capable of identifying goals for therapy; however, recent research has questioned this assumption (Missiuna & Pollock, 2000). While the limitation has been assumed to be children's ability to understand a somewhat abstract process, Curtin (2001) suggested that it may be the methods we use to elicit the goals that are limiting the child. She noted, 'Though occupational therapists tend to be skilled in giving children a voice in treatment activities, involving children in defining the purpose of therapy is more challenging' (p. 301). In a review of self-report assessments used with children, Sturgess, Rodger, and Ozanne (2002) identified several instruments that are valid and reliable when used with children as young as 4 years of age. Particular aspects of the assessment appear to improve validity with younger children including the use of concrete stimuli such as pictures, simplified language, clear response options and the context in which the assessment is conducted (Sturgess et al., 2002).

Instruments exist that allow young children to self-report on constructs such as pain (St-Laurent-Gagnon, Bernard-Bonnin, & Villeneuve, 1999), quality of life (Bouman, Koot, Van Gils, & Verhulst, 1999), perceived competence (Harter & Pike, 1984; Missiuna, 1998) and activity preferences (Hay, 1992; Henry, 2000). Until recently, however, there were no assessments specifically designed for children to enable them to set goals for therapy. Over the past few years, several new instruments have been published that specifically facilitate goal setting for children. As the number of self-report instruments for children increases, so does the evidence that children's perceptions differ from those of the adults around them (Sturgess et al., 2002). This is even more likely to be the case for goal setting, as it involves placing value judgements on the importance of different potential goals (Wigfield & Eccles, 1992). Only the individual can truly do this. Studies conducted with children older than 8 years of age, and particularly with adolescents, have shown that goals are quite different among children, their parents and teachers (McGavin, 1998; Pollock & Stewart, 1998). Missiuna, Pollock, Law, Walter, and Cavey (2006) found that goals set by younger children also differed from those of their parents and teachers. Each of the participants in the therapy process brings very different perspectives, priorities and values and, hence, the goals that they set will also differ.

Goal setting and motivation

> Goals are simply tools to focus your energy in positive directions, these can be changed as your priorities change, new ones added, and others dropped. (Anonymous)

Goal setting can have a powerful impact on the outcome of therapy. Research evidence shows that explicit, challenging goals can enhance and sustain motivation and lead to improved levels of performance (Bandura, 1993; Locke & Latham, 1990). Adopting goals set by someone else has no lasting motivational impact (Bandura, 1997). Poulsen, Rodger, and Ziviani (2006) proposed that understanding self-determination theory (SDT) can help further occupational therapists' understanding of the psychological processes involved in client-centred practice, in particular the importance of goal setting. SDT expands White's (1959 in Deci & Ryan, 2000) model of motivation in which a child's primary motive is perceived to be fulfilment of the need for environmental competence or mastery. Two additional innate psychological needs were identified in SDT, namely autonomy or ownership of one's behaviour and relatedness or the need to feel that one can connect with others and with society in general (Deci & Ryan, 2000).

Occupational therapists aim to support children in acquiring specific skills by planning interventions so that the child's needs for competence, autonomy and relatedness are enhanced (Poulsen et al., 2006). Essential components of client-centred practice, such as the facilitation of empowering environments in which clients actively participate in decision making and attainment of self-managed goals, underpin the promotion of optimal motivation and healthy psychological functioning (Law & Mills, 1998). Client-centred models of practice emphasise the importance of personal choice and self-determination as powerful motivators in shaping behaviour. Identifying goals and establishing the child's motivation for their occupations of choice are critical to occupation-centred practice. Engagement of children and parents in autonomous, self-directed goal setting is the first step to understanding their needs, interests and motivations. Based on information obtained from goal-setting tools, the therapist engages the child and his/her parents in a discussion about the child's activity preferences, engagement patterns (when, where, how and with whom activities occur) and his/her perceptions of competence with these activities leading to collaborative identification of personally meaningful goals. These goals become the basis for occupation-centred intervention. The therapist encourages parental support for the child's decision to select his or her own goals from the outset. Helping parents understand that intrinsically motivated behaviour is sustained by pursuit of child-determined goals is an important aspect of the child–parent–therapist collaboration that is critical to occupation-centred practice.

In summary, in child-centred practice, the child needs to articulate his/her goals for therapy. Use of goals that are elicited from others is likely to be less valid. Goal setting appears to have a positive impact on motivation and the outcomes of therapy. It may be more challenging for younger children to set their own goals due to the reflective and abstract nature of self-assessment; however, there are tools available that can assist the therapist to enable children to set their own occupation-based goals. These will be addressed in the following section.

Tools to facilitate goal setting with children

In this section, six goal-setting tools will be reviewed. Three of these tools, the Canadian Occupational Performance Measure (COPM; Law et al., 2005), the Perceived Efficacy and Goal Setting System (PEGS; Missiuna, Pollock, & Law, 2004) and the Child Occupational Self Assessment (COSA; Keller, Kafkes, Basu, Federico, & Kielhofner, 2006), are specifically designed to facilitate goal setting with children and/or families. Three other tools, the Preferences for Activities of Children (PAC; King et al., 2004), the Paediatric Activity Card Sort (PACS; Mandich, Polatajko, Miller, & Baum, 2004) and the Preschool Activity Card Sort (Berg & LaVesser, 2006), although not specifically designed for goal setting, can be used to facilitate intervention planning.

Canadian Occupational Performance Measure

The COPM (Law et al., 2005) is an individualised measure based on client-centred principles that can be used in initial assessment and in measuring change. The COPM enables the identification and prioritisation of occupational performance issues that are most important to the client. In addition, the client self-evaluates their current performance and their satisfaction with that performance. The COPM was first published in 1991 and has become a well-established occupational therapy measure. It has been translated into 24 languages and is used in over 35 countries (Law et al., 2005). More than 80 studies have been published evaluating the COPM or using the COPM in research (Carswell et al., 2004; McColl et al., 2006).

The COPM takes the form of a semi-structured interview. The therapist interviews the client regarding daily activities in the areas of self-care, productivity and leisure. Clients are asked to identify occupations that they want to do, need to do and are expected to do that they are finding challenging or difficult. The importance of these occupations is rated on a 10-point scale by the client, enabling the identification of the issues that are currently the highest priorities for the client. Self-evaluation of current performance and satisfaction with current performance are then rated separately on 10-point scales. The identified problems or issues can become the goals for therapy and re-assessment can occur at a future time to evaluate the outcomes of therapy and to measure change (see Table 6.1). The COPM fits well within family-centred practice as members of the family can be the respondents and identify their current concerns. It is also clearly an occupation-centred measure as the COPM focuses on daily occupations in which families and/or their children are experiencing difficulties.

Using the COPM with children as the respondents is more challenging. The COPM has been used in studies with children; however, its effectiveness for use with children under 8 years has been questioned due to the abstract level of thought required (Missiuna et al., 2004). In order to identify

Table 6.1 The Canadian Occupational Performance Measure (COPM)

Source	Law et al. (2005)
Purpose	The COPM is a measure that enables the identification and prioritisation of occupational performance issues in the areas of self-care, productivity and leisure. In addition, a client's self-perception of performance and satisfaction with performance are evaluated and measured over time
Type of client	All occupational therapy clients or their parents/carers
Clinical utility	Semi-structured interview administered by an occupational therapist. Some multidisciplinary teams use the COPM. Therapists report that the COPM facilitates client-centred practice and clients report that the COPM helped them to clarify their priorities and to understand the role of the occupational therapist. Administration time: 15–30 min
Reliability	Test–retest reliability has been studied in three populations. Correlation coefficients range from 0.84 to 0.92
Validity	Seventeen validity studies have been published in addition to the original work done by the authors. Strong evidence exists for content, concurrent and convergent/divergent validity

occupational performance issues, the respondent has to be able to reflect on his/her performance and self-evaluate. Attempts have been made to adapt the COPM for use with children in order to facilitate their understanding of the measure. A recent study examining the effectiveness of the Cognitive Orientation to Occupational Performance (CO-OP) approach with children aged 5-7 years who have Developmental Coordination Disorder (DCD) utilised the COPM to enable children to identify three goals (Taylor, Fayed, & Mandich, 2007). The COPM scales were adapted by supplementing numbers with pictorial cues such as happy and sad faces. The COPM was reported to be effectively used with most of these younger children, although one child demonstrated difficulty with understanding the satisfaction scale (Taylor et al., 2007).

The psychometric properties of the COPM have been extensively studied (McColl et al., 2006) (see Table 6.1). Test-retest reliability has been well established and there is good evidence of content, construct and criterion-related validity. The clinical utility of the COPM has been evaluated in 17 studies within a wide variety of settings and with diverse populations. Results of these studies find the COPM to be a clinically useful and responsive measure (McColl et al., 2006) (Figure 6.1).

Perceived Efficacy and Goal Setting System

The PEGS (Missiuna et al., 2004) is a tool designed for children between the ages of 6 and 9 years that enables them to report their perceived competence in performing everyday activities including self-care tasks, school tasks and leisure activities. It is used to collaboratively set goals for therapy, allowing the children to express their concerns, to identify their priorities and to give them a voice.

The PEGS consists of 24 pairs of culturally neutral cards illustrating children performing various everyday activities that would typically be performed by children within and outside school. Each pair consists of one picture depicting a child performing an activity 'more competently' and another card showing a child performing the same activity 'less competently' (see Figure 6.2). The card pairs are presented to the child and he/she is asked to first pick the card that shows the child he/she is most like. The

Initial Assessment:			Reassessment:	
OCCUPATIONAL PERFORMANCE PROBLEMS:	PERFORMANCE 1	SATISFACTION 1	PERFORMANCE 2	SATISFACTION 2
1. _____	☐	☐	☐	☐
2. _____	☐	☐	☐	☐
3. _____	☐	☐	☐	☐
4. _____	☐	☐	☐	☐
5. _____	☐	☐	☐	☐

Figure 6.1 Example of COPM score sheet. Reproduced with permission

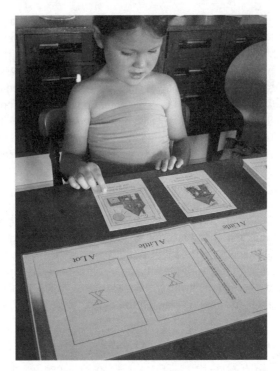

Figure 6.2 Child choosing between two PEGS cards. Reproduced with permission

child then states whether he/she is 'a lot' or 'a little' like the child in the card. Activities in which the child has rated him/herself as being less competent are reviewed and discussed with the child. Opportunity is provided for the child to add activities that he/she finds to be challenging which were not reflected in the set of activities presented on the cards. Goal setting is facilitated by asking the child to choose, among the tasks performed with less competence, which activities he/she would most like to work on in therapy.

The PEGS also includes caregiver and teacher questionnaires which contain the same paired items as written statements. In completing these questionnaires, the adults in the child's environment state their views of the child's competence and then identify the goals that they feel are most important.

The items in the PEGS were originally derived from the *All About Me* (AAM) assessment (Missiuna, 1998) and include typical self-care, school and leisure activities for this age group. Substitute cards are available for use with children with mobility limitations. In a pilot study examining the extension of the AAM as a goal-setting tool, children, parents and therapists provided feedback about the items, and changes and additions were made based on their input (Missiuna & Pollock, 2000).

The original psychometric work conducted with the *AAM* (Missiuna, 1998) showed excellent internal consistency and adequate test–retest reliability, although a small sample size was used for testing the latter (see Table 6.2). To date, there have been no further studies examining the test–retest

Table 6.2 Perceived Efficacy and Goal Setting System (PEGS)

Source	Missiuna et al. (2004)
Purpose	The PEGS is a self-report tool that enables children with disabilities to report their perceived competence in performing everyday activities, and enables children to develop goals for therapy
Type of client	Children with all types of disabilities, who are chronologically or developmentally at a 6–9-year-old level
Clinical utility	Administered by occupational therapists working in the area of paediatrics. Other health care professionals such as physical therapists or school psychologists may also administer the PEGS. Therapists report that the PEGS assists in establishing rapport with the children and that the children enjoy the card sorting activity. Administration time: 20–30 min for the card sort, 5–10 min for the teacher and caregiver questionnaires, and 10 min for summarising results and scoring
Reliability	The *All About Me* (AAM) assessment is the predecessor to the PEGS and includes many of the same items. Cronbach's alpha for the AAM was determined to be 0.85 and 0.91 for the fine and gross motor subscales, respectively Pearson product–moment correlation coefficients for fine motor, gross motor and total scores scales in the AAM were determined to be $r = 0.79$, 0.76 and 0.77 A standardisation study of the PEGS examined goal stability across two test administrations. Results demonstrated that 92% of children selected two to four of the same goals at the second administration
Validity	Items from the AAM were included in the PEGS. Removal and addition of items occurred through pilot testing of the PEGS as well as expert review. A standardisation study demonstrated that items could be grouped into the three categories of self-care, school/productivity and leisure A high correlation between the AAM and the Pictorial Scale of Perceived Competence and the Social Acceptance for Young Children (PCSA) was found ($r = 0.80$). Another study demonstrated moderate correlations ($r = 0.64$ and 0.73) between the AAM and the Developmental Test of Visual Motor Integration, and the Bruininks-Oseretsky Test of Motor Proficiency. A study of 24 children demonstrated that the AAM was able to discriminate between children with and without disabilities. The PEGS showed low correlations with two subscales of the *School Function Assessment* (-0.12 to 0.33) Children with a variety of disabilities showed different profiles on the PEGS. Children with ADHD rated themselves as the most competent and children with physical disabilities the least competent

reliability of the PEGS. A standardisation study demonstrated that goals established through the use of the PEGS were stable across two administrations over a 2-week period (Missiuna et al., 2006). Several aspects of validity were established for the AAM, including content and criterion validity. Content validity has been established for the PEGS through a pilot study as well as through expert review of the items within the PEGS (Missiuna & Pollock, 2000).

In a recent study, Missiuna et al. (2006) found that children consistently rated their competence higher than their parents or teachers; however, there was agreement about specific areas of competence for each child. Little agreement was found between the goals selected by children and those identified by parents and teachers (Missiuna et al., 2006). These results are similar to those found in a recent study by Dunford, Missiuna, Street, and Sibert (2005) that utilised the PEGS to understand the impact of DCD on children's daily activities from their own viewpoints. Results demonstrated that children shared some concerns with their parents and teachers, such as handwriting; however, children identified additional concerns in the areas of self-care and leisure that were not identified by parents or teachers (Dunford et al., 2005). This study highlights the importance of using child self-report tools to truly understand the diversity of children's occupational concerns and reinforces the notion that parent and child goals frequently differ.

A number of research projects have been completed, or are in progress, to validate the use of translated versions of the PEGS in other countries and cultures. Results from a series of reliability and validity studies in Israel are summarised in the manual accompanying the published translation (Missiuna, Pollock, & Law, 2004, 2006). The PEGS has also been shown to be cross-culturally valid in Norway (Sognnaes & Langeland, 2006), Sweden (Nordstrand, 2008) and Brazil (Ruggio, Magalhaes, & Missiuna, in press). In Israel and Sweden, the PEGS was found to be relevant for use with children with disabilities who were up to 12 or 14 years of age, respectively.

Child Occupational Self-Assessment

The COSA (Keller et al., 2006) is a self-report tool that is used to ascertain children's and youth's perception of their own occupational competence as well as the importance of everyday activities. It was designed for use with 8-13-year-olds and accommodations are permitted for children with disabilities. The COSA is based on the Model of Human Occupation (Kielhofner, 2002) and addresses the areas of occupational adaptation and its components – occupational identity and occupational competence (Keller et al., 2006). The COSA is an individualised measure that is consistent with client-centred practice.

The items for the COSA were modelled after the Occupational Self-Assessment (Baron, Kielhofner, Iyengar, Goldhammer, & Wolenski, 2002), a tool developed for adults. The items include self-care tasks, school-related performance, social activities, and items about attention, problem-solving, communication, movement, endurance and behaviour. The COSA may be administered in one of the two formats: the checklist form or the card sort version. Both formats include a list of 25 statements which the child reads and then subsequently rates his/her competence level in performing the activity described. Second, the child rates the degree of importance of the activity or its value to him/her. The four-point scales use statements and visual cues (faces and stars) for each rating (see Figure 6.3).

Myself	I have a big problem doing this	I have a little problem doing this	I do this ok	I am really good at doing this	Not really important to me	Important to me	Really important to me	Most important of all to me
Dress myself	☹☹	☹	☺	☺☺	☆	☆☆	☆☆☆	☆☆☆☆
Do things with my classmates	☹☹	☹	☺	☺☺	☆	☆☆	☆☆☆	☆☆☆☆

Figure 6.3 Example of COSA rating scale. Reproduced with permission

The results of the COSA are reviewed by the therapist and discussed with the child. Particular attention is given to activities that have the largest gap between competence and importance, that is, situations in which the child has indicated an activity is very important but he/she is not able to perform the task very well. This process allows elaboration of the child's strengths and areas of difficulty and the establishment of client-centred goals (Keller et al., 2006). The psychometric properties of the COSA version 1.0 and 2.0 have been investigated in two studies (Keller, Kafkes, & Kielhofner, 2005; Keller & Kielhofner, 2005) (see Table 6.3). The psychometric properties of the COSA version 2.0 were determined in a study of 43 participants, aged 8–17 years. Rasch analysis demonstrated excellent competence and item reliability values, as well as excellent participant reliability on both scales. In addition, rating scales were able to separate clients into distinct groups, indicating the instrument's sensitivity to detect change. Rasch analysis demonstrated internal validity of the competence rating scale as well as unidimensionality of items within the scale, which suggests good construct validity.

Preferences for Activities of Children

The PAC is a companion measure to the Children's Assessment of Participation and Enjoyment (CAPE) (King et al., 2004). The CAPE measures several aspects of participation including the diversity of activities that children participate in outside of school, the intensity of their participation, the enjoyment and with whom and where the children typically perform the activities. The PAC determines children's activity preferences and is suitable for children and youth aged 6–21 years and can be used independently. Although not specifically designed for goal setting, information obtained may be used in planning intervention.

The PAC can be self- or interviewer-administered. The self-administered version involves the completion of the PAC record form by the child, with assistance from a parent or caregiver. The record form contains clear, culturally neutral pictures and written descriptions of various activities, as well as rating scales that require the child to indicate whether he/she would really like to do,

Table 6.3 Child Occupational Self Assessment (COSA) (version 2.1)

Source	Keller et al. (2006)
Purpose	The COSA is an assessment tool and outcome measure that can be used to understand children and youth's perceptions of their own occupational competence as well as the importance of everyday activities. The COSA can be used to involve children in setting goals for therapy
Type of client	Most useful for children and youth between the ages of 8 and 13 years with adequate cognitive abilities for self-reflection and planning, and who have a desire to collaborate in goal setting
Clinical utility	Administered by an occupational therapist either in a checklist form or as cards that the child sorts. Administration time: approximately 20 min for the checklist form version. Time required to complete the card sort version varies depending on the client's abilities and level of assistance required
Reliability	Using Rasch analysis, competence item reliability was 0.85 and values item reliability was 0.82. Participant reliability on the competence scale and values scale was 0.88 and 0.91, respectively
Validity	Rasch analysis demonstrated that competence and value rating scales functioned as intended. A logical hierarchy of items within competence and value scales was apparent, demonstrating internal validity. Items within the competence scale demonstrated unidimensionality, an indicator of construct validity Rating scales were able to separate clients into distinct groups, indicating the instrument's sensitivity to detect change

sort of like to do or not like to do an activity at all. The interviewer-administered version includes 55 pictorial activity cards in which the child rates his/her preference for each activity on rating cards. The range of activities includes formal and informal out-of-school activities in several categories: recreational, physical, social, skill-based and self-improvement.

The CAPE and PAC were initially designed as part of a longitudinal study examining the participation of 427 children with physical disabilities. Several aspects of reliability and validity of the measures were evaluated as part of the study (see Table 6.4 and Figure 6.4). Evidence of internal consistency is present and test–retest reliability studies yielded intra-class correlation coefficients ranging from 0.64 to 0.86. Validity evidence included careful development of the test items through literature review, expert panels and pilot studies. Factor analysis supported the underlying conceptual framework of the PAC. These measures have been recently published, so studies examining reliability and validity are ongoing (King et al., 2007).

Paediatric and Preschool Activity Card Sort

The PACS (Mandich et al., 2004) is a tool that is used to determine a child's current level of occupational engagement. It is an adaptation of the Activity

Table 6.4 Preferences for Activities of Children (PAC)

Source	King et al. (2004)
Purpose	The PAC is used to determine children's preferences for everyday activities excluding school activities. The PAC is an extension of the Children's Assessment of Participation and Enjoyment (CAPE), but may be used independently. Preferences ratings may be used to set client-centred goals
Type of client	Children, adolescents and young adults between the ages of 6 and 21 years
Clinical utility	Self-administered versions as well as interviewer-administered versions are available. The PACS can be administered by professionals in the health and social science fields including occupational therapists, psychologists, recreation therapists, speech and language pathologists, physical therapists, educators, nurses and social workers. Administration time: 15-20 min
Reliability	Cronbach's alpha was calculated for two administrations of the PAC and for the domains and activity types of the PAC. Cronbach's alpha for formal activities ranged from 0.76 to 0.78, and was 0.84 for informal activities. The alpha value for activity types ranged from 0.67 to 0.77. In general, internal consistency ranged from adequate to excellent
Validity	Item generation and placement within domains and activity types was established by review of literature on participation as well as previous measures that included information regarding participation, expert review and pilot testing of children with and without disabilities. Item selection was also based on congruence with the World Health Organization framework Factor analysis supports the conceptual framework of the PAC and the relationships among the activity groupings Evidence for construct validity was found in a study that hypothesised there to be correlations between preference in activity type and perceived competence, age and sex. Several of the predicted correlations were found, thus contributing to the construct validity

Card Sort created for use with adults (Baum & Edwards, 2001) and can be used with children aged 5–14 years. The PACS consists of photographs depicting children engaged in 75 different activities of personal care, school/productivity, hobbies/social activities and sports. Eight additional blank cards allow for the identification of activities not included in the card sort. Progressing through the cards, the child identifies activities in which he/she is currently engaged. If desired, information about the frequency of participation can be requested. Although not explicitly designed as a goal-setting tool, the PACS can be used to identify activities that a child would like to do. In this way, the PACS may be used in setting occupation-focused goals.

The initial development and validation of the PACS was conducted through a series of studies conducted by graduate students working with the authors.

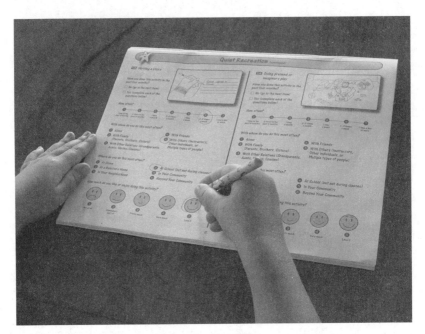

Figure 6.4   Child completing CAPE/PAC. Reproduced with permission

To date, only one study using the PACS has been published. In this project, the PACS was used in conjunction with the COPM to assist children with DCD to set goals and to determine their occupational performance profile at intake (Taylor et al., 2007).

The Preschool Activity Card Sort (Berg & LaVesser, 2006) is another measure derived from the work of Baum and Edwards (2001) designed for children with disabilities from 3 to 6 years of age. The measure includes 85 photographs depicting preschool children engaged in a wide variety of activities. Parents act as the respondents and indicate whether the child participates in the activity and whether he/she requires assistance or environmental modification to participate. The administration process also includes a series of probes to understand why a child may not be participating in an activity (e.g. lack of opportunity, lack of interest and environmental barriers). The process results in an occupational profile for the child across seven categories (self-care, community mobility, high and low demand leisure, social interaction, domestic and education) and identifies barriers to participation. From this profile, therapeutic goals can be discussed with the parents. The content validity of the PACS was determined through literature review, an expert panel of occupational therapists and parent time logs and interviews (Berg & La Vesser, 2006). A Spanish translation has also been completed (Stoffel & Berg, 2008).

Summary

In selecting a tool for goal setting, therapists need to consider the age of the child, the model of service delivery and the context of the activities with which the child is having difficulty. Some tools are comprehensive across areas of occupational performance (such as the COPM, PEGS, COSA and PACS) while others provide more detail regarding participation in extracurricular activities (e.g. PAC). Similarly, some tools are designed to gather information from multiple respondents (e.g. child, parents and teachers such as PEGS) while others elicit information solely from the child (PACS) or parent (preschool ACS).

Goal setting contributes to outcome measurement

Setting explicit, client-centred, occupation-based goals prior to initiating intervention facilitates the measurement of specific intervention outcomes. If the child, the family, the therapist and others involved agree on the desired outcomes, and if these outcomes are expressed in occupational terms, it should be easy to judge if goals have been met. For example, if a goal is that the child will feed himself soft foods using a built-up spoon, this should be obvious through observation.

It may not be enough, however, to have only dichotomous results (i.e. the goals have been achieved or not). It may be important to have a measurement scale that permits degrees of change over time. In order to measure change, assessments that are designed as evaluative tools must be used so that the results are valid. While one could re-administer the tools described previously, most of the child-specific tools have not been validated for use as outcome measures. The exception is the COPM (Law et al., 2005), a tool which has been validated as an outcome measure in a variety of populations (McColl et al., 2006). The problems initially identified on the COPM, which may become the therapy goals, can be rated again using the performance and satisfaction scales in a re-assessment.

An alternative to the use of the COPM is goal attainment scaling (GAS). GAS, a method used to measure change in individuals, was originally developed in the field of mental health (Kiresuk & Sherman, 1968), but has become more commonly used in paediatric rehabilitation. GAS is a criterion-referenced form of measurement where the expected outcome of intervention is articulated as a goal statement and five different levels of goal achievement are specified that range from less than expected to more than expected (typically scored from −2 to +2 with 0 as the expected outcome). The scale can then be used after intervention to evaluate change. Kiresuk and Sherman (1968) provided a formula for converting the scores to a standard score so that multiple scales can be examined and combined for use across goals, clients or programmes.

The first and most critical step in designing a GAS is to clearly articulate the goal statement, adhering to the Specific, Measurable, Acceptable, Relevant and Time-related (SMART) principle. Most of the tools reviewed in this chapter can assist in developing these goal statements, ensuring that they are occupation-based and client-centred as well as SMART. Although intuitively appealing, goal attainment scale development is not easy. McLaren and Rodger (2003) highlighted the fit of GAS with individualised, client-centred practice, the ability of GAS to detect a small but important change, the flexibility for use across performance areas, disciplines and programmes, and the benefit of collaborative goal statement development. The authors caution, however, that many issues remain regarding the reliability and validity of GAS. GAS is very dependent on the skills of the person(s) who design the scales and there is a significant risk of bias. MacKay and Lundie (1998) raised concerns about the statistical methods used to analyse the resulting data. Steenbeek, Ketelaar, Galama, and Gorter (2007), in a critical review of GAS in paediatric rehabilitation, identified outstanding concerns with regard to the psychometric properties. While the evidence is reasonably strong for the responsiveness of GAS, concerns remain about the potential for bias in constructing the scales. Studies have not been conducted to evaluate the reliability of GAS, and the evidence for validity is weak (Steenbeek et al., 2007). King, McDougall, Palisano, Gritzan, and Tucker (1999) used GAS in a programme evaluation study and outlined some important considerations in deciding if GAS is appropriate for use in a specific situation. They emphasised that developing the goal attainment scales is challenging and time consuming and requires training, ongoing coaching and a strong commitment from both team members and the organisation if it is to be used effectively.

In current occupational therapy practice, it is essential that we clearly articulate our contribution to the occupational development of our clients, and that we provide evidence of the effectiveness of our interventions. Setting specific, occupation-based goals is a starting point and using these goals in an individualised system of outcome measurement will provide valuable evidence that can be used in intervention planning with clients, in programme evaluation studies and outcomes research.

This scenario demonstrates the use of COPM to identify child and family goals, as well as to measure outcomes of intervention (performance and satisfaction ratings). While Lachlan's parents wanted him to be able to request appropriately, John was keen to be able to go to the park with Lachlan without him running away or crying when Jacinta was not there. This was important for him as a father and his relationship with his son to have family time together to play and visit the park. Similarly, the goal of sharing/turn taking with his sister during play was important for family harmony as well as establishing sibling play patterns. These goals reflect both meaningful child- and family-centred goals.

Use of the PEGS: Eric

Eric is a 7-year-old boy with DCD. Eric's teacher noted on the referral that he has an awkward pencil grasp and messy handwriting. On the first visit, the therapist spends some time talking with Eric about his interests and then uses the PEGS to help him identify activities that he finds to be challenging. Eric selects cards that suggest that he is 'a lot' like the child who is not good at doing up snaps or zippers, catching a ball, bicycle riding, painting or using cutlery. Eric's priorities are learning to ride a bicycle, finishing his schoolwork so he can go outside at lunchtime and doing up his jeans.

Eric's teacher completes the Teacher PEGS form indicating that Eric has difficulty with most of the productivity items and she lists neater printing, completion of schoolwork and getting his school bag organised so that things do not keep falling out as priorities. The therapist sends home the Caregiver PEGS form for Eric's mother to complete. She indicates that he has a great deal of difficulty with most of the self-care items and some difficulty with most of the leisure items. She adds bottom-wiping as an additional problem

Case examples: goal setting with children and parents

Use of the COPM: John and Jacinta (child with autism, Lachlan)
John and Jacinta participated in the Growing Stronger Families with Autism Project (Rodger, Braithwaite, & Keen, 2004), a research project involving families with a newly diagnosed child 2–4 years of age with autism. Their son Lachlan was 3 years old and had been diagnosed with autism 3 months prior to commencing the programme. They participated in a family-centred early intervention programme designed to provide information and to help parents achieve their goals for their child. It involved a 2-day workshop for parents, followed by 10 home visits, provided twice a week over 5 weeks by a home facilitator. Prior to commencement of the home visits, they completed the COPM.

When working with children (and their parents), it was important to frame occupations as the things children need to do, want to do and are expected to do in their daily lives. For young children with compromised language and communication abilities, parents are in the best position to identify their child's occupational performance issues, prioritise these and, in collaboration with professionals, identify realistic intervention goals. Communication and behaviour are pervasive deficits experienced by children with autism. Parents were asked to consider how their child's communication and behaviour difficulties impacted on the child's ability to engage in their daily occupations. They were asked to reflect on a typical day for their child and then guided to think about potential areas of difficulty experienced by the child, such as communication, behaviour, play, self-care, rest and relaxation. Specifically, parents reflected on their child's ability to have their needs met, express themselves, understand others' communication and interact with others, and identify any concerning behaviour or issues with daily routines, transitions, self-care and play/leisure. In discussing play, parents were asked to reflect on family socialisation, play at home and in early childhood settings, and play likes and dislikes. John and Jacinta identified the goals listed in the following display table

(Continued)

COPM goal	Pre-intervention (1-10)		Post-intervention (1-10)	
	Performance	Satisfaction	Performance	Satisfaction
(1a) For Lachlan to request using sign or photo of food	1	1	6	9
(1b) For Lachlan to request using sign or photo of preferred video	1	1	6	8
(2) To share and take turns with sibling during play	2	2	5	6
(3) To stay beside John when walking to the park (without running away)	2	2	8	9
(4) To play with John at the park (without distress and wanting to go back to mummy)	2	1	6	7

and prioritises improved bottom-wiping, getting dressed quickly and learning to ride his bicycle as her top three goals.

At the meeting to discuss goals and to plan intervention, the teacher expresses surprise at the fact that Eric is struggling so much with self-care activities as she had assumed that his difficulties were solely academic. The teacher agrees to reduce the written requirements and to allow Eric to go outside even when work was incomplete, if he was making an effort. Eric agrees that a goal about printing more neatly would be okay if the expectations are reduced. All recognise that learning how to undo and do up snaps is a priority for Eric and that improvement in this area will likely decrease some of the toileting and dressing issues identified by Eric and by his mother. The strategies used for zippers on jeans will be transferred to the knapsack so that Eric improves his ability to open and close it. Since both Eric and his family are motivated to work on bicycle riding, the therapist books an appointment to see Eric at home to work on this goal. This case illustrates how the use of the PEGS allows the therapist to understand the priorities of the child, the family and in this case the teacher, and facilitates a negotiation around the goals and direction of intervention.

Use of the COSA: Hayden

Hayden is a 12-year-old student who has a diagnosis of Attention Deficit Hyperactivity Disorder (ADHD). He is currently in Grade Seven in his neighbourhood school. Hayden has a history of school difficulties. His teachers consistently report that he has trouble initiating and completing work independently, he is disorganised and his written work is sloppy. He can be disruptive in class and bothers other students. Recently, he has been experiencing more social problems including rejection and some bullying by his peers. In a school conference with his parents present, a referral to occupational therapy is initiated. The occupational therapist decides to use the COSA as the first step in her work with Hayden to assist him in expressing himself so that the therapist can have a clear understanding of Hayden's self-perceptions and values. Hayden was able to complete the self-report version of the COSA and he reported no difficulties on many of the items, particularly those related to self-care. Many of the items Hayden identified as problems were related to schoolwork, for example, 'finish my work in class on time', 'get my homework done' and 'keep working on something even when it gets hard'. However, Hayden did not rate these issues as important. The three items Hayden rated as problems and as very important were 'do things with my friends', 'calm myself down when I get upset' and 'follow classroom rules'. In discussion with the therapist, Hayden revealed that he frequently had trouble keeping himself under control and he recognised that this impulsivity and his tendency towards emotional outbursts was getting him into trouble at school and making other kids stay away from him.

Based on this discussion, the therapist has Hayden complete the Adolescent/ Adult Sensory Profile (Brown & Dunn, 2002). Children with ADHD frequently show sensory processing difficulties that can have an impact on their behaviour. Hayden's profile showed that he is a strong sensory seeker and some of his impulsivity and acting out may be related to his difficulties in modulating sensory input. Together, Hayden and the occupational therapist develop some strategies to make Hayden more aware of his state of neurological arousal and some methods to help keep him calmer and less reactive. Through a combination of cognitive-behavioural and sensory modulation techniques, Hayden now has some tools available to assist him with self-regulation. By learning how to remain calm, Hayden will have less trouble following classroom rules and his peers will be more likely to want to spend time with him.

Conclusion

Forming effective relationships with children and families is the key to family-centred occupational therapy practice. If the service provider and clients have a shared view of the issues and the desired outcomes, they can work in partnership to achieve those outcomes. In this chapter, we have reviewed the importance of goal setting, the link to outcome measurement and six tools available to assist in the process, and have provided examples of the practical use of these tools. The tools and techniques that have been described provide the essential ingredients for a truly client-centred occupational therapist to give children and families a voice.

References

Bandura, A. (1993). Perceived self-efficacy in cognitive development and functioning. *Educational Psychologist, 28*, 117-148.

Bandura, A. (1997). *Self-efficacy: The exercise of control*. New York, NY: W.H. Freeman & Company.

Baron, K., Kielhofner, G., Iyengar, A., Goldhammer, V., & Wolenski, J. (2002). *The Occupational Self Assessment (version 2.1)*. Chicago: Model of Human Occupation Clearinghouse, Department of Occupational Therapy, College of Applied Health Sciences, University of Illinois at Chicago.

Baum, C., & Edwards, D. (2001). *Activity Card Sort*. St. Louis, MO: Simon Enterprises Co.

Berg, C., & LaVesser, P. (2006). The Preschool Activity Card Sort. *OTJR: Occupation, Participation and Health, 26*, 143-151.

Bouman, N., Koot, H. M., Van Gils, A. P., & Verhulst, F. C. (1999). Development of a health-related quality of life instrument for children: The Quality of Life Questionnaire for Children. *Psychology and Health, 14*, 829-846.

Brown, C., & Dunn, W. (2002). *The Adolescent/Adult Sensory Profile*. San Antonio, TX: PsychCorp.

Carswell, A., McColl, M. A., Baptiste, S., Law, M., Polatajko, H., & Pollock, N. (2004). The Canadian Occupational Performance Measure: A research and clinical literature review. *Canadian Journal of Occupational Therapy, 71*, 210-222.

Clark, J., & Bell, B. (2000). Collaborating on targeted outcomes and making action plans. In V. Fearing, & J. Clark (Eds.), *Individuals in context: A practical guide to client-centred practice* (pp. 79-90). Thorofare, NJ: SLACK Inc.

Curtin, C. (2001). Eliciting children's voices in qualitative research. *American Journal of Occupational Therapy, 55*, 295-302.

Deci, E. L., & Ryan, R. M. (2000). The 'what' and 'why' of goal pursuits: Human needs and the self-determination of behavior. *Psychological Inquiry, 11*, 227-268.

Dunford, C., Missiuna, C., Street, E., & Sibert, J. (2005). Children's perceptions of the impact of Developmental Coordination Disorder on activities of daily living. *British Journal of Occupational Therapy, 68*, 207-214.

Harter, S., & Pike, R. (1984). The pictorial scale of perceived competence and social acceptance for young children. *Child Development, 55*, 1969-1982.

Hay, J. (1992). Adequacy in and predilection for physical activity in children. *Clinical Journal of Sports Medicine, 2*, 192-201.

Henry, A. (2000). *Pediatric Interest Profiles*. San Antonio, TX: The Psychological Corporation.

Keller, J., Kafkes, A., Basu, S., Federico, J., & Kielhofner, G. (2006). *A user's guide to Child Occupational Self Assessment (COSA) (version 2.1)*. Chicago, IL: Model of Human Occupation Clearinghouse, Department of Occupational Therapy, College of Applied Health Sciences, University of Illinois at Chicago, and UIC Board of Trustees.

Keller, J., Kafkes, A., & Kielhofner, G. (2005). Psychometric characteristics of the Child Occupational Self Assessment (COSA), part one: An initial examination of psychometric properties. *Scandinavian Journal of Occupational Therapy, 12*, 118–127.

Keller, J., & Kielhofner, G. (2005). Psychometric characteristics of the Child Occupational Self-Assessment (COSA), part two: Refining the psychometric properties. *Scandinavian Journal of Occupational Therapy, 12*, 147–158.

Kielhofner, G. (2002). *A model of human occupation: Theory and application*. Baltimore, MD: Lippincott Williams and Wilkins.

King, G., Law, M., King, S., Hurley, P., Hanna, S., Kertoy, M., et al. (2004). *Children's Assessment of Participation and Enjoyment (CAPE) and Preferences for Activities of Children (PAC)*. San Antonio, TX: Harcourt Assessment.

King, G., Law, M., King, S., Hurley, P., Hanna, S., Kertoy, M., et al. (2007). Measuring children's participation in recreation and leisure activities: Construct validation of the CAPE and PAC. *Child Care, Health and Development, 33*(1), 28–39.

King, G., McDougall, J., Palisano, R., Gritzan, J., & Tucker, M. A. (1999). Goal attainment scaling: Its use in evaluating pediatric practice. *Physical & Occupational Therapy in Pediatrics, 23*, 51–64.

Kiresuk, T. J., & Sherman, R. E. (1968). Goal attainment scaling: A general method for evaluating comprehensive community mental health programs. *Community Mental Health Journal, 4*, 443–453.

Law, M., Baptiste, S., Carswell, A., McColl, M. A., Polatajko, H., & Pollock, N. (2005). *The Canadian Occupational Performance Measure* (4th ed.). Ottawa, ON: CAOT Publications ACE.

Law, M., & Mills, J. (1998). Client-centred occupational therapy. In M. Law (Ed.), *Client-centred occupational therapy* (pp. 1–18). Thorofare, NJ: SLACK Inc.

Locke, E. A., & Latham, G. P. (1990). *A theory of goal setting and task performance*. Englewood Cliffs, NJ: Prentice-Hall.

MacKay, G., & Lundie, J. (1998). GAS released again: Proposals for the development of goal attainment scaling. *International Journal of Disability, Development and Education, 45*, 217–231.

Mandich, A. D., Polatajko, H. J., Miller, L. T., & Baum, C. (2004). *Paediatric Activity Card Sort*. Ottawa, ON: CAOT Publications ACE.

McColl, M. A., Carswell, A., Law, M., Pollock, N., Baptiste, S., & Polatajko, H. (2006). *Research on the Canadian Occupational Performance Measure: An annotated bibliography*. Ottawa, ON: CAOT Publications ACE.

McGavin, H. (1998). Planning rehabilitation: A comparison of issues for parents and adolescents. *Physical and Occupational Therapy in Pediatrics, 18*, 69–82.

McLaren, C., & Rodger, S. (2003). Goal attainment scaling: Clinical implications for paediatric occupational therapy practice. *Australian Occupational Therapy Journal, 50*, 216–224.

Missiuna, C. (1998). Development of the All About Me, a scale that measures children's perceived motor competence. *Occupational Therapy Journal of Research, 18*, 85–108.

Missiuna, C., & Pollock, N. (2000). Perceived efficacy and goal setting in young children. *Canadian Journal of Occupational Therapy, 67*, 101–109.

Missiuna, C., Pollock, N., & Law, M. (2004). *The Perceived Efficacy and Goal Setting System*. San Antonio, TX: PsychCorp.

Missiuna, C., Pollock, N., & Law, M. (2006). *Perceived efficacy and goal setting in young children (PEGS) Hebrew manual* (Translation and research by A. Miller-Hillel). Jerusalem, Israel: PsychTec.

Missiuna, C., Pollock, N., Law, M., Walter, S., & Cavey, N. (2006). Examination of the perceived efficacy and goal setting system (PEGS) with children with disabilities, their parents, and teachers. *American Journal of Occupational Therapy, 60,* 204-214.

Nordstrand, K. V. (2008). *Cross-cultural validation of the Perceived Efficacy and Goal Setting System – PEGS.* Karolinska Institutet, Sweden: Unpublished master's thesis.

Pollock, N., & Stewart, D. (1998). Occupational performance needs of school-aged children with physical disabilities in the community. *Physical and Occupational Therapy in Pediatrics, 18,* 55-68.

Poulsen, A., Rodger, S., & Ziviani, J. (2006). Understanding children's motivation from a self-determination theoretical perspective: Implications for practice. *Australian Occupational Therapy Journal, 53,* 78-86.

Rodger, S., Braithwaite, M., & Keen, D. (2004). Early intervention for children with autism: Parental priorities. *Australian Journal of Early Childhood, 29,* 34-41.

Rosenbaum, P., King, S., Law, M., King, G., & Evans, J. (1998). Family-centred service: A conceptual framework and research review. *Physical and Occupational Therapy in Pediatrics, 18,* 1-20.

Ruggio, C. I. B., Magalhaes, L., & Missiuna, C. (in press). Cross-cultural adaptation of the Perceived Efficacy and Goal Setting System (PEGS) for Brazilian children. *Occupational Therapy International.*

Sognnaes, M., & Langeland, I. (2006). *Perceived efficacy and goal setting system (PEGS): Brukermedvirkning for Norske barn? Rapport fra fou prosjekt.* Norway: St. Olavs Hospital.

St-Laurent-Gagnon, T., Bernard-Bonnin, A. C., & Villeneuve, E. (1999). Pain evaluation in preschool children and by their parents. *Acta Paediatrica, 88,* 422-427.

Steenbeek, D., Ketelaar, M., Galama, K., & Gorter, J. W. (2007). Goal attainment scaling in paediatric rehabilitation: A critical review of the literature. *Developmental Medicine and Child Neurology, 49,* 550-556.

Stoffel, A., & Berg, C. (2008). Spanish translation and validation of the Preschool Activity Card Sort. *Physical and Occupational Therapy in Pediatrics, 28,* 171-189.

Sturgess, J., Rodger, S., & Ozanne, A. (2002). A review of the use of self-report assessment with young children. *British Journal of Occupational Therapy, 65,* 108-116.

Taylor, S., Fayed, N., & Mandich, A. (2007). CO-OP intervention for young children with Developmental Coordination Disorder. *OTJR: Occupation, Participation and Health, 27,* 124-130.

Wigfield, A., & Eccles, J. S. (1992). The development of achievement task values: A theoretical analysis. *Developmental Review, 12,* 265-310.

Wilkins, S., Pollock, N., Law, M., & Rochon, S. (2001). Implementing client-centred practice: Why is it so difficult to do? *Canadian Journal of Occupational Therapy, 68,* 70-79.

Chapter 7

Occupation-centred Assessment with Children

Ted Brown and Chi-Wen Chien

Learning objectives

The objectives of this chapter are to:

- Provide a context for an occupation-centred approach to assessment with children and their families.
- Present a framework for occupational therapists to understand occupation-centred assessment with children.
- Review a range of occupation-centred assessments that can be used with children and their families.
- Illustrate the use of occupation-centred assessment using a case study.

Introduction

Occupational therapists work with children and youth who present with a range of medical, physical, learning, developmental and psychosocial conditions impacting occupational performance and participation. Based on the goals and priorities set with children and families, occupational therapists assess, plan and provide intervention leading to engagement in occupation and enhancing participation. Occupation-centred assessment requires judging, measuring, quantifying, scoring, observing or describing some aspect of occupational performance or the fundamental skills required to engage in occupation (Law & Baum, 2001). Occupational therapy assessment with children and youth ranges from specific to general and from single to holistic issues, all in the context of occupational performance and child- and family-centred practice. Assessment can take place at different stages of the occupational therapy process, such as at initial referral, during the intervention and at follow-up (refer to Figure 7.1 for overview). Occupational therapists

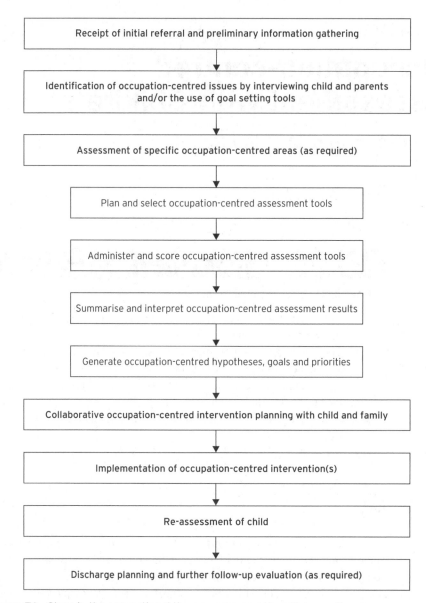

Figure 7.1 Steps in the occupational therapy assessment and intervention process

implement assessment in different settings, such as in a child's home, kinder-garten, childcare centre, school classroom or community.

Bottom-up and top-down approaches to assessment

Approaches to assessment have been generally delineated as either being top-down or bottom-up. Bottom-up assessments have been much more common in occupational therapy practice and fit easily within the traditional medical model. Burke (1997) found that clinicians who used the bottom-up medical model focused on a child's specific pathology, followed standard procedures, asked the child and parents fewer questions and spent less time interacting with the child/parents. Bottom-up assessments tend to assess small, separate components of a child's skills or occupational performance components, rather than taking a global perspective. They focus primarily on body structure and function (impairments) levels of the *International Classification of Functioning, Disability and Health* (ICF) (World Health Organization (WHO), 2001). Moreover, items in bottom-up assessment are frequently administered in rigid, contrived, standardised contexts that may not be meaningful to the child's perspective and are often isolated from meaningful daily environments. Examples of bottom-up assessments often used with children include the *Peabody Developmental Motor Scales – Second Edition* (Folio & Fewell, 2000), the *Sensory Profile* (Dunn, 1999) and the *Test of Visual Perceptual Skills – Third Edition* (Martin, 2006).

By contrast, top-down assessments take a global perspective and focus on the child's participation in his/her contexts to determine what is important to the child and the parents/caregivers. The focus is more aligned with the activities and participation levels of the ICF (WHO, 2001). The top-down assessment approach also fits with client- and family-centred approaches (DeGrace, 2003; Edwards, Millard, Praskac, & Wisniewski, 2003). According to Burke (1997), therapists who used this approach were less concerned with children's medical diagnoses and physical deficits. They interacted more with children and parents, and focused more on their needs in regard to the children's everyday life roles and participation.

Trombly (1993) advised occupational therapists to use top-down assessments that first focus on an individual's occupational performance issues specifically: 'the ability to carry out activities of daily life, including basic activities of daily living (BADL) and instrumental activities of daily living (IADL), education, work, play, leisure, and social participation' (American Occupational Therapy Association (AOTA), 2002, p. 617). Law and Baum (2001) considered occupational performance to be 'the point when the person, the environment, and the person's occupation intersect to support the tasks, activities, and roles that define that person as an individual' (p. 7). Figure 7.2 represents children's occupational performance assessment from both top-down and bottom-up perspectives.

Three frameworks/practice models often referred to in the occupational therapy literature emphasise the importance of assessing children's occupations and participation. All of these also provide valuable theoretical support for the use of a top-down approach in occupation-centred assessment with children (OCAC).

International Classification of Functioning, Disability and Health (ICF)

The ICF model of functioning and disability (WHO, 2001) is a framework that supports a more top-down approach to occupation-centred

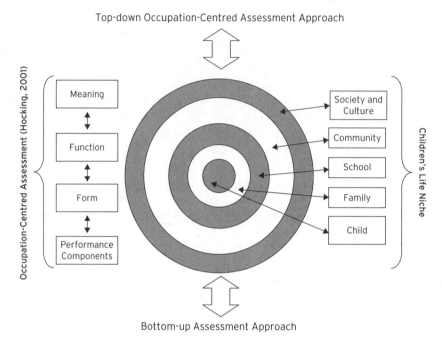

Figure 7.2 Children's occupation-centred assessment from top-down and bottom-up perspectives (Coster, 1998; Hocking, 2001; Nelson, 1996; Trombly, 1993). Reproduced with permission

assessment. Figure 7.3 depicts how the ICF model fits with the *Person-Environment-Occupation* model (Law, Baum, & Dunn, 2005; Law et al., 1996). It is a dynamic model and universal classification that helps describe functioning, disability and health as experienced by the individual in the context of his or her everyday life. Information on functioning and disability is organised into two components: one relating to the *body functions and structures* of people, and one relating to the *activities* people do and the life areas in which they *participate* (WHO, 2001). *Body functions and structures* are referred to as an individual's physiological functions and anatomical parts of body systems, which are the underlying components. *Activity* involves the execution of either a physical or a mental task or accomplishment. *Participation* refers to the individual's involvement in life situations with all environments. The ICF also attributes an individual's functioning, disability and health to *contextual factors*. These comprise the physical, social and attitudinal *environment* in which people live and conduct their lives, and may act as barriers or facilitators to the person's functioning (Law, 2002). The contextual factors also include *personal* factors, or features of an individual that are not part of a health condition yet influence how functioning and disability is experienced by the individual. The ICF *activity*, *participation*, *personal factors* and *environmental factors* provide an invaluable context for the top-down assessment approach to

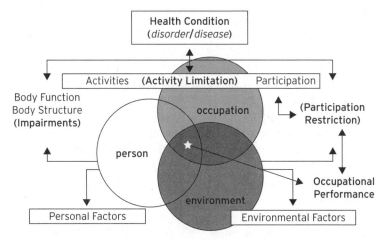

Figure 7.3 Conceptual interaction between the *International Classification of Functioning, Disability and Health* and the *person-environment-occupation model* (Law, Baum, & Dunn, 2005, p. 108). Reproduced with permission from the World Health Organization

children's occupational performance and functioning. The ICF has subsequently influenced the development of the *Occupational Therapy Practice Framework, 2nd Edition* (AOTA, 2008).

Occupational Therapy Practice Framework (OTPF)

The occupational therapy profession has identified the construct of participation within the AOTA *Occupational Therapy Practice Framework, 2nd Edition* (OTPF) (AOTA, 2008), as a research and practice priority. Engagement in occupation to support participation in contexts is the main focus and overall outcome of occupational therapy practice (AOTA, 2008). This view of the OTPF complements the ICF classification system. Both frameworks recognise the limitation or restriction of body systems, activity and participation within an individual's specific environmental contexts, affecting his/her health and well-being (AOTA, 2008; WHO, 2001). Occupational therapists believe that health can be improved and/or maintained when the individual engages in valued and meaningful occupations that allow desired or needed participation in life situations.

In the case of children and youth, both the OTPF and the ICF emphasise three essential occupations of self-care, leisure/play and productivity (e.g. education and learning). In addition, the OTPF and ICF emphasise the interdependence of person and environment factors to achieve participation. It has become a professional priority to develop assessment tools that identify environmental impacts on children's occupational performance and participation (Coster, 1998; Law, 2002; Trombly, 1993).

Based on the OTPF, the assessment process is followed as a top-down approach that begins with identifying an individual's occupational profile, defined as 'occupational history and experiences, patterns of daily living, interests, values and needs' (AOTA, 2002, p. 614). How a profile is developed will vary, based on the questions asked by the therapist who may define the collaborative relationship and scope of therapy at the participation level (e.g. removing barriers to participate in activities at a playground) versus at the impairment level (e.g. sensory processing deficits or fine motor problems). Then an *analysis of occupational performance* is completed to identify facilitating agents and barriers in various aspects of the child's engagement in occupations or participation (AOTA, 2008). This involves identifying skills and patterns in performance as well as evaluating the aspects of engagement in occupation that affect skills and patterns. In the context of supporting a child's participation, Law (2002) acknowledged that there has to be a shift in viewing the child's broader context, looking to community-based interventions if the needs, barriers or affordances lie outside of the child and family. Dunn (2000) referred to this as best practice, defending the child's benefits and rights to full inclusion and community participation.

Canadian Model of Occupational Performance and Engagement (CMOP–E)

The CMOP–E (Townsend & Polatajko, 2007) is a revision of the *Canadian Model of Occupational Performance* (CMOP) (Canadian Association of Occupational Therapists, 1997). The CMOP–E conceptualises occupational performance as the dynamic interaction of person, occupation and environment. The person component of the model comprises four parts: cognitive, affective, physical and spiritual, while the environment component includes four contexts: cultural, institutional, physical and social. Occupation is viewed as the link connecting the person and environment, indicating that people participate in the environment through occupation. The CMOP–E classifies occupation in three ways: self-care, productivity and leisure. In the case of children and youth, productivity includes play or school-related work in learning contexts, whereas leisure includes play in fun contexts. The structure of the CMOP–E promotes a top-down view of health, well-being and justice through occupation (Townsend & Polatajko, 2007). The theoretical underpinnings of the CMOP–E fit with the use of the top-down, occupation-centred approach to assessment with children. In summary, the ICF, OTPF and CMOP–E provide compelling rationales for using top-down assessment in occupational therapy practice with children and youth. The next section introduces OCAC primarily as a top-down assessment approach.

OCAC

OCAC focuses on occupational performance issues most relevant and important to an individual child and his/her family. Using an occupation-centred assessment approach, occupational therapists could decide to assess a child to obtain further information, establish a formal baseline of the child's performance or determine his or her eligibility for intervention or funding. OCAC focuses on the assessment of occupations related to children, including leisure/play, productivity/school, self-care/activities of daily living, as well as time use, roles, habits, routines, social participation, identity, contextual factors (e.g. cultural, temporal, social and physical) and activity patterns. Key features of OCAC are summarised in Table 7.1.

OCAC fits with the top-down approach to assessment since it considers a holistic view of children and their occupational performance within their naturalistic contexts. OCAC also fits with the principles of child- and family-centred practice, because it emphasises an individual or the family as the central element of the assessment process and focuses on only what is identified as important or relevant by them.

OCAC offers several advantages for use in children's occupational therapy. First, it focuses evaluation on a child's valued occupations in naturalistic environments and, therefore, assists therapists to address more realistic and critical occupational issues. Traditional assessment, however, often prescribes artificial or contrived tasks that individuals have to complete, which are largely irrelevant or of little meaning to them. Second, OCAC emphasises ecological assessment that considers different layers of the daily environments such as the home, school, community and society (see Figure 7.2). Third, OCAC provides a holistic top-down approach for evaluation and only utilises traditional, bottom-up assessments if required to determine the underlying reason for performance issues. It helps therapists to refocus on the child's occupational performance issues, rather than the underlying performance components. However, implementing OCAC is also associated with some disadvantages, for example, it can be time-consuming

Table 7.1 Features of occupation-centred assessment with children

- The 'whole child and family' is considered
- The child and family are active agents in the assessment process; their views, perceptions, opinions and priorities are solicited, accepted, integrated and valued
- The child and family are treated with respect, equality and dignity
- The assessment process is child- and family-centred; the assessing therapist works in partnership with the child and family
- The assessment process is responsive, non-invasive and bias-free in relation to the child's age, gender, culture, spiritual beliefs and other related variables
- The items in occupation-centred assessment with children evaluate the interaction of the child, his/her environments and occupations as well as focus on a variety of child-related occupations (such as leisure, play, self-care, rest, time use, education/ school issues, roles, habits, routines, participation, values and work/productivity-related issues)
- The environments/contexts of the child and family are taken into consideration

to complete and at present the number of available occupation-centred instruments is limited.

Implementation of occupation-centred assessment with children: assessment in action

Approaches to and guidelines for the implementation of occupation-centred assessment are gradually being developed. Trombly (1993) advocated a top-down approach that could guide therapists to obtain information about what the client wants or needs to do in the context of what occupations he/she values as well as any impediments to fulfilling these valued occupations. In other words, this approach focuses on the assessment of both the critical roles that the person needs or wishes to fulfil as well as the particular tasks and contexts that define the expectations of these roles for that person.

Coster (1998) focused on a child's overall pattern of occupational engagement in relation to specific contexts of significance, rather than on a child's roles. She concentrated on the extent to which a child's ability allows him/her to engage or participate in occupations in a given environment that is positive and satisfying for the child and acceptable to the adults involved in the child's daily life. Coster suggested four levels of analysis to guide the implementation of occupation-centred assessment in children's occupational therapy practice, namely participation, complex task performance, activity performance and component processes. More recently, Coster and Khetani (2008) advocated that participation and activity can be distinguished by considering the temporal (e.g. routines) and spatial (e.g. specific settings) dimensions of daily life. Participation involves life situations that are characterised by sets of organised sequences of activities directed towards a personally or socially meaningful goal (such as a child dressing to go outdoors in order to participate in outdoor recess time at school). Activities are the units from which such sequences may be constructed, including simple functional actions (e.g. buttoning a shirt, tying shoe laces and pulling up a zipper on a coat) and short sequences of functional actions with a common goal (e.g. putting on a shirt). The School Function Assessment (Coster, Deeney, Haltiwanger, & Haley, 1998) is a tool congruent with occupation-centred assessment.

The other significant discussion of occupation-centred assessment was proposed by Hocking (2001). She provided a conceptualisation of occupation in terms of meaning, function, form and performance components as a guide for assessment. Moreover, she outlined three strategies to assist with selecting occupation-centred assessments. In Hocking's view, occupation-centred assessment is conceptualised as a hierarchy that consists of the meaning of occupation and its importance in creating/maintaining an individual's occupational identity at the top, the function or purpose of the occupation in the individual's life, the form those occupations take and, lastly, *occupational performance components*. Hocking's conceptualisation of occupation-centred assessment is included on the left-hand side of Figure 7.2. From this hierarchical perspective, Hocking stated that occupational therapists' first requirement is to understand clients as occupational beings with unique values, interests, habits, routines and roles that form clients' occupational identity (e.g. understanding *the meaning of the client's occupations*). Framed by this understanding, the *function of the clients' occupations* (e.g. its purpose or importance within the client's daily realm of occupation and the contribution it makes to his or her own and other's lifestyles) should be identified if any problem occurs. The observable characteristics (referred to as the *form*) of the occupations that are problematic need to be subsequently addressed. For example, occupational therapists could assess *where, when and how* frequently the occupations can be observed, what actions or resources are needed for the individual to complete the occupation successfully and whether the environment facilitates or hinders the performance of the occupation. Finally, the individual's *performance components* can be assessed if the cause of his/her occupational dysfunction is not evident and needs to be known.

Regarding the three strategies for analysing the occupational basis of assessments proposed by Hocking (2001), the first strategy is to consider whether the assessment tool measures occupation as well as whether the assessment tool's underlying construct relates to occupational performance. The second deals with what kind of occupation the assessment focuses on. In particular, the occupation-centred assessment process should take cultural and subjective issues into consideration. The final strategy is to find out whether the assessment items involve occupations that are real versus simulated and familiar versus unfamiliar. The use of real occupations that are familiar to the individual is proposed as an important feature within occupation-centred assessment. By following the selection strategies and proposed hierarchical conception of occupation, Hocking believes that 'therapists will be enabled to implement assessments that provide an occupational based, client-centred foundation for practice' (p. 468).

Occupation-centred assessment with children: tools

To help occupational therapists to implement OCAC, 27 tools are reviewed in this section. Some assessment tools provide information about children's perceptions, roles, time use, values and habits, while some instruments explore children's occupations. A few assessments that measure the environmental impacts on children's participation are also included in the review. The 27 assessments are categorised into five areas that assess: (a) children's perceptions of occupational identity, (b) participation in leisure/play, (c) participation in productivity/school, (d) participation in self-care, and (e) environmental impacts on children's participation or occupational performance. Table 7.2

Table 7.2 Assessment tools that measure children's occupational identity

Assessments	Area measured	Reporting format	Age range	Testing time (min)	Scoring	Reliability	Validity
Adolescent Role Assessment[1] (ARA)	Roles	Interview	12-17 years	30	+: appropriate 0: marginal –: inappropriate	Internal consistency: + Inter-rater: – – Test-retest: ++	Content: ++ Criterion: – – Construct: ++
Assessment of Life Habits for Children[2] (LIFE-H)	Life habits	Child-report or interview	5-13 years	NS	Levels of difficulty: 5, assistance: 4, and satisfaction: 5	Internal consistency: – – Inter-rater: ++ Test-retest: +	Content: ++ Criterion: ++ Construct: +
Child Occupational Self Assessment[3] (COSA)	Identity and competence	Child-report	8-13 years	10-20	4-point rating scale	Internal consistency: ++ Inter-rater: NA Test-retest: – –	Content: ++ Criterion: – – Construct: ++
Self-perception Profile[4] (SPP)	Self-concept, efficacy and worth	Child- or teacher-report	Young child version: 4-7 years Child version: 8-12 years Adolescent version: 13-17 years	20	4-point rating scale	Internal consistency: + Inter-rater: NA Test-retest: +	Content: ++ Criterion: ++ Construct: ++
Structured Observation and Report Technique[5] (SORT)	Daily routine	Interview	Children and adolescents	15-45	Descriptive record in activity type, duration and companions, and 3-point rating scale for quality of interaction	Internal consistency: NA Inter-rater: + Test-retest: – –	Content: + Criterion: – – Construct: +

Note: (– –) No evidence reported; (–) limited evidence; (+) some evidence; (++) good evidence; (NA) not applicable; (NS) not specified.
[1]Black (1976).
[2]Noreau et al. (2007).
[3]Keller et al. (2005).
[4]Harter (1985, 1988) and Harter and Pike (1983).
[5]Rintala et al. (1984).

provides a summary of five assessments currently available to measure children's perceptions of their occupational identity, including roles, life habits and daily routines. All of these tools utilise either interview or self-report formats to gather specific information from the individual's perspective, within a reasonable administration time. Occupational therapists could use these tools to target a range of factors to gain a further understanding of individuals. For example, a therapist working with a 6-year-old child who has sustained traumatic brain injury wants to assess the child's social roles, and identify which factors are impeding the child's social participation. The therapist chooses to use the *Assessment of Life Habits for Children* (LIFE-H) (Noreau et al., 2007) since it gathers information about children's life habits including activities of daily life and social roles. All the assessment tools in Table 7.2 were found to have acceptable levels of reliability and validity evidence. It is noted that only the LIFE-H and the young child version of the *Self-perception Profile* (Harter & Pike, 1983) were suitable for use with pre-school age children. The remaining tools are applicable for children 8 years or older.

Table 7.3 lists six existing assessment tools that measure children's participation in leisure/play occupations including play behaviour, experiences, interests and/or playfulness. The selected tools cover a wide age range, from infancy to adolescence, as well as use various administration formats (e.g. child-report, interview or rated observation). For example, the *Paediatric Activity Card Sort* (PACS) (Mandich, Polatajko, Miller, & Baum, 2004) requires therapists to conduct an interview using picture cards, but this may present a time burden for therapists in busy clinics (see Chapter 6 for more information). The use of child self-report questionnaires is thus one possible solution for this situation to reduce demands on the therapist's time. Most of the tools listed in Table 7.3 have acceptable evidence of their reliability and validity report to support their clinical use. The *Paediatric Interest Profiles* (Henry, 2000) and the PACS, however, have limited validity evidence, and the PACS in particular has no published reliability evidence to date. The *Test of Playfulness* (ToP) (Bundy, 2003) requires specialised training and certification for administration.

Table 7.4 provides a review of six assessment tools that measure children's participation in productivity/school occupations. The *Children Helping Out: Responsibilities, Expectations and Supports* (CHORES) (Dunn, 2004) is a tool that measures school-age children's participation in household tasks (including self-care and family-care activities), while the remaining five instruments focus on children's school-related participation. Except for the *School Outcome Measure* (SOM) that takes less than 15 min, the other four school-related assessment tools each take at least 40 min to complete. The SOM was developed by McEwen, Arnold, Hansen, and Johnson (2003) as a minimal data set to measure outcome (including self-care, mobility, assuming a student's role, expressing learning and behaviour) of students who receive school-based occupational therapy. The *School Function Assessment* (Coster et al., 1998) consists of 26 subscales, each one taking approximately 5–10 min

Table 7.3 Assessment tools that measure children's participation in leisure and play occupations

Assessments	Area measured	Reporting format	Age range	Testing time (min)	Scoring	Reliability	Validity
Children's Assessment of Participation and Enjoyment/ Preferences for Activities of Children[1] (CAPE/PAC)	Participation in, enjoyment of and preferences for activities other than school activities	Child-report	6-21 years	30-45 (CAPE) 15-20 (PAC)	Each activity: yes or no, 7- and 5-point rating scales (CAPE) or 3-point rating scale (PAC)	Internal consistency: + Inter-rater: + Test-retest: +	Content: ++ Criterion: + Construct: ++
Paediatric Activity Card Sort[2] (PACS)	Engagement in a range of activities (including play)	Interview	5-14 years	20-25	Each activity: yes or no and frequency Identify five important and five desirable activities	Internal consistency: NA Inter-rater: − Test-retest: NA	Content: ++ Criterion: −− Construct: −
Paediatric Interest Profiles[3] (PIP)	Play interests	Child-report	6-21 years	15-30	Each activity: yes/no or 3-point rating scale and levels of enjoyment: 3 or 5 (depending on versions used), frequency: 3, competence: 3, and with whom: 3	Internal consistency: + Inter-rater: NA Test-retest: +	Content: ++ Criterion: −− Construct: −
Play History[4] (PH)	Play experiences and opportunities	Interview	Infancy to adolescence	NS	NA	Internal consistency: NA Inter-rater: ++ Test-retest: +	Content: ++ Criterion: ++ Construct: −
Revised Knox Pre-school Play Scale[5] (PPS-R)	Play behaviour	Rated observation	0-6 years	60	Yes/no binary choice	Internal consistency: ++ Inter-rater: ++ Test-retest: ++	Content: ++ Criterion: ++ Construct: +
Test of Playfulness[6] (ToP)	Playfulness during free play	Rated observation	6 months to 18 years	30-40	4-point rating scale	Internal consistency: ++ Inter-rater: ++ Test-retest: +	Content: ++ Criterion: + Construct: ++

Note: (−−) No evidence reported; (−) limited evidence; (+) some evidence; (++) good evidence; (NA) not applicable; (NS) not specified.
[1]King et al. (2004).
[2]Mandich et al. (2004).
[3]Henry (2000).
[4]Takata (1969) and Bryze (2008).
[5]Knox (2008).
[6]Bundy (2003).

Table 7.4 Assessment tools that measure children's participation in productivity and school occupations

Assessments	Area measured	Reporting format	Age range	Testing time (min)	Scoring	Reliability	Validity
Children Helping Out: Responsibilities, Expectations and Supports[1] (CHORES)	Household task performance	Parent- or caregiver-report	6-11 years	NS	Each task: yes/no Levels of assistance: 7 and importance/ satisfaction: 6	Internal consistency: – – Inter-rater: NA Test-retest: ++	Content: ++ Criterion: – Construct: – –
Occupational Therapy Psychosocial Assessment of Learning[2] (OTPAL)	Psychosocial skills and student-environment fit	Rated observation and interview	6-12 years	40 (observation) 45 (interview)	4-point rating scale	Internal consistency: – – Inter-rater: – – Test-retest: – –	Content: + Criterion: – – Construct: – –
School Function Assessment[3] (SFA)	Functional performance in school	Teacher-report	5-12 years	90-120	Levels of participation: 4, assistance: 4, and performance: 4	Internal consistency: ++ Inter-rater: NA Test-retest: ++	Content: ++ Criterion: ++ Construct: ++
School Outcome Measure[4] (SOM)	Functional performance in school	Rated observation	3-18 years	10-15	6-point assistance rating scale	Internal consistency: – – Inter-rater: + Test-retest: +	Content: ++ Criterion: – – Construct: – –
School Setting Interview[5] (SSI)	Student-environment fit	Interview	≤10 years	40	4-step rating scale	Internal consistency: ++ Inter-rater: ++ Test-retest: +	Content: ++ Criterion: – – Construct: ++
School Version of the Assessment of Motor and Process Skills[6] (School AMPS)	Skilfulness of school-related activities	Interview and rated observation	≤3 years	30 (interview) 30-40 (observation)	4-point rating scale	Internal consistency: ++ Inter-rater: ++ Test-retest: – –	Content: ++ Criterion: + Construct: ++

Note: (– –) No evidence reported; (–) limited evidence; (+) some evidence; (++) good evidence; (NA) not applicable; (NS) not specified.
[1]Dunn (2004).
[2]Townsend et al. (1999).
[3]Coster et al. (1998).
[4]McEwen et al. (2003).
[5]Hemmingsson et al. (2005).
[6]Fisher et al. (2005).

to complete. Therapists do not have to administer all 26 subscales and may choose applicable individual subscales to address the specific circumstance and needs of a child.

The *School Setting Interview* (SSI) (Hemmingsson, Egilson, Hoffman, & Kielhofner, 2005) is an assessment of student–environment fit, based on the *Model of Human Occupation*. Its development was influenced by focusing on the problems of a student's actual doing, where both the student's participation in school tasks and the influences of the school environment are captured. Therefore, the SSI provides occupational therapists the opportunity not only to obtain data about the child's participation in school tasks, but also to identify needs for task or environmental accommodations to his/her participation in the school setting. In terms of the measurement properties, all but two assessment tools in Table 7.4 have reasonable reliability and validity. The two assessments that currently have no published validity evidence (except for content validity) are the SOM and the *Occupational Therapy Psychosocial Assessment of Learning* (OTPAL) (Townsend et al., 1999). Moreover, the OTPAL has no accessible reliability evidence to date. The only tool that requires therapists to complete formal training and obtain certification to administer it is the *School Version of the Assessment of Motor and Process Skills* (Fisher, Bryze, Hume, & Griswold, 2005).

Table 7.5 presents six instruments that assess children's participation in self-care occupations. All the self-care assessment tools are well-developed, commonly used instruments that have reasonable administration times and acceptable evidence of reliability and validity. The latest editions of both the *Adaptive Behavior Assessment System* (Harrison & Oakland, 2003) and the *Vineland Adaptive Behavior Scales* (Sparrow, Cicchetti, & Bella, 2005), although purporting to assess an individual's general adaptive skills or behaviour, include the assessment of basic and instrumental activities of daily living (BADL and IADL). The *Pediatric Evaluation of Disability Inventory* (Haley, Coster, Ludlow, Haltiwanger, & Andrellos, 1992) and the *Functional Independence Measure for Children* (Uniform Data System for Medical Rehabilitation, 2006) have been largely used to assess children's functional status (including self-care).

Unlike the tools that focus on the broad assessment of children's adaptive behaviours or functional status, the *Activities Scales for Kids* (ASK) (Young, 1996) is designed to specifically measure a child's physical function including personal care, dressing and locomotion. The *Assessment of Motor and Process Skills* (Fisher, 1995) also assesses the quality (or skilfulness) of an individual's performance specifically in BADL activities, and requires specialised administration training and certification. The PACS and CHORES, presented earlier, also include a few self-care assessment items, which may also be used to assess components of children's self-care performance.

Table 7.6 provides a summary of four tools that consider the environmental impacts on children's participation or occupational performance. Each

Table 7.5 Assessment tools that measure children's participation in self-care occupations

Assessments	Area measured	Reporting format	Age range	Testing time (min)	Scoring	Reliability	Validity
Activities Scales for Kids[1] (ASK)	BADL and IADL	Child- or parent-report	5-15 years	10-30	5-point rating scale	Internal consistency: ++ Inter-rater: ++ Test-retest: ++	Content: ++ Criterion: ++ Construct: ++
Adaptive Behavior Assessment System – second edition[2] (ABAS-II)	BADL, IADL, communication, functional academics, social, leisure, self-direction and work	Interview, rated observation or parent-teacher report	0-89 years	15-20	4-point Likert scale	Internal consistency: ++ Inter-rater: ++ Test-retest: ++	Content: ++ Criterion: ++ Construct: ++
Assessment of Motor and Process Skills[3] (AMPS)	Skilfulness of BADL activities	Rated observation	≤3 years	3-40	4-point rating scale	Internal consistency: ++ Inter-rater: ++ Test-retest: ++	Content: ++ Criterion: ++ Construct: ++
Functional Independence Measure for Children[4] (WeeFIM)	BADL, IADL and social cognition	Rated observation	6 months to 7 years	15	7-level rating scale (for 3-7-year version) or 3-level rating scale (for 0-3-year version)	Internal consistency: ++ Inter-rater: ++ Test-retest: ++	Content: ++ Criterion: ++ Construct: ++
Pediatric Evaluation of Disability Inventory[5] (PEDI)	BADL, IADL and social function	Interview and caregiver-report	6 months to 7 years	45-60	Levels of functional skills: 2, assistance: 6, and modification: 2	Internal consistency: ++ Inter-rater: ++ Test-retest: ++	Content: ++ Criterion: ++ Construct: ++
Vineland Adaptive Behavior Scales - Second Edition[6] (Vineland-II)	BADL, IADL, cognition, language, play and social competency	Interview or caregiver-teacher report	0-90 years	20-60	3-point rating scale	Internal consistency: ++ Inter-rater: + Test-retest: ++	Content: ++ Criterion: ++ Construct: ++

Note: (−−) No evidence reported; (−) limited evidence; (+) some evidence; (++) good evidence; (NA) not applicable; (NS) not specified.
[1]Young (1996).
[2]Harrison and Oakland (2003).
[3]Fisher (1995).
[4]Uniform Data System for Medical Rehabilitation (2006).
[5]Haley et al. (1992).
[6]Sparrow et al. (2005).

Table 7.6 Assessment tools that measure the environmental impacts on children's participation or occupational performance

Assessments	Area measured	Reporting format	Age range	Testing time (min)	Scoring	Reliability	Validity
Children's Physical Environments Rating Scale[1] (CPERS)	Childhood educational facility	Educator- or therapist-report	Early childhood	NS	5-point Likert scale	Internal consistency: ++ Inter-rater: ++ Test-retest: ++	Content: ++ Criterion: −− Construct: +
Craig Hospital Inventory of Environmental Factors[2,3,4] (CHIEF)	Physical, attitudinal, service, productivity and policy barriers	Self/proxy-report or interview (original) and being adapted to children as parent-report[4]	16–95 years (original) 6–14 years (adapted)	10–15	Levels of frequency: 5 and magnitude: 2	Internal consistency: ++ Inter-rater: + Test-retest: ++	Content: ++ Criterion: −− Construct: ++
Home Observation for Measurement of the Environment[5] (HOME)	Home	Interview and rated observation	0–15 years	45–60	Yes/no binary choice	Internal consistency: ++ Inter-rater: ++ Test-retest: ++	Content: ++ Criterion: ++ Construct: +
Test of Environmental Supportiveness[6] (TOES)	Play environment	Rated observation	6 months to 18 years	15–20	4-point rating scale	Internal consistency: ++ Inter-rater: ++ Test-retest: −−	Content: ++ Criterion: −− Construct: ++

Note: (−−) No evidence reported; (−) limited evidence; (+) some evidence; (++) good evidence; (NA) not applicable; (NS) not specified.

[1]Moore and Sugiyama (2007).

[2]The reliability and validity evidence of the CHIEF are based on previous studies with adults, because it has not yet been validated with children.

[3]Whiteneck et al. (2004).

[4]Law et al. (2007).

[5]Caldwell and Bradley (1984).

[6]Bundy (1999).

of the assessments quantifies different physical environments such as the child's home, school and play environments. Besides physical environments, the *Craig Hospital Inventory of Environmental Factors* (CHIEF) (Whiteneck et al., 2004) considers other environmental factors including attitudinal or policy factors that may impact on an individual's participation. The CHIEF was originally developed as a self-report tool for people aged over 16 years, but it has been recently adapted to a parent-report format appropriate for use with 6–14-year-old children (Law, Petrenchik, King, & Hurley, 2007). However, the validity and reliability of the CHIEF has not yet been established when used with parents; therefore, the CHIEF's measurement evidence reported in Table 7.6 is based on previous studies with adults. In addition to the CHIEF, the other three assessment tools exhibited acceptable reliability and validity evidence to support their use with children.

The *Home Observation for Measurement of the Environment* (HOME; Caldwell & Bradley, 1984) consists of four versions appropriate for use with children from infancy and toddlerhood, early and middle childhood, and early adolescence. The use of the appropriate age versions could facilitate therapists to make correct interpretations of the levels of environmental support in a child's home context. The *Test of Environmental Supportiveness* (TOES)

Case study: application of the occupation-centred assessment with children to a child with juvenile idiopathic arthritis

Jill is an 8-year-old girl diagnosed with pauciarticular juvenile idiopathic arthritis (JIA), 2 weeks ago. This is the most common and generally mildest form of JIA, where four or fewer joints are involved. The most commonly affected joints are the knee, ankle, wrist and elbow. The clinical course of pauciarticular juvenile arthritis may involve flares and remissions, but with appropriate treatment, there is rarely permanent damage to the joints.

The primary methods of treating JIA include medications to control the inflammation, exercises to keep the joints moving well and the muscles strong, splints to support the joints, steroid injections to reduce inflammation in particular joints and pain management strategies. The goals of medical and rehabilitation intervention are: to reduce inflammation, to reduce pain (usually due to inflammation), to minimise damage to the joints, to ensure that the joints keep working at an optimal level, to get the child diagnosed with JIA back to his or her normal activities, to prevent JIA from interfering with the child's routine lifestyle and to provide information and education for the family of the child with JIA as needed. The first line of treatment involves a non-steroidal anti-inflammatory drug (NSAID) while disease modifying drugs (DMARDs) are added as a second-line treatment when arthritis remains active despite NSAID therapy.

(Bundy, 1999) is a companion scale of the ToP and explores elements (e.g. caregivers, playmates, objects and space) of a particular environment that supports or inhibits a child's play engagement (Bronson & Bundy, 2001).

Besides the four assessment tools shown in Table 7.6, the SSI, presented earlier, may be used to ascertain the fit between the child's and his/her school environment. Moreover, Ziviani and Rodger (2006) also provided a summary of tools that focus on environmental assessment, where the *Environment Rating Scales* and *Classroom Environment Scale* are also potential instruments that therapists can use to measure childcare environment or classroom social climate, respectively.

Medical history

Jill was referred by her general practitioner to a paediatric rheumatology clinic at a regional children's hospital, after she presented with a 6-week history of morning stiffness, spiking fevers and sore swollen joints that included her left knee, both wrists and right elbow. About 1 week before Jill developed her painful swollen joints, she had a mild flu for 3 days. Jill had also tripped going up the stairs at home and hit her left knee during this time. When she started complaining about having a sore knee, elbow and wrists, Jill was seen by her family physician. Jill's mother reported that Jill's joints usually felt sore in the morning, but seemed to become more comfortable and mobile as the day progressed. The family doctor noted that Jill's wrists, right elbow and left knee were visibly swollen and warm to touch. Furthermore, Jill complained of pain, did not want to walk, go up and down stairs or perform any self-care or school-related activities that involved flexing and extending her wrists.

Family history

Jill's father works as a brick layer in the construction industry and her mother works as a teaching assistant in a neighbourhood pre-school classroom. Jill has a 16-year-old sister and 10-year-old twin brothers. The family rent a two-storey townhouse with three bedrooms in a new housing development on the outskirts of a large metropolitan area.

Education and developmental history

Jill attends Grade Three at the local state primary school. Her teacher reported that Jill is an average student at school, but has difficulties with mathematics. However, Jill enjoys art, creative writing and social studies. Jill was born at 39 weeks with a birth weight of 2.5 kg. She attained her developmental milestones at expected ages and has had no previous history of significant health problems. There is no previous family history of autoimmune type diseases.

Clinical assessment results

When the rheumatologist saw Jill, he completed an initial physical examination and ordered X-rays, and blood tests. It was reported that both of Jill's wrists, left knee and right elbow exhibited limited active range of motion due to swelling and pain. Based on the presenting symptoms, Jill was prescribed oral medication for pain as well as monthly intra-muscular injections of methotrexate (*Rheumatrex*), a type of DMARD. Meanwhile, Jill was also referred to a physiotherapist and an occupational therapist in the rheumatology clinic. The physiotherapist completed the traditional assessment based on physical measurements of Jill's joint range of motion, grip strength, manual muscle testing and subjective pain measures.

Paul, the occupational therapist, used an occupation- and client-centred approach to assessment. Initially, he interviewed Jill and her parents to find out what issues and factors were important to Jill, and her parents in relation to Jill's participation in her routine life and to develop of profile of Jill's daily occupations. The interview results are summarised in Table 7.7.

Based on the discussion with Jill and her mother, it was decided that the following four occupation-centred assessment tools would be used to obtain further information. The first tool Jill completed with Paul was the *Child Occupational Self Assessment* (COSA) (Keller, Kafkes, Basu, Federico, & Kielhofner, 2005). The COSA was used to elicit Jill's perceptions regarding her sense of occupational competence and the value that she placed on completing occupational performance tasks. The use of the COSA also assisted Paul in identifying the differences between Jill's perceived occupational competence and valued occupations. On the COSA, Jill identified four items as being 'Really important to me' but 'I have a problem doing this'. They were: 'Dress myself', 'Get my chores done', 'Have enough time to do things I like' and 'Use my hands to work with things'. The results indicate that Jill identified several of the occupations she valued as being difficult to complete. The COSA results also confirmed Jill's initial interview results, where she reported completing her chores, using her hands to complete homework tasks on the computer and playing the piano were challenging for her, but those were also occupations she highly valued. Therefore, Paul could utilise the information from Jill's COSA results to establish the priorities for his intervention process.

Second, the *Kids Play Survey* (KPS) of the *Paediatric Interest Profiles* (Henry, 2000) was selected by Paul to measure Jill's interest, enjoyment and participation in age-appropriate play activities. Jill's KPS results indicated that she liked to participate in *sports activities* (such as soccer), *summer activities* (such as gardening), *indoor activities* (such as listening to music and using the computer), *creative activities* (such as singing), *lessons/classes* (such as music lessons) and *socialising activities* (such as hanging out with friends). However, she did not like to participate in *outdoor activities* or *winter activities*. In addition, Jill's KPS results showed

Table 7.7 Issues identified by Jill and her parents using the occupation-centred assessment approach

1. Perceptions of occupational identity:
   - reported feeling frustrated, angry and anxious about not being able to do many daily tasks herself
   - reported that her role as a student was challenging, since she could not keep up with her peers and felt that she was not able to complete her work within specified time periods
   - reported feeling left out, since she was not able to play her favourite sport and take part in her favourite hobby (e.g. playing soccer and piano)
   - reported feeling anxious that she was not able to complete her assigned household chores

2. Participation in leisure/play occupations:
   - likes to play piano and takes weekly piano lessons, but now finds it difficult to play longer than 5 min
   - likes to play soccer at school with friends and plays on neighbourhood girls' soccer team, but now finds it hard to keep up with her friends and team mates
   - likes to play computer games with her two older brothers, but now finds it difficult

3. Participation in productivity/school occupations:
   - finds grasping and holding a pencil when printing for longer than 5 min challenging, when performing writing tasks that have to be completed within specific time periods (such as dictation or tests)
   - finds it difficult to use keyboard to complete homework tasks for longer than 10 min
   - finds carrying school materials in backpack difficult
   - finds it difficult to open/close heavy doors at school and go up/down stairs from the playground to her classroom
   - finds it challenging to keep up with peers during physical education activities that involve high-impact movements, such as jumping, running, catching and throwing
   - finds completing assigned household chores difficult, such as walking pet dog daily, vacuuming first floor of house once per week and loading/unloading dishwasher every second day

4. Participation in self-care occupations:
   - finds taking the lid off and putting it back on the toothpaste tube and squeezing toothpaste onto brush difficult; also finds holding tooth brush to clean her teeth and turning water taps on and off difficult
   - finds grasping and pulling on tights and socks difficult; also finds putting on shoes and tying shoelaces challenging

5. Environmental factors:
   - home environment: found opening and closing the door difficult to get in or out; also found going up and down stairs to her bedroom difficult
   - school environment: found it exhausting to climb the stairs from the ground floor of the school to her classroom on the second floor
   - classroom environment: found not being able to stretch out her left leg challenging to her sitting posture; also found her desk being located at the back of the room made it challenging for her to pay attention
   - playground environment: had to limit her activities on the playground to avoid high-impact activities
   - community environment: found the field where her soccer team practiced challenging to access

that she preferred to participate with her friends in sports, summer, indoor and socialising activities, whereas she liked to take part in creative and lessons/classes with adults. In combination with the results of the initial interview, Paul concluded that, due to Jill's sore joints, two play activities that she liked the most but had difficulty participating in (e.g. playing soccer and practicing her piano lessons) should be prioritised for intervention to enhance her participation with peers in out-of-school leisure and piano playing.

Third, the ASK, as a self-report measure, was used to describe both Jill's participation and capability primarily in self-care activities. The domains that the ASK measures include personal care, dressing, eating and drinking, miscellaneous, locomotion, stairs, play, transfers and standing skills. There are two ASK versions that can be used. The performance measure (ASKp) queries what the child 'did do' in the past week and the capability measure (ASKc) queries what the child 'could do' during the past week. Therefore, Paul used the ASKp to determine from Jill's perspective what she did during the last week and compared it to the ASKc where Jill reported what she could have really done. The results indicated that Jill's mean performance score was markedly lower than her capacity score. This reflected that Jill could likely participate to a larger degree in self-care occupations, but her participation was being limited possibly by the impact of the JIA or environmental factors.

Finally, Paul considered both Jill's role of being a student and also that Jill school's environment may be impacting on her occupational performance. Therefore, he conducted the SSI to assess student-environment fit and to identify the need for accommodations required for Jill in her school setting. The SSI focuses on not only the classroom, but also the playground, gymnasium, corridors and school excursions. Using the SSI, Paul asked Jill about past, present and future management of the 16 SSI context areas. The SSI results revealed that there was a *perfect fit/no need for adjustments* in relation to seven areas: read, speak, remember things, social break activities, get assistance and interact with staff. However, there was a *partial fit* for the following nine contexts: write, do mathematics, do homework, take exams, do sport activities, practical subjects, getting around the classroom, go on field trips, get assistance and access the school. The SSI results provided helpful information for Paul about the improved fit between Jill and her school setting by environmental adjustments. In summary, the four occupation-centred assessment tools (COSA, KPS, ASK and SSI) provided Paul with relevant, valuable, client-centred information about Jill's participation and occupational engagement. The assessment results further confirmed the issues that were identified in the initial interview with Jill and her parents, and also offered objective data and evidence for occupational therapy service planning. The results indicated that there were several environmental factors impacting Jill's participation in her home, school and community environments. Based on the information gathered, Paul determined the areas that Jill wanted to improve, designed a therapeutic programme, recommended accommodations appropriate to her and was able to evaluate the effectiveness of the intervention provided.

Conclusion

In this chapter, bottom-up and top-down approaches to assessment as well as the ICF, OTPF and CMOP-E were used to contextualise *OCAC*. The occupational-centred assessment frameworks proposed by Coster (1998) and Hocking (2001) were discussed in the context of *OCAC*. Specific tools that assess children's self-care occupations, play occupations, school occupations and environmental influence on daily occupations were reviewed and discussed. Finally, a case study was presented illustrating the use of *OCAC* as a means to ground occupational therapy practice in children's occupational performance and participation.

References

American Occupational Therapy Association. (2002). Occupational therapy practice framework: Domain and process. *American Journal of Occupational Therapy, 56,* 609–639.

American Occupational Therapy Association. (2008). *Occupational therapy practice framework: Domain and process, 2nd edition*. Bethesda, MD: American Occupational Therapy Association.

Black, M. M. (1976). Adolescent role assessment. *American Journal of Occupational Therapy, 30,* 73–79.

Bronson, M., & Bundy, A. C. (2001). A correlational study of the Test of Playfulness and the Test of Environmental Supportiveness. *Occupational Therapy Journal of Research, 21,* 223–240.

Bryze, K. (2008). Narrative contributions to the play history. In L. D. Parham, & L. S. Fazio (Eds.), *Play in occupational therapy for children* (pp. 43–54). St. Louis, MO: Mosby Elsevier.

Bundy, A. (1999). *Test of Environmental Supportiveness*. Fort Collins, CO: Colorado State University.

Bundy, A. (2003). *Test of Playfulness*. Lidcombe, NSW: University of Sydney.

Burke, J. P. (1997). *Frames of meaning: An analysis of occupational therapy evaluations of young children*. Philadelphia, PA: Penn Libraries, University of Pennsylvania.

Caldwell, B., & Bradley, R. (1984). *Home observation for measurement of the environment* (Revised ed.). Little Rock, AR: University of Arkansas.

Canadian Association of Occupational Therapists. (1997). *Enabling occupation: An occupational therapy perspective* (Revised ed.). Ottawa, ON: CAOT Publications ACE.

Coster, W. (1998). Occupation-centered assessment of children. *American Journal of Occupational Therapy, 52*(5), 337–344.

Coster, W., Deeney, T., Haltiwanger, J., & Haley, S. (1998). *School Function Assessment*. San Antonio, TX: Harcourt Assessment.

Coster, W., & Khetani, M. A. (2008). Measuring participation of children with disabilities: Issues and challenges. *Disability and Rehabilitation, 30*(8), 693-648.

DeGrace, B. W. (2003). Occupation-based and family-centered care: A challenge for current practice. *American Journal of Occupational Therapy, 57*(3), 347-350.

Dunn, W. (1999). *The Sensory Profile.* San Antonio, TX: Psychological Corporation.

Dunn, W. (2000). The screening, referral, and pre-assessment processes. In W. Dunn (Ed.), *Best practice occupational therapy: In community service with children and families* (pp. 55-77). Thorofare, NJ: SLACK Incorporated.

Dunn, L. (2004). Validation of the CHORES: A measure of school-aged children's participation in household tasks. *Scandinavian Journal of Occupational Therapy, 11,* 179-190.

Edwards, M., Millard, P., Praskac, L. A., & Wisniewski, P. A. (2003). Occupational therapy and early intervention: A family-centred approach. *Occupational Therapy International, 10*(4), 239-252.

Fisher, A. G. (1995). *Assessment of Motor and Process Skills.* Fort Collins, CO: Three Star Press.

Fisher, A. G., Bryze, K., Hume, V. H., & Griswold, L. A. (2005). *School AMPS: School Version of the Assessment of Motor and Process Skills* (2nd ed.). Fort Collins, CO: Three Star Press.

Folio, M. R., & Fewell, R. R. (2000). *Peabody Developmental Motor Scales: Examiner's manual* (2nd ed.). San Antonio, TX: Psychological Corporation.

Haley, S. M., Coster, W. J., Ludlow, L. H., Haltiwanger, J. T., & Andrellos, P. J. (1992). *Administration manual for the Pediatric Evaluation of Disability Inventory.* San Antonio, TX: Psychological Corporation.

Harrison, P., & Oakland, T. (2003). *Adaptive behavior assessment system – Second edition manual.* San Antonio, TX: Psychological Corporation.

Harter, S. (1985). *Manual for the self-perception profile for children.* Denver, CO: University of Denver.

Harter, S. (1988). *Manual for the self-perception profile for adolescents.* Denver, CO: University of Denver.

Harter, S., & Pike, R. (1983). *The pictorial scale of perceived competence and acceptance for young children.* Denver, CO: University of Denver.

Hemmingsson, H., Egilson, S., Hoffman, O., & Kielhofner, G. (2005). *A user's manual for the School Setting Interview version 3.0.* Chicago, IL: MOHO Clearinghouse.

Henry, A. D. (2000). *Pediatric Interest Profiles.* San Antonio, TX: Harcourt Assessment.

Hocking, C. (2001). Implementing occupation-based assessment. *American Journal of Occupational Therapy, 55*(4), 463-469.

Keller, J., Kafkes, A., Basu, S., Federico, J., & Kielhofner, G. (2005). *A user's guide to Child Occupational Self Assessment version 2.1.* Chicago, IL: MOHO Clearinghouse.

King, G., Law, M., King, S., Hurley, P., Hanna, S., Kertory, M., et al. (2004). *Children's Assessment of Participation and Enjoyment and Preferences for Activities of Children.* San Antonio, TX: Harcourt Assessment.

Knox, S. (2008). The Revised Knox Preschool Play Scale. In L. D. Parham, & L. S. Fazio (Eds.), *Play in occupational therapy for children* (pp. 55-70). St. Louis, MO: Mosby Elsevier.

Law, M. (2002). Participation in the occupations of everyday life. *American Journal of Occupational Therapy, 56*(6), 640-649.

Law, M., & Baum, C. (2001). Measuring in occupational therapy. In M. Law, C. Baum, & W. Dunn (Eds.), *Measuring occupational performance: Supporting best practice in occupational therapy* (pp. 3-19). Thorofare, NJ: SLACK Incorporated.

Law, M., Baum, C., & Dunn, W. (Eds.). (2005). *Measuring occupational performance: Supporting best practice in occupational therapy* (2nd ed.). Thorofare, NJ: SLACK Incorporated.

Law, M., Cooper, B. A., Strong, S., Stewart, D., Rigby, P., & Letts, L. (1996). The person-environment-occupation model: A transactive approach to occupational performance. *Canadian Journal of Occupational Therapy, 63,* 9-23.

Law, M., Petrenchik, T., King, G., & Hurley, P. (2007). Perceived environmental barriers to recreational, community, and school participation for children and youth with physical disabilities. *Archives of Physical Medicine and Rehabilitation, 88*(12), 1636-1642.

Mandich, A., Polatajko, H., Miller, L., & Baum, C. (2004). *Pediatric Activity Card Sort.* Ottawa, ON: CAOT Publication ACE.

Martin, N. A. (2006). *Test of Visual Perceptual Skills - Third edition.* Novato, CA: Academic Therapy Publications.

McEwen, I. R., Arnold, S. H., Hansen, L. H., & Johnson, D. (2003). Interrater reliability and content validity of a minimal data set to measure outcomes of students receiving school-based occupational therapy and physical therapy. *Physical and Occupational Therapy in Pediatrics, 23*(2), 77-95.

Moore, G. T., & Sugiyama, T. (2007). The Children's Physical Environment Rating Scale (CPERS): Reliability and validity for assessing the physical environment of early childhood educational facilities. *Children, Youth and Environments, 17*(4), 24-53.

Nelson, D. L. (1996). Therapeutic occupation: A definition. *American Journal of Occupational Therapy, 50*(10), 775-782.

Noreau, L., Lepage, C., Boissiere, L., Picard, R., Fougeyrollas, P., Mathieu, J., et al. (2007). Measuring participation in children with disabilities using the Assessment of Life Habits. *Developmental Medicine and Child Neurology, 49*(9), 666-671.

Rintala, D. H., Uttermohlen, D. M., Buck, E. L., Hanover, D., Alexander, J. L., & Norris-Baker, C. (1984). Self-observation and report technique: Description and clinical applications. In A. S. Halpern, & M. J. Fuhrer (Eds.), *Functional assessment in rehabilitation* (pp. 205-221). Baltimore, MD: Paul H. Brookes.

Sparrow, S. S., Cicchetti, D. V., & Bella, D. A. (2005). *The Vineland Adaptive Behavior Scales, second edition.* Circle Pines, MN: AGS Publishing.

Takata, N. (1969). The play history. *American Journal of Occupational Therapy, 23,* 314-318.

Townsend, S., Carey, P., Hollins, N., Helfrich, C., Blondis, M., Hoffman, A., et al. (1999). *A user's manual for Occupational Therapy Psychosocial Assessment of Learning.* Chicago, IL: Model of Human Occupation Clearinghouse.

Townsend, E. A., & Polatajko, H. J. (2007). *Enabling occupation II: Advancing an occupational therapy vision for health, well-being, & justice through occupation.* Ottawa, ON: CAOT Publications.

Trombly, C. (1993). Anticipating the future: Assessment of occupational function. *American Journal of Occupational Therapy, 47*(3), 253-257.

Uniform Data System for Medical Rehabilitation. (2006). *WeeFIM II system clinical guide. Version 6.0.* Amherst, NY: Uniform Data System for Medical Rehabilitation.

Whiteneck, G. G., Harrison-Felix, C. L., Mellick, D. C., Brooks, C. A., Charlifue, S. B., & Gerhart, K. A. (2004). Quantifying environmental factors: A measure of physical, attitudinal, service, productivity, and policy barriers. *Archives of Physical Medicine and Rehabilitation, 85*(8), 1324-1335.

World Health Organization. (WHO). (2001). *International classification of functioning, disability, and health: ICF*. Geneva: WHO.

Young, N. L. (1996). *The Activities Scale for Kids manual*. Toronto, ON: The Hospital for Sick Children.

Ziviani, J., & Rodger, S. (2006). Environmental influences on children's participation. In S. Rodger, & J. Ziviani (Eds.), *Occupational therapy with children: Understanding children's occupations and enabling participation* (pp. 41-66). Oxford, UK: Blackwell.

Chapter 8

Cognitive Orientation for Daily Occupational Performance (CO-OP): A Uniquely Occupation-centred Intervention created for Children

Sylvia Rodger and Helene Polatajko

Learning objectives

The objectives of this chapter are to:

- Provide an overview of Cognitive Orientation to daily Occupational Performance (CO-OP) as an intervention that uses dynamic performance analysis (DPA), global and domain-specific strategies (DSSs) and guided discovery.
- Illustrate how CO-OP meets the characteristics of an occupation-centred approach for children and families, enabling occupational performance and participation, by drawing on its theoretical underpinnings and empirical research.
- Present a short case study regarding the use of CO-OP with a child with Asperger's syndrome (AS) to illustrate its applicability to children with participation issues related to social skills and anger management difficulties.

Introduction

Cognitive Orientation for daily Occupational Performance (CO-OP) (Polatajko & Mandich, 2004; Polatajko, Mandich, Missiuna et al., 2001) is an occupation-centred intervention that enhances children's skill acquisition, enables engagement in relevant occupations and hence promotes participation in the activities of daily life. CO-OP was developed originally for children identified with developmental co-ordination disorder (DCD) (Polatajko, Mandich, Missiuna et al., 2001). Over time it has been used and researched with a variety of populations, both child and adult, including: Asperger's syndrome (AS) (Rodger, Ireland, & Vun, 2008; Rodger, Pham, & Mitchell, 2009; Rodger, Springfield, & Polatajko, 2007), cerebral palsy (Samonte, Solish, Delaney, & Polatajko, 2004), traumatic brain injury (Dawson et al., in press; Dawson, Polatajko, & Cameron, 2007; Dawson, Polatajko, & Levine, 2007; Solish, Samonte, & Polatajko, 2005) and stroke (McEwen, Polatajko, Huijbregts, & Ryan, 2008). It has its origins in learning theory, viewing DCD from a motor learning rather than a neuro-developmental perspective (Polatajko, Mandich, Miller, & Macnab, 2001). It arose from the integration of a verbal, educational, cognitive and occupationally based approach to DCD intervention.

The focus of this chapter will be on the use of CO-OP with children who have a range of occupational performance and participation issues that primarily impact on their ability to 'do' the things they need to, want to or are expected to do.

CO-OP: a brief overview

CO-OP is a client-centred, problem-solving approach that is performance-based in which child (or child and parent) specified goals are addressed from a learning perspective. The primary objective of the CO-OP approach is skill acquisition through strategy use. The approach has seven key features:

- Client-centred goal setting, where the child, in consultation with the parents, is asked to identify specific skills he/she wants to improve upon;
- Cognitive strategies, both global and domain-specific: the former, *goal-plan-do-check*, is a strategy to support problem-solving and the latter supports the acquisition of the particular skill in question in the particular context;
- Session format, which includes collecting data to establish performance levels before and after the intervention, setting session by session goals and homework;
- Dynamic performance analysis (DPA), where the specific performance breakdowns are identified and addressed using the problem-solving structure of goal-plan-do-check;
- Enabling principles, that are designed to support skill acquisition, generalisation and transfer;
- Guided discovery, where the therapist uses a variety of techniques to enable the child to identify solutions to the performance problems the child is experiencing;
- Parent/teacher participation, which ensures that those in the child's world that play a significant role in the transfer and generalisation of

skills and strategies have the ability to support the child and enable success (Polatajko & Mandich, 2004). Accordingly, CO-OP can be considered a uniquely occupation-centred approach.

In this chapter, we will illustrate how CO-OP exemplifies each of the characteristics of occupation-centred interventions proposed in Chapter 2. We will illustrate its theoretical underpinnings, its salient features and the research demonstrating its utility and effectiveness. Table 8.1 provides a summary of the key occupation-centred characteristics of CO-OP. When using the CO-OP approach, children are taught a global problem-solving framework (goal, plan, do and check) and are assisted to discover the specific and individualised cognitive strategies known as domain-specific strategies (DSSs) that are necessary to master their chosen goals (Polatajko & Mandich, 2004). Table 8.2 describes the key features of CO-OP and Figure 8.1 maps these features within the CO-OP protocol.

CO-OP: an occupation-centred intervention

In this section, we will address each of the characteristics of occupation-centred interventions described in Chapter 2 and demonstrate, from a theoretical perspective and an empirical basis, how CO-OP meets each of these characteristics (see Table 8.1 for illustration).

Child- and family-centred orientation

CO-OP is consistent with McLaughlin Gray's (1997) characteristic of occupation-centred interventions, that is, it is child- and family-centred. In so doing, CO-OP intervention targets occupations, performance and participation that are purposeful and meaningful to the child in context. As suggested in Chapter 3, there is a need to acknowledge both the child and the parents (family members) as clients. CO-OP is grounded in client-centredness as espoused by the Canadian Occupational Therapy Association (CAOT) in its guidelines for client-centred practice (Polatajko & Mandich, 2004) and is consistent with the Canadian Model of Client-Centred Enablement (CMCE) (Townsend & Polatajko, 2007). Whilst the focus of CO-OP is primarily on the child's mastery of occupational goals, the crucial role of parents is recognised in terms of their perspectives regarding the child's occupational concerns and strengths, and their role in assisting with strategy generalisation and transfer of strategies and skills learned.

Collaborative partnerships

Occupational therapists using CO-OP aim to create collaborative relationships with clients that engage them by fostering motivation and commitment. Indeed, the very name of the approach is intended to capture the co-operation that

Table 8.1 CO-OP: a uniquely occupation-centred intervention

Characteristics of occupation-centred interventions	Cognitive Orientation to daily Occupational Performance (CO-OP)
Client-centred orientation (child- and/or family-centred)	Child (and parent)-chosen goals used Child is client and focus of intervention Child's perspective and goals are central to the intervention
Based on collaborative partnerships	Collaborative relationships with child and parents are critical to CO-OP and developed from the outset with goal setting
Client-chosen goals	Focus of assessment and intervention is on child's and parent's goals for child
Contextually relevant	Approach relevant to child's occupational performance and participation in relevant environments/life situations Parents/teachers assist to generalise strategies in home/community/school setting
Active engagement of child and parent/s	Child is actively engaged in problem-solving throughout intervention Parents are actively engaged in generalisation and transfer in home/community environments
Individualised intervention	Child-specific strategies and goals are the focus of intervention
Focus on occupational performance and participation – at all stages of OT process	COPM used for goal setting, DPA during assessment, child's occupational performance goals form the basis of intervention
Information gathering focuses on roles, occupations, occupational performance and environment	Focus is on assessing child's occupations and occupational performance and understanding the impact of this on participation
Intervention focuses on roles, occupations, occupational performance and environment	Focus is on child's occupations and occupational performance to enhance participation in valued life roles such as player, student and self-carer
Interventions are 'whole' or 'finite', have a beginning, middle and end	End point of intervention is defined by the child's goal achievement and is clear at outset of intervention
Occupation-centred evaluation of intervention outcomes	Utilises COPM, PQRS and can use GAS as pre/post-intervention measures. These focus on goal achievement and performance quality. Child and parent report on COPM ratings of performance and satisfaction

COPM: Canadian Occupational Performance Measure; PQRS: Performance Quality Rating Scale; DPA: dynamic performance analysis; GAS: Goal Attainment Scaling.

Table 8.2 Summary of key features of CO-OP (Polatajko & Mandich, 2004)

Features of CO-OP	Explanation
Global problem-solving strategy	'Goal-plan-do-check' • *Goal*: What do you want to achieve? • *Plan*: How do you want to get there? What do you need to try/alter/do differently? • *Do*: Have a go and do it! • *Check*: Did the plan work? These steps are referred to continually during therapy, reinforcing to the child where he/she is in the sequence
Domain-specific strategies (DSSs)	Strategies that are specific to the child and the task and are developed by the child and therapist together as they are problem-solving various solutions: • *Supplementing task knowledge*: providing information to the child about the task if this is lacking • *Body position*: relates to shifting of the body, whole or in part, relative to the task • *Attention to the task*: relates to attending to the task or appropriate aspects of the task • *Task specification or modification*: attending to the specifics of the task or modifying aspects of the task to enable performance • *Feeling the movement*: focuses on the movements required for completion of the task • *Verbal Rote Scripts*: guide the child through doing of the task (using a rote pattern of words to guide the motor sequence) • *Verbal mnemonics*: assist the child to imagine a visual picture of part of the task or how it should be done, or an acronym that would help them remember what or how to do the task
Guided discovery	The concept is unique to CO-OP and reflects the process of engagement between the therapist and child which focuses on asking rather than telling, demonstrating rather than doing for the child and assisting the child to find his/her own solution to a problem and experiment with that solution
Generalisation and transfer	Generalisation of task performance to other contexts Transfer of strategies learned to other skills/tasks

is fundamental to the approach (Polatajko & Mandich, 2004). Therapists employ a number of strategies to facilitate such relationships (Mattingly & Fleming, 1994; Turpin, 2004) as described in Chapter 2. When using the CO-OP approach, *choice* is created in terms of identifying the child-chosen goals that become the focus of intervention, determining which goal/s will be addressed during individual sessions and assisting the child to identify

Key features of the CO-OP approach

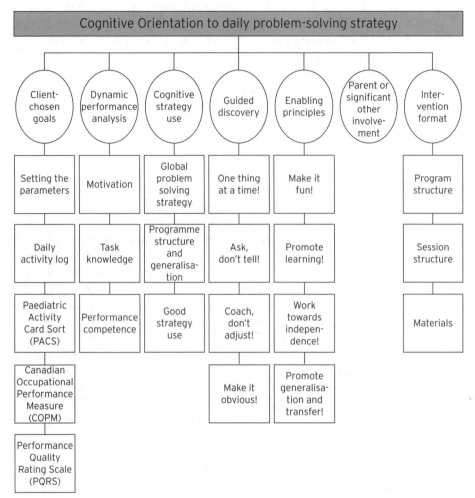

Figure 8.1 Key features of CO-OP. With permission from CAOT Publications ACE

the most useful cognitive strategies to support successful performance. *Individualisation* of treatment will be addressed in a subsequent section. *Structuring success* is pivotal during CO-OP as the therapist uses DPA (Polatajko, Mandich, & Martini, 2000) and decides where to start intervention, given numerous points of performance breakdown. The therapist then facilitates the child to discover what strategies might assist him/her to overcome the breakdowns and gradually master performance. For example, when learning to ride a bike there are many things a child needs to learn, some more critical than others (e.g. checking on the child's knowledge of how the brakes work). *Exchanging stories* may be utilised to share other children's narratives about intervention successes with the child and his parent/s. Sharing stories may also assist with the development of rapport, as often a child feels that he/she is the only one who cannot tie his shoes at 9 years or do her own hair at 11 years. Finally, *joint problem-solving* is pivotal to CO-OP as the therapist and the child work together to solve the mystery of occupational performance. Typically, the therapist and the child experiment with various strategies, evaluating their success and deciding which ones to employ. This empowers the child by acknowledging his/her expertise, analytical skills and decision-making capacity.

Child-chosen goals

CO-OP is also consistent with McLaughlin Gray's (1997) characteristic of occupation-centred intervention being goal-directed. Occupation-centred interventions focus on child- and/or family-chosen goals that emphasise skill acquisition, modification to occupations/tasks and/or environments to enhance the child's performance of meaningful and purposeful occupations. Goal setting and working with child-chosen goals is a key feature of CO-OP (Polatajko & Mandich, 2004). Each child chooses individual goals to accomplish, which increases motivation, transfer of learning (Polatajko, Mandich, Missiuna et al., 2001) and self-efficacy (Mendes & Polatajko, 2004).

When using CO-OP, the Canadian Occupational Performance Measure (COPM) (Law et al., 1998) is used to establish the child's intervention goals. Polatajko and Mandich (2004) also recommended the use of a daily log to facilitate administration of the COPM and discussion about the child's productivity (e.g. school work and chores), play/leisure and self-care occupations. The COPM can be administered to the child alone or to the child in conjunction with the parent. The COPM is also used to enable prioritisation of goals and ensures an emphasis on the child's ratings of performance and satisfaction, prior to and after intervention. Other goal-setting tools such as the Perceived Efficacy and Goal Setting System (PEGS) (Missiuna, Pollock, & Law, 2004) or Paediatric Activity Card Sort (PACS; Mandich, Polatajko, Miller, & Baum, 2004), described in Chapter 6, can be utilised along with the COPM to determine intervention goals.

It is acknowledged that goal prioritisation may require some negotiation between child, parent/s and therapist. This might be resolved by the therapist and child agreeing to work on two of the child's goals (e.g. using a knife and fork to cut meat and playing handball) and one parent's goal (e.g. neater writing). This can be effective as long as the child acknowledges that handwriting is challenging and he/she has some interest and motivation to improve this skill (even just to appease parents or to avoid completing work during recess). One example of these different perspectives is illustrated by the following quote:

> I didn't think that learning to be a goalie was a good goal for therapy. I thought writing was the important thing. Well I have to tell you that he learned to be a good goalie with you, and then he made the school floor hockey team. They went to the championships and won. He is living his dream! (Mandich, Polatajko, & Rodger, 2003, p. 584)

Therapists may also find that goal choice is limited to what can reasonably be addressed given the context and available resources. For example, in a study by Rodger and Brandenburg (2009), Bob, a 9-year-old boy with AS, had a goal to remember his gymnastic routines. Whilst expertise in gymnastics was beyond the therapist's skills and the therapy environment did not contain complex gymnastic equipment, the parent was able to videotape a number of his routines. This enabled the therapist to observe Bob's performance and discuss his performance during sessions. Together they generated plans for each routine. Some floor routines were practiced in the clinic using gym mats, enabling immediate implementation of plans and checking of success, whilst others were written on index cards that were taken to gym sessions. Primarily therapy sessions focused on discussing videotapes of real gym sessions and refining plans. Whilst not as ideal as using *plan, do and check* in situ, videoing performance for later analysis is an option. In this case, the child and therapist collaboratively engaged in analysis of performance breakdown whilst watching the videos. This requires the child to be able to focus on what is happening in real time (i.e. when watching the videotape) and then remembering to use plans prior to embarking on a particular routine at gym at a later time.

Contextual relevance

Contextual relevance refers to an emphasis on the human as an occupational being within his/her environmental context (McLaughlin Gray, 1997). The ultimate objective of occupation-centred interventions is to enhance the child's participation in relevant life occupations. Occupational therapists understand children's roles and occupations, as well as the environments that support or hinder their occupational performance. CO-OP focuses on the child (in particular, the child's performance issues and goals), the occupation (relevant tasks such as handwriting and shoelace tying) and the environment in which the performance is located (facilitating the child's discovery of features of the environment that hinder or support successful task performance and how these can be altered).

The environment is an important consideration throughout CO-OP in terms of its impact on the child's performance and the transfer and generalisation of skills. For example, in the task of bike riding or rollerblading, the therapist might discuss with the child how different surfaces affect performance. Accordingly the therapist might commence in the clinic room on a carpeted floor, then move to a smooth floor, then to a quiet outdoor vacant car park with minimal distractions and a relatively smooth surface, then to a bike track at a quiet time of day and finally at a busy time. Parents have a crucial role in assisting with practising bike riding between sessions and generalisation to home and neighbourhood environments.

Active engagement of children and parent/s

What we have to learn to do, we learn by doing. (Aristotle)

Children's engagement

CO-OP involves active participation by both the child and his/her parents (Polatajko, Mandich, Missiuna et al., 2001). The child is actively engaged in setting the goal and then using a global problem-solving strategy to discover DSSs relevant to his/her task performance throughout CO-OP sessions. One of the therapist's key roles is using process questions that lead the child to discover new and refine existing strategies. The child's active participation is seen in planning the task, 'doing' the task whilst focusing on the execution of newly developed plans, and checking the success of the strategies in achieving the goal. The focus is always on child-chosen goals which are determined at the outset of intervention and attended to during individual sessions.

Investigation of cognitive strategy use during CO-OP intervention with children with DCD (Banks, Rodger, & Polatajko, 2008; Bernie & Rodger, 2004; Rodger & Liu, 2008) and AS (Rodger et al., 2009; Rodger & Vishram, in review) has demonstrated the significant amount of time spent by the child actively discussing the performance plan, identifying possible solutions and trying them out. One study found that four boys with DCD, all engaged in handwriting goals, spent significant amounts of time, across 10 one-hour sessions, talking about the task (58%) (i.e. describing the goal, planning and checking) compared to 31% of time spent practicing the task (doing) and only 1% dual tasking (talking and doing together) (Banks et al., 2008). In this study, across the four boys over the 10 sessions, 28% of total session time was spent checking, 25% doing handwriting and 15% planning or developing strategies. It should be noted that 28% of time was coded 'other' (i.e. activity preparation, set up or off task). These data reinforce the collaborative nature of the CO-OP approach, in which the crux of the intervention involves the therapist and child engaging together in collaborative discussions prior to and after practising or doing the task in question.

Similar findings were revealed for two children with AS with motor-based goals who were both actively engaged for approximately 75% of sessions (Rodger et al., 2009). For these children, between approximately one-third (34%) and half (50%) of the total time coded in CO-OP sessions was spent in the global strategy of 'do', whilst 17% and 17%, respectively, were spent on 'plan' and 24% and 6%, respectively, were spent on 'check'. This illustrates the focus on enhancing occupational performance through developing strategies that support task performance (*plan*), applying and testing these strategies/plans (*do*) and then evaluating the strategies (*check*) (Polatajko, Mandich, Miller et al., 2001). The study also highlighted considerable therapist–child interaction compared to self-guidance or therapist-directed activity during 'plan' and 'check', which further reinforces the collaborative nature of CO-OP and the centrality of the active involvement of the child. During CO-OP, the therapist aims to facilitate rather than dictate the production, refinement and evaluation of the planning process.

Parent involvement

Parents are encouraged to observe as many CO-OP sessions as possible to assist their children in generalising their learning to home, school and community environments and transferring them to other skills. Generalisation requires the practice of the tasks or activities required for goal achievement across different environments (Polatajko & Mandich, 2004). For example, the culture of the classroom encompasses school and class teacher's expectations of handwriting legibility standards and speed, presence of peers, physical set up of desk, blackboard, etc., whilst the home environment where homework is completed comprises different people, expectations regarding completion of written tasks and physical spaces. Both of these environments are different to the clinic environment where typically the occupational therapist and the child engage one-on-one in a child-friendly room with minimal distractions.

Transfer refers to the use of skills, including cognitive strategies, across different tasks/activities (Polatajko & Mandich, 2004). For example, the strategy of utilising a 'helper' and 'doer' hand can be discovered during handwriting: holding down the page with non-dominant hand whilst the dominant hand grasps the pencil and writes; holding the paper steady whilst the dominant hand manipulates the scissors; holding the ruler still whilst drawing a line with a pencil; and holding a cup steady whilst pouring a drink from a jug. Parents are important facilitators of this additional learning but need to be assisted to make this strategy transfer overt to the child during relevant tasks.

Rodger et al. (2007) reported two case studies of siblings with AS. The children's mother kept a detailed diary from the start of the 10–1h weekly intervention sessions for each child and continued for 2 months after intervention ceased. Thematic analysis of the diary entries revealed multiple detailed accounts of the children's spontaneous use of the global problem-solving framework to assist with acquisition of new skills and to overcome organisational and social difficulties, as well as numerous examples of generalisation and transfer. One of the children (Alice, aged 11 years) used her eating and shoelaces plans at Guide camp after five sessions. Her mother reported:

> She was happy to go to Guide camp knowing she can manage cutlery, shoes and hair. She talks about it being good now she can do these things easily and appears keen and confident to go and motivated to get herself organized to go – she even packed her things by herself. (Rodger et al., 2007, p. 13)

She also identified new goals not addressed during sessions, namely getting organised at school and home. She independently transferred the global strategy to this organisational task. Skill transfer was also demonstrated from eating with a knife and fork:

> Alice has attempted new activities and was able to talk about her plans for doing these. She tried eating with chopsticks for the first time (stir fry meat and rice) and persisted for the entire meal. (Rodger et al., 2007, p. 14)

As well as providing evidence for generalisation and transfer, these accounts provide evidence regarding how parents are engaged in CO-OP and how effective their engagement can be in guiding the child's discovery and use of strategies at home.

In some cases, parents have been taught to use CO-OP (Polatajko & Mandich, 2004), suggesting that parents are able (with support) to engage in analysis of performance breakdown and to guide the child's discovery of appropriate strategies. In a Hong Kong study, Donna (2007) demonstrated that parents could be taught how to implement the key features of CO-OP to realise performance gains in their children.

Individualisation of intervention

CO-OP intervention is very child-specific. One challenge, especially for novices, is that it is not possible to *fully* plan a session prior to the child arriving (Copley, Rodger, Hannay, & Graham, in review). The therapist must work in situ to find out how the child's plans succeeded since the last session, and determine the child's current level of performance. DPA occurs throughout the session and plans evolve. These can neither be pre-planned nor session direction but determined entirely at the outset (Copley et al., in review). CO-OP is individualised, iterative and dynamic. Whilst children may have similar goals, the specific points of performance breakdown are unique as are the different strategies and plans the children identify using their own words/images. Based on the child's interests, therapists tailor intervention to capitalise on themes such as cartoons, favourite TV program characters, etc.

In published case studies of CO-OP with children with DCD and AS, the pattern of DSS use across motor-based goals has been found to be distinct for each child, indicating that DSS use was specific to the child and goal being addressed (Banks et al., 2008; Bernie & Rodger, 2004; Rodger et al., 2009; Sangster, Beninger, Polatajko, & Mandich, 2005). Further, Rodger and Liu (2008) investigated changes in cognitive strategy and session time use by children over the course of 10 sessions. Some trends were observed, including the use of the global strategy 'goal' in earlier sessions and shifts in the use of DSSs for particular goals over time. Evolution of DSSs was also noted in that *Verbal Rote Script* always originated from another previously used DSS. Although fluctuations in strategy use between sessions were noted, it was observed that overall there was more stability than change over time for each of the four boys studied. These patterns of strategy and session time use confirm the individualised nature of CO-OP and highlight the unique three-way interaction between the child, task and therapist that is encompassed in this approach (Rodger & Liu, 2008).

Finally, a study specifically related to strategy use during handwriting (Banks et al., 2008) demonstrated that even when all four boys with DCD had a handwriting goal, the nature of the goals (e.g. writing letters or numbers correctly versus writing more neatly or faster) and the strategies used were individual and often unique. Whilst the predominant DSS used by all four boys to improve their handwriting was *task specification/modification*, each boy employed different plans within this DSS. Examples of the individual nature of DSSs used for writing can be found in Table 8.3.

Focus on occupational performance and participation

CO-OP, by definition, is occupation-centred – it focuses on using strategies to acquire the occupational skills that the child identifies as important for day-to-day living.

The following quote is from an interview with a parent whose child with DCD engaged in CO-OP intervention:

There is no doubt about it, that for R, bike riding has been a lifeline, a lifeline into the social community, and a lifeline so far as his self-esteem has

Table 8.3 Cognitive strategies used to master handwriting by four boys with DCD

Handwriting goal	Domain-specific strategy	Examples
To write letters and numbers accurately	Task specification	'Join 3 dots to make a "3"'; 'Start on the left side of the page and work right'; starting letters at the top
	Verbal mnemonic	'"S" looks like a dollar sign'; '"3" looks like a B, check to see if a line makes a B'; '2 looks like a "z"'; 'S looks like a dollar sign'
	Body position	'Helper hand holds the paper still'; '3 goes away from the helper hand'
	Verbal Rote Script	'"Across and down" for 7'; '"g" looks like an "a" with a tail'
	Feel the movement	Tracing letters in the air
	Attention to do	'Look at the "w"'
To write more neatly and faster	Task specification	Writing letters on the lines; leave spaces between words; use a sharp pencil; use same size letters; write on the lines
	Feel the movement	'We need to make the pencil lighter'; pressure on the pencil
	Body position	Paying attention to posture; 'Hold the paper still with your other hand'
	Verbal mnemonic	'k looks like an r with a longer neck'
	Verbal Rote Script	'Along, down and cross for 4'

Adapted from Banks et al. (2008, p. 105) (reproduced with permission from The American Occupational Therapy Foundation).

definitely grown. It sort of was a rite of passage, a real marker for him. It has built his confidence to do other things and to keep trying. (Mandich et al., 2003, p. 588)

It highlights the importance of being able to 'do' in enhancing children's self-esteem and sense of belonging within their peer group. The boy's father uses the metaphor that learning to ride a bike (acquiring a motor skill) was a 'life line' for his son, opening up opportunities for participation with peers in his community (i.e. optimising his occupational role of player and social role of friend). Not only was this the case for bike riding, but also the resulting self-efficacy provided the confidence to master other activities not previously attempted and therefore broadened participation opportunities. Clearly, CO-OP focuses on the International Classification of Functioning, Disability and Health (ICF) (WHO, 2001) levels of activities (or in occupational therapy context, occupations and occupational performance) and participation.

Information gathering about roles, occupations, performance and environments

Approaches that are occupation-centred are characterised by an information gathering process that:

(1) Focuses on the child's occupational and social roles, occupations and the environmental context for performance;
(2) Emphasises occupational performance and participation;
(3) Promotes assessment that identifies aspects of the child, occupation and environment that both facilitate and impede performance.

When interviewing the parent/s and child using the COPM (Law et al., 1998), the therapist focuses on the child's roles and relevant occupations, the environments where these take place, the child's strengths and the child's and parent's concerns.

Subsequent assessment that is specific to the goals set (e.g. writing and getting organised for school) focuses on the specifics of the performance and the performance breakdown, that is, when and where a child encounters difficulty (e.g. knows the shape of some of the letters but does not know the shape of others; starts writing with letters on the line, but drifts with each successive letter and does not drop letters with lower loops below the line) using DPA (Polatajko et al., 2000). There is no need to undertake assessment of performance components of writing such as hand use, tone, visual motor integration, etc., that are characteristic of a bottom-up approach.

Intervention is occupation-focused, 'whole' or 'finite'

The evidence that CO-OP is occupation-centred draws from its focus on child-identified goals related to children's roles, occupations and performance as previously discussed. McLaughlin Gray (1997) also described occupation-centred interventions being 'whole (or finite) or as having a beginning, middle and end'. CO-OP has a suggested individual session outline as well as a protocol for 10 intervention sessions (as used in CO-OP research). The protocol includes pre-intervention goal setting, followed by sessions focusing initially on teaching the global strategy and then applying this to child-chosen goals over remaining sessions. These sessions entail analysing performance breakdown, developing strategies to enhance performance, trialling these strategies and evaluating their success (Polatajko & Mandich, 2004). Typically, individual sessions have a beginning (connecting with the child and parent and reviewing use of plans/strategies during the week, and their success or otherwise), a middle (working on specific goals using the global strategy and applying DSSs) and an end (summarising the new plans for each goal, documenting these in a note book or on PowerPoint ® and considering opportunities during the coming week for generalisation and transfer with the child and parent/s). Figure 8.2 shows some plans developed by a child with AS for cutlery use/eating.

Occupation-centred evaluation of intervention outcomes

In occupation-centred evaluation of intervention, the focus is on the use of outcome measures that consider occupational performance, roles and participation as well as the child's and family's satisfaction with the intervention process and outcomes. A key aspect of CO-OP is that it is evidenced-based, starting and ending with the administration of the COPM and the Performance Quality Rating Scale (PQRS) – both direct measures of occupational performance, the former a client self-report and the latter a therapist evaluation of quality of the child's goal performance. Examples of this can be seen in research studies such as those by Miller, Missiuna, Macnab, Malloy-Miller, and Polatajko (2001) and Polatajko, Mandich, Miller et al. (2001), demonstrating improvement in the performance of 7-12-year-old children with DCD; Ward and Rodger (2004) and Taylor, Fayed, and Mandich (2007) in younger children with DCD (5-7 years); Rodger and Brandenburg (2009) and Rodger et al. (2008, 2009) in children with AS; and Samonte et al. (2004) in children with cerebral palsy (CP) and acquired brain injury (ABI). These studies have used the

Eating

- Use a plate
- Put my plate in front of me
- Have my chair in front of my plate
- Put my cup at the other side of my plate and to the side so I don't knock it
- Use my knife by sawing back and forwards
- Stick out pointer finger along the blade of the knife
- Hold the carrot firmly.

Figure 8.2 Plans for using cutlery (11-year-old girl with AS)

COPM (Law et al., 1998) to measure pre- and post-intervention task/goal performance and satisfaction from the perspective of either the child, parent or both and observational evaluation of the performance.

Studies using post-intervention parent interviews (e.g. Mandich et al., 2003; Rodger & Mandich, 2005) and parent diaries (Rodger et al., 2007) provide evidence that CO-OP leads to enhanced participation for their children in various contexts. These have also attested to parents' satisfaction with the process of CO-OP, as well as the outcomes of the intervention. Other measures described in Chapter 3 may provide information for occupational therapists about how family-centred parents have found the therapist and the intervention. It is important that clinicians using CO-OP consider the measures they use to evaluate outcomes to ensure that these focus on occupations and participation.

Anger management using CO-OP with a child with Asperger's syndrome

AS is a pervasive developmental disorder (PDD) characterised by:

(1) severe and sustained impairment in social interaction
(2) restricted, repetitive patterns of behaviour, interests and activities
(3) impaired social, occupational or other important areas of functioning
(4) no clinically significant delays or deviance in language acquisition, although more subtle aspects of social communication may be affected
(5) no clinically significant delays in cognitive development during the first 3 years of life (American Psychiatric Association (APA), 2000)

The presence of motor clumsiness and difficulties with organisational skills, whilst not diagnostically significant, are also common (Attwood, 1998). These children commonly lack insight into accepted social protocols, and have difficulties in interpreting and understanding social cues and the rules of social behaviour (Attwood, 1998; Barnhill, 2001; Myles & Simpson, 2001). They have a limited ability to engage in reciprocal communication and often lack micro-level (i.e. tone of voice, volume and rate; facial expression, posture, use of gestures and social distance) and macro-level (i.e. starting conversations and greeting people) social skills (Barnhill, 2001; Woodyatt & Rodger, 2006).

Lack of social and emotional reciprocity and impaired theory of mind are thought to contribute to difficulties with social relationship formation and maintenance (Attwood, 1998; Barnhill, Cook, Tebbenkamp, & Myles, 2002; Gutstein & Whitney, 2002; Myles & Simpson, 2001).

Children with AS have been found to utilise both global and DSSs effectively to solve not only motor-based (Rodger & Brandenburg, 2009; Rodger et al., 2009), but also social and organisational occupational performance problems (Rodger et al., 2008). Some of the goals addressed in these studies included organisational tasks such as getting ready for school or extracurricular activities, completing homework and getting to sleep at night, and social issues such as managing anger. We have identified that children with AS utilise additional strategies to those identified initially by Mandich, Polatajko, Missiuna, and Miller (2001). These additional strategies (Rodger et al., 2008) have been classified as:

(1) *transitional supports* that help children manage change or transition from one activity/context to the next
(2) *motivational supports* to assist with motivation to do including the use of rewards
(3) *affective supports* that help children manage overwhelming emotions
(4) *understanding the context*

These are defined and explained with examples in Table 8.4. The following case study illustrates the use of some of these strategies.

Case study: Thomas

Thomas was aged 12 years and in Year 7 when he was referred to occupational therapy. He lived with his mother, father and 10-year-old brother. He was diagnosed with AS when he was 5 years old. He had difficulties in asserting himself in an acceptable manner, coping with criticism/teasing and dealing with peer aggression. One of his goals was managing playground anger (Rodger et al., 2008). He was a keen soccer player and athlete and one of the best players in the team. However, he had frequent altercations with the coach during practice sessions and referee during matches. Leading up to the school sports day, he exhibited fiercely competitive behaviour towards a peer who was his rival at track and field. The pair frequently exchanged jibes and taunts regarding who would win the upcoming heat or selection for competition, often resulting in a physical scuffle.

Over a number of weeks, he worked with his therapist to develop anger management strategies to help him deal with concrete situations he described on the playground or sports field. First, the therapist needed to *understand the context*, so she would ask him to describe any tricky playground or sporting situations he encountered during the week, and to verify the situation with his mother so that she could understand all sides of the story. One of Thomas's difficulties was not being able to see the other's perspective. Using drawings and Power Point® to depict the situations he had regularly to deal with, Thomas and the therapist developed a series of plans/strategies using a modified approach to Social Stories® (Gray & White, 2002).

Typically social stories are written by an adult to clearly and directly inform the child with AS what he/she must do and how he/she needs to respond in a given situation. However, during CO-OP the therapist facilitated Thomas to author his own story, based on the situations he encountered each week and the strategies he planned and solutions he discovered. An anger thermometer was used to help him to describe his anger (a concrete image) based on his description of angry feelings 'like you are boiling hot'. The therapist introduced the thermometer as a way of measuring anger and how hot it was getting. Thomas understood and was interested in this image. Weekly angry situations were mapped on one side of the thermometer and his responses and strategies to manage these on the other.

Some of his anger story is illustrated in the sequences in Figure 8.3 and the DSSs used are described and classified in Table 8.4. The story, some of which is illustrated using Power Point® and Thomas's own words, was written over about 6 weeks. Each new page depicted a new situation encountered and the corresponding new plans devised, or checking activities completed during each session to see how the previously developed plans were working.

Conclusion

This chapter has described CO-OP as an occupation-centred intervention that meets all of the characteristics of occupation-centred approaches introduced in Chapter 2. In so doing, we have drawn from research undertaken by ourselves and by others using CO-OP to provide evidence of the claims we have made about its utility and to provide data to demonstrate how it meets these characteristics. Specifically, a case study was provided to illustrate the use of CO-OP with children with AS, who often struggle with anger management in social situations. A number of additional DSSs are introduced based on research that has investigated strategy use during CO-OP by children with different conditions and occupational performance problems. Whilst CO-OP is a relatively new intervention approach, a considerable amount of research is being amassed about its use, the children with whom it is effective, how change is affected, the specifics of strategy used by children with various conditions and performance difficulties, and ultimately its efficacy. Whilst to date many of these studies have utilised case studies and small samples, they have explored in detail the key features of CO-OP and demonstrated positive outcomes from the perspectives of both children and their parents. There is still much research to be conducted, however, that which has been completed to date continues to provide evidence of its utility with children and their families.

One of my goals is:

TO AVOID ANGRY SITUATIONS

This is a picture of Andrew giving the finger to me. This makes me feel angry.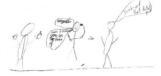

My plans to avoid angry situations are:

- Avoid Andrew in the playground. Stay away from kids who get me in trouble.

- Play with Callum, Billy and Luke. They help keep me out of trouble.

Sometimes I get into angry situations before I realise it!

- When I am getting angry, I need to recognise what is happening.

- I need to notice what I am feeling and what my body is telling me.

- When I get a little bit angry I get sweaty palms and tense muscles and feel like yelling, shouting and swearing

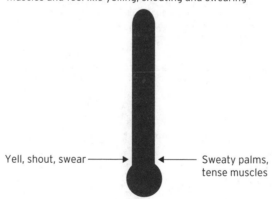

Yell, shout, swear ⟶   ⟵ Sweaty palms, tense muscles

When I get a little bit angry.

- I can turn around and walk away.
- I can think about something else like football.
- I can think about playing my computer. That makes me feel calm.

Figure 8.3 Part of Thomas's story illustrating his strategies for managing anger

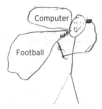

- Last week when I played soccer I got angry and yelled at my coach, because he told me to "Stop". I obeyed him but I missed saving the goal.

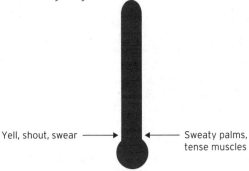

When I feel angry with my coach and feel like yelling and swearing at him

- I can "shut up and take it"
- I can calm down:
  - I can kick the ball (but not at somebody) or ground
  - I can think about something that helps me calm down
    - Think about saving a goal
    - Think about playing computer
    - Think about lying under palm tree in Hawaii

- At presentation at the end of the sport's day, I felt really angry with Andrew.

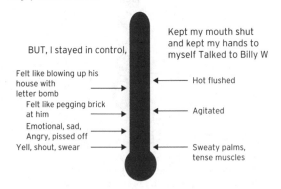

Figure 8.3   (Continued)

Table 8.4 Additional DSSs used by children with AS for social and organisational goals

Name of domain-specific strategy (DSS)	Explanation	Examples
Transitional supports	Strategies to help manage change or transition from one activity/context to the next	Choose a toy from box near door to take in the car to go out
Motivational supports	Strategies to assist with motivation to do	Reward charts and stickers, reward such as apastry at the end of the week if five stickers for getting dressed on time each morning
Affective strategies	Strategies that help children manage overwhelming emotions	
Affective avoid	Strategies to help the child remove himself/herself from the emotionally charged situations/conflict/anger to prevent uncontrolled emotional outburst	Stay away from kids who get me angry and play with kids who keep me out of trouble Turn around and walk away
Affective distract	Strategies used by the child to help him calm down in emotionally charged situations/conflict/anger	Think about something to calm down: lying under a palm tree, playing computer games, think about cool ice
Affective physical	Strategies to manage/redirect physical intensity of emotions that enable the child to discharge physical energy	Recognise when I am feeling angry and what my body is telling me such as sweaty palms, tense muscles and feel like yelling. Then use physical activity such as kicking soccer ball, hitting punching bag, going outside for a run
Understanding the context	Strategy used by the therapist to enhance the therapist's understanding of the social/environmental context of relevance to the goal. Often seen in relation to social issues	Discussions about social happenings at school and in the playground during the week

Adapted from Rodger et al. (2008). Reproduced with permission from The British Association of Occupational Therapists and College of Occupational Therapists

References

American Psychiatric Association (APA). (2000). *Diagnostic and statistical manual of mental disorders (DSM-IV-TR)* (4th ed.). Washington, DC: Author.

Attwood, T. (1998). *Asperger's syndrome: A guide for parents and professionals.* London, UK: Jessica Kingsley Publishers Ltd.

Banks, R., Rodger, S., & Polatajko, H. (2008). Mastering handwriting: How children with DCD succeed with CO-OP. *Occupational Therapy Journal of Research: Occupation, Participation and Health, 28*(3), 100-109.

Barnhill, G. (2001). What is Asperger syndrome? *Intervention in School and Clinic, 36*(5), 259-265.

Barnhill, G., Cook, K., Tebbenkamp, K., & Myles, B. (2002). The effectiveness of social skills intervention targeting nonverbal communication for adolescents with Asperger syndrome and related pervasive developmental delays. *Focus on Autism and Other Developmental Disabilities, 17*(2), 112-127.

Bernie, C., & Rodger, S. (2004). Cognitive strategy use in school-aged children with developmental coordination disorder. *Physical & Occupational Therapy in Pediatrics, 24*(4), 23-45.

Copley, J., Rodger, S., Hannay, V., & Graham, F. (in press). Students' experiences in learning top down approaches to working with children. Canadian Occupational Therapy Journal.

Dawson, D. R., Gaya, A., Hunt, A., et al. (2009). Using the Cognitive Orientation to Occupational Performance with adults with traumatic brain injury. *Canadian Journal of Occupational Therapy, 76*(2), 115-127.

Dawson, D., Polatajko, H., & Cameron, D. (2007). A contextualized, meta-cognitive rehabilitation approach for enhancing participation in adults and children with acquired brain injury. Course presented at the *2007 Joint Education Conference of the American Congress of Rehabilitation Medicine and American Society of Neurorehabilitation*, Washington, DC, October 5.

Dawson, D., Polatajko, H., & Levine, B. (2007). Naturalistic rehabilitation for executive dysfunction. *Journal of the International Neuropsychological Society, 13*(1, Suppl. 1), 120. Retrieved 5 June 2009 from http://journals.cambridge.org/download.php?file=%2FINS%2FINS13_S1%2FS1355617707079969a.pdf&code=e43bf4363c29360379829c68c457666d.

Donna, Y. K. (2007). The application of cognitive orientation to daily occupational performance (CO-OP) in children with developmental coordination disorder (DCD) in Hong Kong: A pilot study. *Hong Kong Journal of Occupational Therapy, 17*(2), 39-44.

Gray, C., & White, A. (2002). *My social stories book.* London, UK: Jessica Kingsley Publishers Ltd.

Gutstein, E., & Whitney, T. (2002). Asperger syndrome and the development of social competence. *Focus on Autism and Other Developmental Disabilities, 17*(3), 161-183.

Law, M., Baptiste, S., Carswell, A., McColl, M., Polatajko, H., & Pollock, N. (1998). *Canadian Occupational Performance Measure manual* (3rd ed.). Ottawa, ON: CAOT Publications ACE.

Mandich, A., Polatajko, H., Miller, L., & Baum, C. (2004). *The Paediatric Activity Card Sort (PACS).* Ottawa, ON: Canadian Association of Occupational Therapists.

Mandich, A. D., Polatajko, H. J., Missiuna, C., & Miller, L. T. (2001). Cognitive strategies and motor performance in children with developmental coordination disorder. *Physical & Occupational Therapy in Pediatrics, 20*(2/3), 125-143.

Mandich, A. D., Polatajko, H. J., & Rodger, S. (2003). Rites of passage: Understanding participation of children with developmental coordination disorder. *Human Movement Science, 22*(4-5), 583-595.

Mattingly, C., & Fleming, M. (1994). *Clinical reasoning: Forms of inquiry in a therapeutic practice.* Philadelphia, PA: F.A. Davis.

McEwen, S. E., Polatajko, H. J., Huijbregts, M. P., & Ryan, J. D. (2008). Exploring the effectiveness of a cognitive-based treatment approach to improve motor skill performance in chronic stroke: Results of 3 single case experiments. *Archives Physical Medicine & Rehabilitation, 89*(10), e36.

McLaughlin Gray, J. (1997). Application of the phenomenological method to the concept of occupation. *Journal of Occupational Science, 4*(1), 5-17.

Mendes, J., & Polatajko, H. (2004). Shifting self-efficacy in children: The impact of the Cognitive Orientation to daily Occupational Performance approach. Student paper presented at the *Canadian Association of Occupational Therapists Conference*, Charlottetown, P.E.I., June 25.

Miller, L. T., Missiuna, C. A., Macnab, J. J., Malloy-Miller, T., & Polatajko, H. J. (2001). Clinical description of children with developmental coordination disorder. *Canadian Journal of Occupational Therapy, 68*(1), 5-15.

Missiuna, C., Pollock, N., & Law, M. (2004). *PEGS. The Perceived Efficacy and Goal Setting system.* San Antonio, TX: PsychCorp.

Myles, B., & Simpson, R. (2001). Understanding the hidden curriculum: An essential social skill for children and youth with Asperger syndrome. *Intervention in School and Clinic, 36*(5), 279-286.

Polatajko, H. J., & Mandich, A. D. (2004). *Enabling occupation in children: The Cognitive Orientation to daily Occupational Performance (CO-OP) approach.* Ottawa, ON: CAOT Publications ACE.

Polatajko, H. J., Mandich, A. D., & Martini, R. (2000). Dynamic performance analysis: A framework for understanding occupational performance. *American Journal of Occupational Therapy, 54*(1), 65-72.

Polatajko, H. J., Mandich, A. D., Miller, L. T., & Macnab, J. J. (2001). Cognitive Orientation to daily Occupational Performance (CO-OP): Part II - The evidence. *Physical & Occupational Therapy in Pediatrics, 20*(2/3), 83-106.

Polatajko, H. J., Mandich, A. D., Missiuna, C., Miller, L. T., Macnab, J. J., Malloy-Miller, T., et al. (2001). Cognitive Orientation to daily Occupational Performance (CO-OP): Part III - The protocol in brief. *Physical and Occupational Therapy in Pediatrics, 20*(2/3), 107-123.

Rodger, S., & Brandenburg, J. (2009). Cognitive Orientation to (daily) Occupational Performance (CO-OP) with children with Asperger's syndrome who have motor based occupational performance goals. *Australian Occupational Therapy Journal, 56*(1), 41-50.

Rodger, S., Ireland, S., & Vun, M. (2008). Can Cognitive Orientation to daily Occupational Performance (CO-OP) help children with Asperger syndrome master social and organisational goals? *British Journal of Occupational Therapy, 71*(1), 23-32.

Rodger, S., & Liu, S. (2008). Cognitive Orientation to daily Occupational Performance (CO-OP): Changes in strategy and session time use over the course of intervention. *OTJR: Occupation, participation and health, 28*(4), 168-179.

Rodger, S., & Mandich, A. (2005). Getting the run around: Accessing services for children with developmental coordination disorder. *Child: Care, Health and Development, 31*(4), 449-457.

Rodger, S., Pham, C., & Mitchell, S. (2009). Cognitive strategy use by children with Asperger's syndrome during intervention for motor-based goals. *Australian Occupational Therapy Journal, 56*, 103–111.

Rodger, S., Springfield, E., & Polatajko, H. J. (2007). Cognitive Orientation for daily Occupational Performance approach for children with Asperger's syndrome: A case report. *Physical & Occupational Therapy in Pediatrics, 27*(4), 7–22.

Rodger, S., & Vishram, A. (in press). Mastering social and organisational goals: Strategy use by children with autism spectrum disorder during Cognitive Orientation to daily Occupational Performance (CO-OP). *Physical and Occupational Therapy in Pediatrics*.

Samonte, S., Solish, L., Delaney, L., & Polatajko, H. (2004). Cognitive Orientation to daily Occupational Performance: Beyond developmental coordination disorder. Student paper presented at the *Canadian Association of Occupational Therapists Conference*, Charlottetown, P.E.I., June 25.

Sangster, C. A., Beninger, C., Polatajko, H. J., & Mandich, A. (2005). Cognitive strategy generation in children with developmental coordination disorder. *Canadian Journal of Occupational Therapy, 72*(2), 67–77.

Solish, L., Samonte, S., & Polatajko, H. (2005). Cognitive Orientation to daily Occupational Performance (CO-OP): A six month follow-up. Poster presentation at the *Canadian Association of Occupational Therapists Conference*, Vancouver, BC, May 26.

Taylor, S., Fayed, N., & Mandich, A. (2007). CO-OP intervention for young children with developmental coordination disorder. *OTJR: Occupation, Participation & Health, 27*(4), 124–130.

Townsend, E., & Polatajko, H. (2007). *Enabling occupation II: Advancing an occupational therapy vision for health, well-being & justice through occupation.* Ottawa, ON: Canadian Association of Occupational Therapists.

Turpin, M. (2004). *Clinical reasoning and reflective practice: Postgraduate practicums.* Brisbane, Qld: Division of Occupational Therapy, University of Queensland.

Ward, A., & Rodger, S. (2004). The application of Cognitive Orientation to daily Occupational Performance (CO-OP) with children 5–7 years with developmental coordination disorder. *British Journal of Occupational Therapy, 67*(6), 256–264.

Woodyatt, G., & Rodger, S. (2006). Communication and social skills for occupational engagement. In S. Rodger, & J. Ziviani (Eds.), *Occupational therapy with children: Understanding children's occupations and enabling participation* (pp. 158–176). Oxford, UK: Blackwell.

World Health Organisation (WHO). (2001). *International Classification of Functioning, Disability and Health (ICF)*. Geneva, Switzerland: WHO.

Chapter 9

Perceive, Recall, Plan and Perform (PRPP): Occupation-centred Task Analysis and Intervention System

Christine Chapparo

Learning objectives

The purpose of this chapter is to:

- Describe the Perceive, Recall, Plan and Perform (PRPP) System of Task Analysis (Chapparo & Ranka, 1997b) and Intervention (Chapparo & Ranka, 2007).
- Describe aspects of information processing theory and apply these to occupational performance.
- Illustrate the use of the PRPP System of Task Analysis and Intervention through a case example of a young child, David, with autism spectrum disorder (ASD).

Introduction

Occupational performance is based on the interaction between people and their environments, with effective performance thought to be supported by a number of cognitive capacities including the ability to process salient information for use (Chapparo & Ranka, 1997a). Of particular relevance to this chapter is the child's ability to apply cognitive information processing strategies during everyday task performance. These include attending, perceiving, recognising, remembering, judging, learning and problem-solving. The ability to apply cognitive strategies to sensing, thinking and monitoring also contributes to self-regulation of emotions, mood, affect and appropriate behaviour during task performance (Chapparo & Ranka, 1997a; Kielhofner, 2004; Nott, Chapparo, & Heard, 2008).

The following three assumptions underlie use of the Perceive, Recall, Plan and Perform (PRPP) system. First, the way information is processed and used during task performance is determined by the processing capacity of the child, the processing demands of the task that is being performed and the processing demands of the context of performance. Second, the application of some information processing strategies can be behaviourally observed during everyday tasks. Third, application of information processing strategies can be taught within the context of task instruction to improve performance.

Information processing and occupational performance

Information processing is one explanatory model of cognitive behaviour that has been used to guide educational programming for children with learning disabilities (Lerner, 2000; Singer-Harris, Weiler, Bellinger, & Waber, 2001; Swanson, 2001), and as a basis for explaining disorders in motor learning (Schmidt & Wrisberg, 2000). Using principles from information processing theory, occupational therapists can structure their observations of how children do everyday tasks, and plan interventions to enhance the child's *capacity to* both *learn* and *perform everyday occupations*. Information processing is an ecological, inclusive model of cognition that can be used to explain errors that may be made by all children including those with processing disabilities.

Information processing is conceptualised as a self-organised cycle. Children gather information from people, things and events in their environment. They organise this information in their minds, and code it in ways that keep it usable and easily understood. They match the information with what they have learned before, noticing similarities and differences, and store the information for future use. Once this process is complete, children behave in ways that suggest that learning has taken place. They develop a large repertoire of automatic thinking skills, making performance quick and easy. These automatic skills are *used strategically* to solve problems and contribute to new learning, allowing children to become 'independent learners of occupational performance'.

Models of information processing such as the one illustrated in Figure 9.1 (white boxes and associated arrows) trace the staged flow of information from initial reception, processing and response to it (Bohannon & Bonvillian, 2005). The human brain or information processor takes in information (sensation), stores and re-locates it (memory or recall), organises the information by means of various strategies for problem-solving and decision making (planning) and generates responses to the information (planning and output monitoring). This processing system is controlled by an executive system, which is generally considered to have two main functions: *awareness* of the skills, strategies and resources needed to perform each task; and *self-regulatory strategies* to monitor thinking processes, and engage in corrective strategies when processing is not going smoothly (Huitt, 2003). Central to applying the theory to occupational performance is that successful occupational

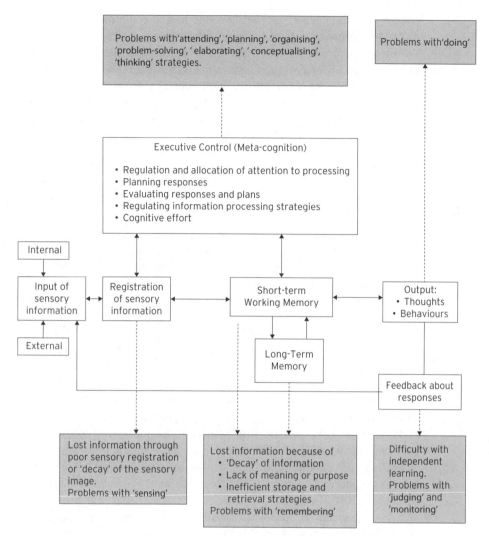

Figure 9.1 A model of information processing and associated difficulties with strategy application

performance requires deliberate information processing, and that disordered performance emerges when there are persistent processing errors at any point in this process. Examples of such difficulties are found in the grey boxes in Figure 9.1.

The Perceive, Recall, Plan and Perceive (PRPP) System of Task Analysis and Intervention

The flow of information processing during occupational performance is determined largely by the processing demands of *the task*, the performance *context* and the processing *capacity* of the person doing the task. At times, all children experience temporary difficulty in processing information from the environment and learning from it as a result of stress, illness, environmental conditions or being required to undertake a task that is too difficult. However, while most recover from these events, some children experience a persistent processing disorder, resulting in a long-term impact on occupational performance. In this part of the chapter, the various stages of information processing and how this information can be applied to occupational therapy observation and intervention using the PRPP System of Task Analysis and Intervention will be explored.

PRPP assessment

Each task undertaken by a child at home or school demands particular information to be chosen, constructed, processed, stored, recalled, organised and used for a particular purpose. Children have their own particular way of doing everyday activities. Increasingly, we are beginning to understand the limitations of traditional deficit-specific approaches to assessment and intervention (Chapparo & Ranka, 1997b; Fisher, 1992; Larkin & Parker, 2002; Losardo & Notari-Syverson, 2001). While test scores in one information processing domain alone (such as a child's visual perception scores) give us information about a specific set of abilities, there is little evidence to suggest that test results in a single domain correlate with overall function in context. There has been a shift towards incorporating a more ecological approach to assessment (Cermak & Larkin, 2002; Dunn, 2000; Law, Baum, & Dunn, 2001; Puderbaugh & Fisher, 1992). With respect to cognitive function, observational measures of the way children *use cognitive information strategically* in everyday performance is becoming a target of contemporary assessment practices (Chapparo & Ranka, 1997b; Miller, Missiuna, MacNab, Malloy-Miller, & Polatajko, 2001).

The PRPP System of Task Analysis is conducted in two stages. Stage One is an overall measure of mastery for specific and relevant occupations. Using a standard *behavioural* task analysis, relevant tasks that are the targets of assessment are broken down into steps and errors in performance recorded (Kirwan & Ainsworth, 1992). A mastery score can be derived by calculating the number of 'error-free' steps within the total number of task steps, and then converting that fraction to a percentage score. Stage Two focuses on information processing strategies required for performance by using a *cognitive* task analysis. Cognitive task analysis is a family of assessment methods that describe the cognitive processes that underlie performance of tasks and the cognitive strategies used to respond adeptly to complex situations (Militello & Hutton, 1998; Schraagen, Chipman, & Shalin, 2000). This chapter focuses on the use of Stage Two of the PRPP assessment.

The PRPP conceptual model (Figure 9.2) (Chapparo & Ranka, 2005) is centred on four processing quadrants with multidirectional arrows that mirror the

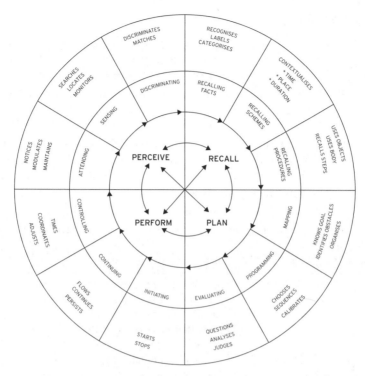

Figure 9.2 The Perceive, Recall, Plan, and Perform System of Task Analysis (Chapparo & Ranka, 2005)

multistaged flow of information in theoretical models of information process-ing in Figure 9.1. These quadrants include attention and sensory perception (Perceive), memory (Recall), response planning and evaluation (Plan) and performance monitoring (Perform).

The four central quadrants are further divided into 12 subcategories as found in the middle ring of Figure 9.2. Key descriptive words used to name and frame information processing strategies that are observable during task performance are termed 'descriptors'. These form the outer layer of the system (see Figure 9.2). The assessment format yields either a descriptive or a quantitative processing score based on the therapist's judgement about how effectively the child is observed to demonstrate application of each of the 'descriptor' strategies during task performance.

An underlying assumption of the assessment system is that a person's capacity to process the cognitive demands inherent in everyday tasks can be observed, identified and used to determine the need for occupational therapy intervention (Chapparo & Ranka, 1997b; Chrenka, Hutton, Klinger, & Aptima, 2001). The purpose of the assessment is to identify difficulties in application of specific information processing strategies during task performance and to provide a focus for intervention (Fry & O'Brien, 2002; Nott & Chapparo, 2008; Nott et al., 2008).

PRPP intervention

The PRPP intervention is a task-oriented information processing approach that simultaneously focuses on task and strategy training within the context of everyday performance (Chapparo & Ranka, 2007; Nott et al., 2008). It is an extension of the 'Stop Think Do' programme developed for use with children and adolescents with intellectual disability (Beck & Horne, 1992), self-harm tendencies, and impulsivity and anger management issues (Murphy & Cooke, 1999). Table 9.1 defines the core intervention principles in the PRPP System of Intervention.

Children learn to apply a sequence of processing strategies to 'Stop/Attend, Sense, Think, Do', that is, gain the required level of arousal/attention for the task (*Stop/Attend*), perceive sensory information relevant to the task (*Sense*),

Table 9.1 Core principles of intervention of the PRPP System of Intervention

Principles	Definition
Intervention goal is task mastery	• Expected outcome is improved functional performance in everyday tasks required by the child's occupational roles and context • Intervention success is therefore measured by increased functional performance
Application of evidence-based principles for systematic instruction	• Goal of intervention is clear to child/parent/teacher • Least to most prompt hierarchy is used • Multiple opportunities for practice of the task and target cognitive strategies are offered and performance errors are prevented • Learning occurs across natural contexts and tasks to promote generalisation • Feedback is specific to task mastery and the cognitive strategy that is the target of intervention
Target descriptors (cognitive strategies) are behaviourally defined and measurable	• Descriptors required for task performance are identified using the PRPP System of Task Analysis (outer ring in Figure 9.2) and their effectiveness measured before and throughout intervention
'Chunking' of descriptors across all PRPP quadrants is planned	• Starting with 'Stops' to correct errors, one or two descriptors only are targeted from each processing quadrant for 'Attend/Sense' (Perceive quadrant), 'Think' (Recall and Plan quadrants) and 'Do' (Perform quadrant) • Training in single descriptors is not used • A line of processing required for the task mirrors the direction of arrows in the centre of the PRPP System (Figure 9.2)
Focus of intervention is on application of cognitive strategies (descriptors) to real-world performance	• The descriptor behaviours form the central verbal, physical or visual prompts given during performance and are modelled by the therapist if required • The child is taught to self-instruct in the strategies if possible

engage in recall (*Think to remember*) or planning strategies to develop a plan of action (*Think to problem-solve*), and then implement the plan (*Do/monitor*). Children learn to apply these strategies to their task performance by initially observing and modelling the therapist, parent or teacher. The therapist's participation in the task performance fades as the child internalises the strategies and applies them across a range of tasks and settings. The prompts of 'Stop, Attend, Sense, Think, Do' (given via verbal, visual, gestural and/or physical modes) are initially used as content-free 'meta-prompts' to alert children to process information required for task performance. Content-free prompts have been shown to improve executive dysfunction by enhancing monitoring of current and future goals in performance, as well as the strategies necessary to achieve them (Fish et al., 2007). These global prompts are followed up with more specific content-based behavioural prompts selected by the therapist, based on findings from the assessment component of the system. One or two descriptor strategies from each processing quadrant for 'Stop, Attend, Sense, Think, Do' are selected by the therapist to prompt a sequence of information processing. For example, Table 9.2 illustrates the type of prompts that could be given by a mother as she prompts her child to process information required for buttoning his shirt.

Using the PRPP System of Task Analysis and Intervention: David

Before observing children, therapists should have a clear understanding of the type and level of processing required to perform the particular tasks involved. The goal of observation is to determine whether children are able to process information required by a particular task in a particular context, rather than in comparison to other children. In other words, successful observation is referenced to particular *criteria* that are determined by the task and the

Table 9.2 'Stop/attend, sense, think, do' verbal prompting example using 'chunks' of PRPP descriptors

Strategy	Prompt (verbal)	Target quadrant	Target descriptor
Stop/attend	'Stop, David. Look at my hands'	Perform/Perceive	*Stops/modulates (re-focus)*
Sense	'Use your fingers to find the button and the button hole'	Perceive	*Searches Locates*
Think	'Think how you did your buttons yesterday' Ask yourself 'does this look/feel right? How should I push the button through the hole?'	Recall Plan	*Uses body Recalls steps Analyses*
Do	'Keep going until the buttons are all done'	Perform	*Continues*

task context, and may be different for each child. This approach differs from a norm-referenced model of assessment that specifies one general standard of performance against which all children's capacities are measured.

Three questions guide therapists' observations of ability in information processing:

- What type of processing does this task demand?
- What type of processing does the performance context demand?
- Is there evidence that the child is processing to the level needed?

David's story is used throughout this chapter to illustrate how observations of everyday function can be interpreted using the PRPP System of Task Analysis.

David

David is 8 years old and has ASD. He is in his second year of formal schooling.

His teacher is worried about his school performance in many areas. His written work is never completed in the allotted time and his ability to concentrate is at best 5 min for any one task before he gets out of his chair and wanders around the classroom. When he has to go to the toilet or it is his turn to get the class lunches from the canteen, he gets lost and is often found walking around the perimeter of the schoolyard. No one wants to sit next to him at school because he rocks continuously or fiddles with his pencil and does not help with group tasks. He often loses his pencil case and has to 'borrow' pencils and work tools from the other children or the teacher. Although he can read and verbally recount a factual story, he finds writing about events difficult. His work is illegible to anyone but himself. His letters are too big to fit the worksheet given to him, and words and letter formations are incomplete, despite repeated practicing. When the teacher gives the class verbal instructions, his eye contact is poor and he often stares at the ceiling fan. The teacher has indicated that he prefers to follow instructions when she puts them on the board, or on the children's worksheets. He prefers to play by himself and does not have friends.

David's parents have indicated that he has difficulty sitting still for mealtimes and other activities at home. This has stopped them from taking him out to eat, and attending family gatherings can be a nightmare. His use of a spoon and fork is poor, and he prefers to eat with his fingers while he walks around. He is not allowed to use a knife. He can dress himself but needs help with shoe fastenings and buttons. His favourite clothes are track pants, t-shirts and sneakers without laces, which he can put on quickly. David was referred to occupational therapy to improve his ability to participate in academic and social activities at school.

ASD is a behaviourally based developmental disability that is present at birth or develops within the first 30 months of a child's life (Jordan, 2002). It is a life-long neurobiological disorder that affects how people perceive and interpret their world. Researchers theorise that the behaviour of children with ASD occurs as a result of a complex variety of impairments in the physiology and chemistry of brain function that culminate in a functional disorder of information processing (Jordan, 2002; Sigman & Capps, 1997). Therapists often rely on assessments that can be used within the child's natural environment, as they have been found to produce more useful information for intervention than norm-referenced tests (Case-Smith & Bryan, 1999; Kientz & Dunn, 1997; Stuhec & Gisel, 2003; Watling, Deitz, & White, 2003). The following section of the chapter illustrates how best practice assessment criteria (Kientz & Miller-Kuhaneck, 2001) can be operationalised using the PRPP System of Task Analysis.

'Perceive': observing and prompting sensory processing behaviours during task performance

Once sensory input captures our attention, and we focus on it, details of the information are registered and we create sensory pictures of events. Sensory registration serves to interpret and maintain the information from the input receptors long enough for it to be perceived and analysed. It becomes *sensory perception*, registered sensory input that is meaningful. Information processing research has demonstrated how copies of sensory images are stored very briefly, for seconds only (Huitt, 2003). Unless there is an effort to pay attention to sensory images, the information is lost from the sensory register.

The top left-hand quadrant (Perceive) in Figure 9.3 outlines some specific behaviours from the PRPP System of Task Analysis associated with this first stage of information processing. These behaviours are observable signs that children are attending to and purposefully dealing with sensory input that is needed for task performance (Chapparo & Ranka, 1997b).

Assessment: 'perceive'

When we observe David performing the task of writing in the particular classroom context described, he has difficulty:

- *noticing* when the teacher is talking to him
- *shifting* his attention from what the teacher says to writing in his book
- *maintaining* his attention for the length of the task
- *purposefully listening* to all the instructions, or *looking* through his book in a systematic way
- *searching for and finding the tools* he needs for the task (pencil and place in his book)
- *monitoring* how tightly he is holding the pencil

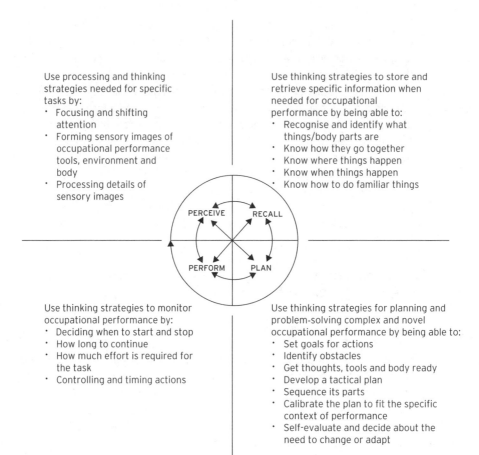

Use processing and thinking strategies needed for specific tasks by:
* Focusing and shifting attention
* Forming sensory images of occupational performance tools, environment and body
* Processing details of sensory images

Use thinking strategies to store and retrieve specific information when needed for occupational performance by being able to:
* Recognise and identify what things/body parts are
* Know how they go together
* Know where things happen
* Know when things happen
* Know how to do familiar things

PERCEIVE   RECALL

PERFORM   PLAN

Use thinking strategies to monitor occupational performance by:
* Deciding when to start and stop
* How long to continue
* How much effort is required for the task
* Controlling and timing actions

Use thinking strategies for planning and problem-solving complex and novel occupational performance by being able to:
* Set goals for actions
* Identify obstacles
* Get thoughts, tools and body ready
* Develop a tactical plan
* Sequence its parts
* Calibrate the plan to fit the specific context of performance
* Self-evaluate and decide about the need to change or adapt

Figure 9.3 Some processing strategies associated with the Perceive, Recall, Plan and Perform (PRPP) system quadrants (Chapparo and Ranka, 1997a,b)

We can hypothesise that part of the reason David is not performing to his teacher's expectations is because he is not processing some of the necessary information in the first stage of information processing. He does not have some of the critical attention and sensory processing strategies in place to give him updated information about what he has to do and how.

'Recall': observing strategies used for storage and retrieval of information during task performance

In the second stage of information processing, incoming sensory images are transferred to temporary short-term information processing storage. This working memory is what we are thinking about at any given time. It is created when we pay deeper attention to sensory input, or a thought that 'comes to mind'. Children become consciously aware of the information in working memory and begin to manipulate it purposefully. Working memory has a limited capacity, so incoming information continually replaces information that is already in this short-term storage. It will initially last somewhere around 15–20 s unless it is repeated, at which point it may be available for use for up to 20 min, the length of a typical learning session in early grades at school. If information is not placed into long-term storage for use at a later time, it fades. We also retrieve information from long-term memory storage and bring it back into working memory for use when we need it (Smith, 1999; Thagard, 2005). This allows us to compare present and past information for solving problems requiring recognition and discrimination.

Memories of our experiences are configured efficiently into long-term memory structures called schemas. Schemas serve as filters for ongoing experience, allowing us to come to conclusions about what we see, hear or do automatically (Sodorow & Rickabaugh, 2002). For typical children, these long-term schemas become a platform of knowledge from which information is retrieved for learning. Some children have gaps in this knowledge platform, distorted schemas or trouble retrieving information. They have to engage in the process of learning the same things over and over, while their typical peers move ahead to learn new skills.

Assessment: 'recall'

For occupational performance, memories of occupational performance that are stored for use serve as our 'functional reference system' (Ranka, 2005). The purpose of this functional reference system is to enable us to interpret the *present* based on experience from *the past*. It grounds us, gives us direction for responses, provides behavioural templates (rules) for future planned action and answers the question, 'Do I know ...?' The purpose of occupational therapy assessment is, in part, to determine what children have learned (know), how their knowledge is constructed and how functional it is for everyday living.

Three broad categories of information are stored and retrieved for use during every task we do. These are:

● Factual information (facts) – 'Do I know WHAT ...?' The storing and recalling of facts enables children to recognise sensory experiences, attach meaning to sensory experiences and retrieve useful memories about sensory experiences that are used for future planning. Combinations of sensory information and language are coded to form the basis for organising coherent action. When factual information is not stored or coded correctly, children either do not recognise sensory images or make mistakes of recognition. They will call things by the wrong name, put things together the wrong way or use things the wrong way. These are all common errors that are made by children with learning difficulties during performance of school tasks that can be traced to this stage of information processing.

- Schematic information (schemes) – 'Do I know WHERE …?'; 'Do I know WHEN …?'; 'Do I know HOW LONG …?' Schematic memory represents what we have learned about where, when and how long something happens. This type of memory is based on particular experiences that are located in *personal* time and space. It keeps us anchored and stable in everyday situations. Schematic information provides us with a personally constructed 'map' or a model for how, when and where to act. When children are unable to develop stable schematic memory, their behaviour will not match the context. Claims of inappropriate behaviour, immaturity, social ineptitude and poor social skills that are often levelled at children with learning disorders may often be the result of a difficulty with processing schematic information. Although children may be able to *do* what is required, they are unable to either retrieve the contextual rules for behaviour (now/not now; here/not here) or use meta-cognitive strategies to assess the appropriateness of behaviours across different contexts (e.g. talking now/not now; write here/not there). Children with combinations of learning and social disabilities are often described as doing the wrong thing at the wrong time in the wrong place.
- Procedural information – 'Do I know HOW …?' Procedural memory enables us to perform certain actions 'automatically' based on past experience. Procedural memory has been shown to be the most resistant to forgetting in people with CNS disorders (Sodorow & Rickabaugh, 2002). Examples of tasks we use every day that rely on procedural memory are dressing, brushing teeth and walking along a daily route. We can usually do these things without thinking because we have learned them so well. Children with difficulty storing and retrieving procedural knowledge may forget how to use tools such as pens, pencils, toys, cutlery and play equipment. Their movements may seem clumsy, even when doing familiar tasks, because they are unable to remember how to use their bodies in the most efficient manner. They may consistently forget steps of what should be well-learned tasks, such as brushing teeth, doing up buttons and shoelaces, and have to be shown many times how to do the same task.

Intervention: 'recall'

A significant focus of intervention for children with learning disorders involves helping them establish functional memory stores of successful occupational performance that they can use automatically when needed. This has been referred to as 'skills training' or 'task-specific instruction' (Larkin & Parker, 2002). The process starts with careful and detailed observation of a child's ability to store, retrieve and use what they have learned within the parameters listed in the top right-hand quadrant in Figure 9.3 (Recall).

There are two major strategies that are important for getting information into working memory: repetition and organisation (Thagard, 2005). This may explain why children who have learning disorders need and actively seek repetition of instruction in order to understand what has to be learned, and respond better to information that is presented in an organised way. Let us review David's performance again to see how this aspect of information processing is causing him difficulty.

It is David's turn to collect the lunches from the canteen. The task requires David to manipulate many things in his working memory. He has to remember the teacher's instruction. He has to retrieve information about where his classroom is, and the route to the canteen in the form of sensory snapshots and language from his long-term memory and place it in working memory for use. Along with those images, he has to remember what to say to the lady in the canteen when he gets there. While he is able to remember the teacher's instruction about what has to be done (*facts*), he has difficulty remembering how to do it (*schemes and procedures*). He is unable to access his schematic memories of the route to and from the classrooms and requires help from another student.

'Plan': processing information for organising and problem-solving

Organisation, problem-solving, decision making, insight and purposeful allocation of attention are all referred to as executive functions within the information processing system. This third stage of information can be thought of as the 'rules of operation' that we apply to problem-solving and analysing information in any learning situation. They are not linked to any particular type of sensory information or ability, but are applied to all information that has to be organised for use. Every day, we rely on our executive skills by applying thinking strategies to what we do. Strategy application allows us to orchestrate multiple tasks and parts of tasks into a seamless whole. Findings from several studies suggest that children with learning difficulties do not self-instruct as often, or as well, as other children (Berry & West, 1993; Bohannon & Bonvillian, 2005; Missiuna, 1998; Polatajko, Mandich, Miller, & McNab, 2001; Schunk, 1990).

Assessment: 'plan'

Daily, children have to engage in new and complex learning. Information flows into the processing system and presents it with a problem to solve. *What is that word? What did Mum say to do? How can I do it differently? How much do I need to do? How can I do it without making a mistake? How does my work compare with others? Did I do what was expected?* These are just a few of the typical problems children have to solve in most tasks they do, requiring the use of higher order information processing such as critical thinking, decision making and planning. While some children with learning difficulties are able to develop strong procedural memories, they almost universally have difficulty with some aspect of planning and problem-solving, giving rise to difficulties coping with transition and change.

To engage in problem-solving, planning and self-evaluation, children must construct and evaluate their own goal-oriented strategies for action. This means that they process information with reference to a particular goal, an idea, and an understanding of an outcome. Children with processing problems may have no idea of how to construct an idea or a goal; they may have an incomplete idea of the expected outcome; or the idea may fade when they begin to act, as performance becomes increasingly influenced by other motivations. When an outcome is kept in mind, children who are independent learners initiate executive thinking operations that prepare them to put a plan into action. These strategies are different to mere memory retrieval, and involve 'figuring out' extensions or elaborations to habitual responses that may be demanded by the task, or by what is happening around them in the learning context. Children have to solve the following problems before, during and on review as they learn to do complex tasks:

- What *obstacles* might/did get in the way?
- How can I *get ready* for action?
- What is the *best choice* of action, place and tool to use for *this specific task*?
- How do I have to *sequence* the task?
- What do I have to do to make my responses *fit* the expectation/context/my abilities?

Intervention: 'plan'

Children are, and want to be, responsible for their own learning. This happens when they can reflect on, evaluate their own plans and performance, and make considered decisions about satisfaction, effectiveness and the need for correction or change. This evaluative thinking involves meta-cognition, where children think about their thinking. It is a type of cognitive monitoring that involves questioning, analysing their performance and ideas, and making final judgements about their worth. Three thinking strategies appear to be critical for being able to evaluate our own performance:

- being able to question whether our performance matched the expected outcome
- being able to further analyse the reasons why we did or did not meet our goals
- being able to make decisions about the need to carry on, or change the goal and the plan

Observations of children's planning, problem-solving and decision making can be guided by asking how well a given child seems to know the answers to questions in the bottom right-hand quadrant of Figure 9.3 (Plan).

Writing a creative story requires David to undertake a number of executive processing tasks. David's ability to remember facts (Recall) is strong, enabling him to recount events with great accuracy. When he has to write a story about a 'made up' event, he cannot rely on memory alone. He has to make an overall mental plan for what has to be done that will draw many sensing and thinking strands together into a coherent whole. He has to get all the tools needed for the task (e.g. pencil and writing book). He has to figure out where he has to write (e.g. page in the book and the right line). He has to make a mental story plan that involves bringing information into working memory. He has to purposefully shift his attention between each one of these operations and keep each one in his working memory so that there are no gaps in the story. The story has to be sequenced. He must not be distracted by the noise in the class, the boy next to him or thinking about how good it would be to get up and walk around outside. He has to make an effort to concentrate on his thinking. The task must be done within a specified time. David has difficulty with the basic executive functions required for this task:

(1) He is unable to generate an imagined story or select from many story-writing ideas provided by the teacher.
(2) He has difficulty modifying the timing of his performance to fit the time constraints.
(3) He has difficulty ignoring other information and persisting with the task at hand.
(4) He is unable to simultaneously keep track of what he has to do, what he has done, what he is doing and what he will do next.

'Perform': processing output and performance feedback

The last stage of information processing focuses on using thinking strategies to perform, or create output responses. Numerous researchers have linked reduced thinking strategies and reduced speed of processing to inefficient response control and timing (e.g. Giuffrida, 2001; Rothi & Heilman, 1997; Schmidt & Wrisberg, 2000). Actively responding to information that is processed requires being able to plan and initiate both starting and stopping of action. Responses generate further input into the information processing system and result in 'learning through doing'. For this feedback to be effective for learning, children must have a response goal in mind and be able to bring the goal back into focus for review as they *do*.

Assessment: 'perform'

Guidelines for identifying information processing behaviours which may indicate a difficulty with monitoring actions in children with learning disorders are listed in the bottom left-hand quadrant in Figure 9.3. They are dependent on formation of an adequate plan, knowing the purpose of responses and rapid and accurate processing of the changing body and contextual sensory details that are critical to task performance.

David has difficulty working with his learning group at school. Similarly, he is unable to join groups of children at play and has no friends. Playing different games with the other children and working in groups are situations that are novel or complex. Based on observations listed in Figure 9.3, this scenario suggests that David has difficulty with the following information processing strategies:

- He has difficulty figuring out the rules of the game/work project (*understanding the goal*).
- He is unable to come up with an effective plan to join in the group game (*knowing how to play the game and its sequence/knowing what to do and the sequence*).
- His self-evaluation confirms that he does not 'fit in' (*questions*), but he does not know why (*analyses*), or what he can do about it (*choosing solutions and alternative solutions*).
- He does not know when to start playing/working (*choosing when to act and when not to act*).
- He does not finish (*continues and persists*).

Intervention: 'perform'

While David's therapist and teacher can investigate ways to make his school environment more conducive to his participation, David can also learn more effective ways of thinking that might assist him in solving the problems that arise for him every day. Expert modelling of thinking from the therapist, together with scaffolding of thinking skills required to solve problems, is viewed as a 'best practice' direct instruction technique. In this approach, the therapist can instruct the child's parent or teacher to guide the child by serving as a model who overtly and explicitly verbalises the strategic meta-cognitive strategies needed for successful performance. This is done through teaching David how to process information strategically, and figure out solutions to problems and complexities that arise while he is with other children. David's therapist/mother and teacher will have to model a process of sensing and thinking, rather than simply directing David's action.

The following are examples of how the 'Stop/Attend, Sense, Think, Do' PRPP intervention process can be used by David's teacher and mother to prompt both task performance and improved information processing:

Teacher: The teacher's goal is for David to engage in writing independently and to finish his work. Instead of asking the class to 'get out your book and write about ...', the teacher could additionally prompt specific processing strategies that will help David get started and keep going with the task as summarised in Table 9.3.

Table 9.3 Example of PRPP intervention prompts for teacher to use during writing

Strategy	Prompt (verbal)	PRPP quadrant	PRPP descriptor
Stop/attend	'David. Stop looking at the fan. Look and listen to what I say (indicate face)'	Perform/Perceive	*Stops/modulates (re-focus)*
Sense	'Get your eyes ready to look for the place to write' (begins visual search strategy)	Perceive	*Searches Locates*
Think	'Remember what you did yesterday' 'Use your eyes to look at all your pages until you reach the work you did yesterday' (systematic purposeful search strategy) 'Look until you find the line with the green dot. That is where you will start' 'Use your finger on the page to help your eyes to look'	Recall Plan	*Uses body Recalls steps Chooses* (right place)
Do	'Start writing and keep writing until you reach the red dot'	Perform	*Continues*

Mother: One of David's mother's goals is for him to do up his shoelaces. Prompts outlined in Table 9.2 for buttoning could be used by her to achieve the goal of tying shoelaces.

Conclusion

This chapter described elements of the PRPP System of Task Analysis and Intervention. An example of how this system could be employed as an observational assessment format was provided. Information processing theory was coupled with notions of occupational performance to demonstrate how difficulty with learning new skills impacts on occupational performance. All children who have such difficulty are different and require individual consideration. In this chapter, the story of one child, David, was used to illustrate just some of the problems that children with reduced processing capacity may encounter at home and school, and brief examples of intervention were given. The approach presented in this chapter is consistent with contemporary shifts in education and therapy towards a more ecological and dynamic style of intervention where assessment and intervention are ongoing and mutually informative, and where the focus is on the particular occupational needs of particular children and families in particular contexts.

References

Beck, J., & Horne, D. (1992). A whole school implementation of the stop, think, do! Social skills training program. In B. Willis, and J. Izard (Eds.), *Student behaviour problems: Directions, perspectives and expectations*. Hawthorne, Vic.: Australian Council for Educational Research.

Berry, J., & West, R. (1993). Cognitive self efficacy in relation to personal mastery and goal setting across the life span. *International Journal of Behavioral Development, 16*(2), 351–379.

Bohannon, J. N., & Bonvillian, J. D. (2005). Theoretical approaches to language acquisition. In J. B. Gleason (Ed.), *The development of language* (6th ed., pp. 230–291). Boston, MA: Pearson.

Case-Smith, J., & Bryan, T. (1999). The effects of occupational therapy with sensory integration emphasis on preschool-age children with autism. *American Journal of Occupational Therapy, 53*(5), 489–497.

Cermak, S., & Larkin, D. (2002). Developmental coordination disorder. Albany, NY: Delmar Thomson Learning.

Chapparo, C., & Ranka, J. (1997a). *Occupational performance model (Australia): Monograph 1*. Sydney: Total Print Control.

Chapparo, C., & Ranka, J. (1997b). The perceive, recall, plan and perform system of task analysis. In C. Chapparo, and J. Ranka (Eds.), *Occupational performance model (Australia): Monograph 1* (pp. 189–198). Sydney: Total Print Control.

Chapparo, C., & Ranka, J. (2005). *The PRPP training manual: Research edition 7*. Lidcombe, NSW: Discipline of Occupational Therapy, Faculty of Health Sciences, The University of Sydney.

Chapparo, C., & Ranka, J. (2007). *The PRPP system: Intervention*. Lidcombe, NSW: Discipline of Occupational Therapy, Faculty of Health Sciences, The University of Sydney.

Chrenka, J., Hutton, R. J., Klinger, D. W., & Aptima, D. A. (2001). Focusing cognitive task analysis in the cognitive function model. Proceedings of the *Human Factors and Ergonomics Society 45th Annual Meeting, 5*: 1738–1742.

Dunn, W. (2000). *Best practice in occupational therapy in community service with children and families*. Thorofare, NJ: CB Slack Publishers.

Fish, J., Evans, J. J., Nimmo, M., Martin, E., Kersel, D., Bateman, A., et al. (2007). Rehabilitation of executive dysfunction following brain injury: "Content-free" cueing improves everyday prospective memory performance. *Neuropsychologia, 45*(6), 1318–1330.

Fisher, A. (1992). Functional measures, part 1: What is function, what should we measure, and how should we measure it? *American Journal of Occupational Therapy, 46*(2), 183–185.

Fry, K., & O'Brien, L. (2002). Using the Perceive, Recall, Plan and Perform System to assess cognitive deficits in adults with traumatic brain injury: A case study. *Australian Occupational Therapy Journal, 49*(2), 182–187.

Guiffruda, C. (2001). Praxis, motor planning and motor learning. In S. S. Roley, E. I. Blanche, & R. C. Schaaf (Eds.), *Understanding the nature of sensory integration with diverse populations* (pp. 133–154). San Antonio, TX: Therapy Skill Builders.

Huitt, W. (2003). The information processing approach to cognition. *Educational Psychology Interactive*. Valdosta, GA: Valdosta State University. Retrieved 8 May 2009 from http://chiron.valdosta.edu/whuitt/col/cogsys/infoproc.html.

Jordan, R. (2002). *Autistic spectrum disorders in the early years: A guide for practitioners*. Staffordshire, UK: Lichfield Publishers.

Kielhofner, G. (2004). *Conceptual foundations of occupational therapy*. Philadelphia, PA: F.A. Davis Company.

Kientz, M. A., & Dunn, W. (1997). A comparison of the performance of children with and without autism on the Sensory Profile. *American Journal of Occupational Therapy, 51*(7), 530–537.

Kientz, M. A., & Miller-Kuhaneck, H. (2001). Occupational therapy evaluation of the child with autism. In H. Miller-Kuhaneck (Ed.), *Autism: A comprehensive occupational therapy approach* (pp. 55–84). Bethesda, MD: American Occupational Therapy Association.

Kirwan, B., & Ainsworth, L. K. (1992). *A guide to task analysis*. London, UK: Taylor and Francis.

Larkin, D., & Parker, H. (2002). Task-specific intervention for children with developmental coordination disorder: A systems review. In S. Cermak, & D. Larkin (Eds.), *Developmental coordination disorder* (pp. 234–247). Albany, NY: Delmar.

Law, M., Baum, C., & Dunn, W. (2001). *Measuring occupational performance: Supporting best practice in occupational therapy*. Thorofare, NJ: SLACK Inc.

Lerner, J. (2000). *Learning disabilities. Theories, diagnosis, and teaching strategies* (8th ed.). Boston, MA: Houghton Mifflin.

Losardo, A., & Notari-Syverson, A. (2001). *Alternative approaches to assessing young children*. Baltimore, MD: Paul H. Brookes Publishing Co.

Militello, L. G., & Hutton, R. J. B. (1998). Applied cognitive task analysis (ACTA): A practitioner's toolkit for understanding cognitive task demands. *Ergonomics, 41*(11): 1618–1641.

Miller, L. T., Missiuna, C. A., Macnab, J. J., Malloy-Miller, T., & Polatajko, H. J. (2001). Clinical description of children with developmental coordination disorder. *Canadian Journal of Occupational Therapy, 68*(1), 5–15.

Missiuna, C. (1998). Development of "All about me", a scale that measures children's perceived motor competence. *Occupational Therapy Journal of Research, 18*(2), 85–108.

Murphy, D. P., & Cooke, J. (1999). Traffic light lessons: Problem solving skills with adolescents. *Community Practitioner, 72*, 322–324.

Nott, M. T., & Chapparo, C. (2008). Measuring information processing in a client with extreme agitation following traumatic brain injury using the perceive, recall, plan and perform system of task analysis. *Australian Occupational Therapy Journal, 55*(3), 188–198.

Nott, M. T., Chapparo, C., & Heard, R. (2008). Effective occupational therapy intervention with adults demonstrating agitation during post-traumatic amnesia. *Brain Injury, 22*(9), 669–683.

Polatajko, H., Mandich, A., Miller, L., & McNab, J. (2001). Cognitive orientation to daily occupational performance (CO-OP): Part II – The evidence. *Physical & Occupational Therapy in Pediatrics, 20*(2/3), 83–105.

Puderbaugh, J. K., & Fisher, A. (1992). Assessment of motor and process skills in normal young children and children with dyspraxia. *Occupational Therapy Journal of Research, 12*, 195–216.

Ranka, J. (2005). The recall quadrant. In C. Chapparo, & J. Ranka (Eds.), *PRPP training manual: Research edition 7*. Lidcombe, NSW: Discipline of Occupational Therapy, Faculty of Health Sciences, The University of Sydney.

Rothi, L., & Heilman, K. (Eds.). (1997). *Apraxia: The neuropsychology of action*. Hove, UK: Psychology Press.

Schmidt, R., & Wrisberg, C. (2000). *Motor learning and performance*. Champaign, IL: Human Kinetics Books.

Schraagen, J. M., Chipman, S. F., & Shalin, V. (2000). *Cognitive task analysis*. Mahwah, NJ: Lawrence Erlbaum Associates.

Schunk, D. (1990). Goal setting and self efficacy during self-regulated learning. *Educational Psychologist, 25*(1), 71–86.

Sigman, M., & Capps, L. (1997). *Children with autism: A developmental perspective*. Cambridge, MA: Harvard University Press,

Singer-Harris, N., Weiler, M., Bellinger, D., & Waber, D. P. (2001). Children with adequate academic achievement scores referred for evaluation of school difficulties: Information processing deficiencies. *Developmental Neuropsychology, 20*(3), 593–603.

Smith, E. E. (1999). Storage and executive processes in the frontal lobes. *Science, 12*(5408), 1657–1661.

Sodorow, L. M., & Rickabaugh, C. A. (2002). *Psychology* (5th ed.). Boston, MA: McGraw Hill.

Stuhec, V. K., & Gisel, E. G. (2003). Standardized procedure in the administration of tests for children with pervasive developmental disorders: Do they exist? *Canadian Journal of Occupational Therapy, 70*, 33–41.

Swanson, H. L. (2001). Searching for the best model for instructing students with learning disabilities. *Focus on Exceptional Children, 34*, 1–14.

Thagard, P. (2005). *Mind: Introduction to cognitive science*. Cambridge, MA: The MIT Press.

Watling, R. L., Deitz, J., & White, O. (2003). Comparison of Sensory Profile scores of young children with and without autism spectrum disorders. In C. B. Royeen (Ed.), *Pediatric issues in occupational therapy* (pp. 130–139). Bethesda, MD: American Occupational Therapy Association.

Chapter 10

Occupational Performance Coaching: Enabling Parents' and Children's Occupational Performance

Fiona Graham and Sylvia Rodger

> ### Learning objectives
>
> The objectives of this chapter are to:
>
> - Briefly outline the theoretical and philosophical basis of occupational performance coaching (OPC) with reference to other interventions which support the use of OPC.
> - Describe the domains, session format and some of the techniques used during OPC.
> - Illustrate the application of OPC through case vignettes.

Introduction

This chapter describes occupational performance coaching (OPC) (Graham, Rodger, & Ziviani, 2009), an intervention for working with parents to achieve occupational performance goals for themselves and their children. OPC is an occupational therapy intervention suitable to situations when: (1) children's performance is highly dependent on the context where performance occurs; (2) parents seek ways to support their children's performance of occupational roles, tasks and routines; and (3) parents have goals relating to their own occupational performance. OPC is suitable for parents of children with mild to severe performance issues and for goals in any areas of occupational performance. OPC is not suitable when children are medically compromised or when parents themselves have significant mental health or learning issues.

Therapists using OPC coach parents to identify adjustments within the home or community performance context (e.g. changes to the sequence of tasks in the morning routine or the arrangement of seating during mealtimes). Improved occupational performance is facilitated by creating a better match between the person, occupation and environment (Law et al., 1996). OPC is based on the premise that a better match leads to successful practice and subsequently improved occupational performance and transferable skills. Through collaborative analysis of child and/or parent performance, parents learn to identify actions which facilitate goal achievement.

Theoretical and philosophical basis

OPC is grounded in enablement perspectives of health, and occupation- and family-centred practices which are described in detail elsewhere (Graham et al., 2009). Disability is viewed as resulting from a mismatch between individuals' specific impairments and their environments (World Health Organisation, 2001). Performance in home and community contexts is the focus of OPC since these are the environments that parents can influence most directly.

OPC is an occupation-centred intervention in that occupation is central to all stages of the therapeutic exchange. Hence, the goals of OPC intervention describe observable occupational performance improvement in the lived or naturalistic environment of children and parents. An important principle is that parents have the most influence on children's environments (Bronfenbrenner, 1979), and therefore play a critical role in enabling children's occupational performance. Using OPC, the therapist guides parents through a collaborative process of performance analysis to improve performance. Occupational performance is re-evaluated by parents throughout intervention to determine the effectiveness of OPC for their families. Hence, occupation is central at all stages of OPC.

OPC is a family-centred intervention (see Chapter 3 for a more detailed discussion on family-centred practice). OPC goals are parent-generated and describe expected improvement in occupational performance by children, parents or the family. While goals usually refer to children's performance, parents are also invited to describe goals for themselves in relation to their role as parents. When applying OPC, there is a two-fold intention to: (1) enable occupational performance in the areas identified by parents as goals, and (2) improve parents' ability to manage future occupational performance challenges.

Three enabling domains

To assist parents' construction of more enabling performance contexts, the therapist utilises three *enabling domains*: (1) *emotional support*, (2) *information exchange,* and (3) a *structured process* (see Figure 10.1). The emphasis on each domain varies among parents and at different stages of the intervention process. An awareness of each of these three domains during OPC

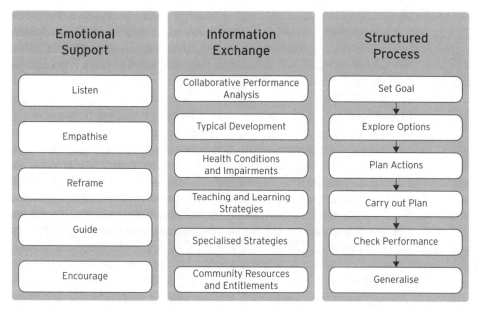

Figure 10.1 Three enabling domains

interactions assists the therapist to notice parents' responses and learning needs and thereby effectively coach parents in implementing change. Each domain will be described with techniques illustrated through case examples.

Emotional support

The emotional support domain includes the specific intentions to listen, empathise, reframe, guide and encourage parents to enable goal achievement. Emotional support is at times critical to parents' goal achievement, particularly during initial sessions when parents may need to express their frustration and confusion about situations before they are ready to discuss potential solutions to performance dilemmas. Within OPC, emotional support is an enabling domain because of its role in facilitating parents' shift from an emotional (reactive) orientation to a solution-finding (proactive) orientation in which they can discuss actions to improve performance (for further discussion on this transition, see Nezu, Palmatier, & Nezu, 2004).

Listen

Listening to parents is critical to understanding home and community performance contexts and children's performance. When coaching parents to facilitate improved performance at home, it is essential to know what parents perceive happens in the process of normal family routines rather than when performance of a task is demonstrated to the therapist. Listening to parents' descriptions informs the therapist about parents' interpretation of performance, motivators for change, learning needs in implementing change and previous successes in enabling performance. The therapist consciously listens for examples of effective problem-solving, improved performance and possibilities for further action (De Jong & Kim Berg, 2008). Through listening without judgement, the therapist validates parents' experiences and knowledge and builds trust in the relationship (Dunst, Trivette, & Deal, 1994).

Empathise

Genuine empathy has long been recognised as essential to therapeutic relationships (e.g. Rogers, 1951) as it builds parents' trust that the therapist understands and respects their perspectives. Trust in the therapist is essential before parents will engage in solution-focused discussions about anything more than superficial performance difficulties. By expressing genuine empathy, the therapist positions her/himself alongside the parent and begins the process of problem-solving collaboratively (e.g. Murphy & Dillon, 2008).

Reframe

Assisting parents to reframe (Geldard & Geldard, 2005) their perceptions of performance is an important way in which therapists guide parents to develop more enabling performance contexts. Reframing situations by paraphrasing or gently offering alternative interpretations can open the way for learning new information or techniques to support children's performance. For example, suggesting that a child who spills food often during dinner may have difficulty attending to multiple task demands or instructions leads parents to different support strategies than when a child's difficulties are framed as motor skill issues.

Guide

The therapist focuses on enabling performance as directly as possible while guiding parents' reflections and choices of action. Therapists' guidance has a 'coaching' style as parent's knowledge, judgement and ability is emphasised within discussions. Therapists 'lead from behind' by seeking and providing information (by guiding conversation) while encouraging parents to make choices about specific actions or changes. Direct advice giving is minimised as this discourages independent future problem-solving.

Encourage

The therapist deliberately encourages parents through commenting on specific progress; complimenting parent actions, insights or new learning; and reiterating goal scenarios or relaying inspiring short stories of other families who have succeeded in similar situations. When parents begin implementing changes within the performance context, considerable effort is often required by them before performance improvement is apparent. Encouragement can be critical to parents' persistence through the early stages of OPC sessions while in the later stages the successful performance becomes the inherent encouragement to continue with alternative actions. In summary, *emotional support* is an essential enabling domain within OPC because it:

- Facilitates parents' readiness to engage in exploring and implementing performance solutions;
- Builds partnership and trust, allowing deeper exploration of performance issues and solutions;
- Motivates parents to persist with implementing change in the initial stages of intervention.

Information exchange

The second enabling domain of OPC refers to the process of reciprocal *information exchange* between parent and therapist and includes the areas of collaborative performance analysis: typical development, health conditions and impairments, teaching and learning strategies, specialised strategies and provision of information about community resources and entitlements. Information sharing is a two-way process with information from parents (e.g. about what they have already tried and what works for their children) seen as equally essential to improving performance as information shared by the therapist (e.g. developmental norms).

Information is shared by the therapist, not as an assumed first step, but when additional specialist information is needed for parents to identify ways of enabling performance. Information is limited to what parents *need to know* in order to plan and carry out actions. The content of information relates directly to parents' capacity to implement changes or strategies within the performance context. At times, parents may need background information in order to reframe their understanding of children's behaviour. For example, in order to support his/her child more effectively, a parent may need to know that a child's social interactions are very affected by his/her awareness that other people can have different feelings from oneself. At other times, information needs will be quite specific, for example, how to write a Social Story (Gray & Arnold, 2000). To target information provision, the therapist needs to investigate what the parent *already knows* (e.g. about the relevant condition and about typical development or strategies that assist performance), with an emphasis on highlighting existing knowledge rather than knowledge gaps (e.g. see Knowles, Holton, & Swanson, 2005; McKenna & Tooth, 2006). While information provided by the therapist is important within OPC, information provided by the parent is equally important. Information from parents is essential to discussions, reinforces parents' expertise and minimises perceptions of the therapist as the exclusive expert, a disempowering perspective for parents. Some examples of the ways in which parent knowledge is emphasised are by:

- Asking how the parent managed other similar difficulties in the past, what they have already tried and what they think might work;

- Asking the parent to describe a time when the goal activity was less of a problem or less likely to occur;
- Relating the situation to parents' other roles in which they have skills or knowledge that is relevant but not yet applied to this situation.

Collaborative performance analysis

Collaborative Performance Analysis (CPA) is a goal-specific examination of occupational performance based on information exchanged between the parent and the occupational therapist. CPA occurs during the *explore options* stage of the structured problem-solving process (see Table 10.1). It is a step-wise process for exploring what *actually happens* as the parent and child attempt to engage in the occupation and *what would happen* when performance has improved. As such, CPA is based on observable events during performance (or parents' report of observed events) as they occur in the natural context in which performance of the task is required. CPA involves exchanging information about the person (child or parent), task and the proximal (i.e. social and physical) environment. For an example of how CPA could be

Table 10.1 Collaborative Performance Analysis

1. *Identify what currently happens*
   (a) Child's actions
   (b) Parent and significant others' actions
   (c) Background and immediate environment
   (d) Strategies one parent and accommodations used/tried
   (e) Performance outcomes

2. *Identify what the parent would like to happen*
   (a) Child's actions
   (b) Parent and significant others' actions
   (c) Background and immediate environment
   (d) Strategies one parent and accommodations used/tried
   (e) Performance outcomes

3. *Explore barriers and bridges to enabling performance*
   (a) In the child's
       (i)   Motivation
       (ii) Knowledge
       (iii) Ability
   (b) In the task's
       (i)   Steps
       (ii) Sequence
       (iii) Standard
   (c) In the environment's
       (i)   Physical aspects
       (ii) Social aspects

4. *Identify parents' needs in implementing enabling change*
   (a) Interpretation
   (b) Motivation
   (c) Learning needs

applied to a child's performance when eating a meal see Table 10.2. The therapist's objectives are to: (1) determine what needs to be different in order for the child to be successful at this task, (2) determine what needs to be different in order for the parent to enable change, and (3) develop parents' ability to find solutions to their children's performance challenges. Each step of CPA will now be explained in detail.

Identify what (the parent perceives) currently happens

CPA is initiated by asking parents to describe what normally happens when the task is performed. The therapist may ask parents to describe a 'typical scenario' or a 'typical day' regarding the goal. The intention is to gain a clear, shared understanding of each step in performance as it *currently occurs*. In relation to performance of the goal, the therapist notes: the actions of the child, parent (i.e. the adult leader in the situation) and significant others (e.g. siblings); the background and immediate physical environment; any strategies or task accommodations employed; and performance outcomes (e.g. how far the child actually rode the bike and how long the child remained at the dinner table). This first step of CPA is largely an information gathering phase. The parent is questioned to obtain or clarify the information needed to understand performance in detail. For example, the therapist may guide the parent's description by asking: *Is anyone else at the dinner table? Where are you while James is getting dressed?* Information about what currently happens is only required insofar as it relates to performance of the goal with the most obviously influential factors probed initially (Table 10.2).

By beginning CPA with a description of what currently happens, the therapist invites the parent to focus on the problem rather than solutions. Talking about the problem can make the transition to solution (enablement)-oriented thinking and discussion more difficult because it often amplifies the current view of being in a negative and hopeless situation. However, occupational therapists often work with children with atypical responses to everyday situations; hence, there is usually important information in observation or discussion of the child's current performance and responses, that is, the problem. The therapist minimises the problem-focus of the discussion about what currently happens by guiding parents to describe specific recent examples and to remain focused on known rather than assumed information. Historical descriptions (e.g. reports of performance examples from more than a month ago) are avoided as these provide less accurate information for performance analysis and encourage problem-focused rather than solution-focused conversation.

Identify what the parent would like to happen, step by step

Similar to step 1, the therapist guides the parent in a stepwise description about how the parent would prefer performance to occur. This description includes information about: the actions of the child, parent and significant others; the background and immediate physical environment; potential strategies or task accommodations; and anticipated performance outcomes as they relate to achievement of the goal. This description contains more detail than goal statements. The detailed description assists in identifying possible

Table 10.2 Collaborative Performance Analysis for goal: eating tidily at the dinner table

Collaborative Performance Analysis steps	Example parent's response
1. *Identify what currently happens* (a) Child's actions (b) Parent's and significant others' actions (c) Background and immediate environment (d) Strategies and accommodations used/tried (e) Performance outcomes	• Child comes to table when called • Busy time, lots of noise, 2 siblings + dog • Usually spills drink, puts it near elbow • Plate slides around • Fingers slide down cutlery into food • Food spilt on table, child and floor • Takes 30–40 min to finish dinner • Use a heavy plate, bought sticky matting, tell child + + to use manners • Expect child to eat with no mess on fingers, table or floor
2. *Identify what the parent would like to happen* (a) Child's actions (b) Parent's and significant others' actions (c) Background and immediate environment (d) Strategies and accommodations used/tried (e) Performance outcomes	• Dinner time will be calm and quiet enough to talk about our day • My voice will be steady and calm • Child will keep hands free of food and hold cutlery effectively • Drink will stay in cup • Food will stay on the plate until eaten

3. *Explore barriers and bridges to enabling performance*
(a) In the child's
   (i) Motivation
   (ii) Knowledge
   (iii) Ability
(b) In the task's
   (iv) Steps
   (v) Sequence
   (vi) Standard
(c) In the environment's
   (vii) Physical aspects
   (viii) Social aspects
	• Does the child want dinner to be calm and hands to be free of food?
	• Does the child know how to keep hands in position on cutlery; how to keep plate still; where to put cup?
	• Can the child cope with co-ordinating cup, plate and conversation at this stage?
	• What would need to change for dinner time to be calm?
	• Does the chair/table arrangement provide sufficient support for the child?
	• What would help you to keep your voice calm and steady?

4. *Identify parents' needs in implementing enabling change* (a) Interpretation (b) Motivation (c) Learning needs	• What does the parent suspect is limiting the child's mealtime performance: motor skills? Motivation? Information overload? • Does the parent feel able or willing to try something different during mealtimes? • What does the parent know of alternative ways of cuing the child during mealtimes?

strategies or adjustments as well as helping parents to visualise the occurrence of the preferred performance. Step 2 of CPA is a transition point in the intervention as the tone of the conversation changes from discussing the problem to an enablement-oriented discussion of future performance of the goal. The therapist prompts this transition through solution-oriented (De Jong & Kim Berg, 2008) questions such as:

- Tell me about his best ever performance, step by step.
- If there was a miracle overnight that took the problem away, talk me through what you would notice?

Again, the therapist guides the description to a level of detail that prompts insight into possible performance solutions rather than exploring all possible information about the child, task and environment. The level of detail is also restricted to parents' capacity to adopt new insights or information within one session. An effective way of judging this is by asking parents if they feel they have enough to act on or to attend to regarding this goal situation until the next session. For example, the therapist may say, 'Does the plan to ask Jayden what he thinks when he gets stuck during Lego play feel like enough to focus on for this week?', or 'Would you like to cover more in today's session?'

Explore barriers and bridges to enabling performance

At each step of performance, the therapist notes *barriers* and potential *bridges* to the enablement of performance. Important barriers and bridges are points of flexibility (e.g. things that could be done differently), variability (e.g. stages of performance with fluctuating success) or transitions in performance or the performance context (e.g. changes in the setting, such as a new school term or moving from the bedroom to the lounge). Flexible, variable or transition points in the child's performance context are often more amenable to change and hence of interest when enabling performance. Examples of cues to investigate barriers and bridges to performance include when the parent describes:

- the child moving from being successful to unsuccessful
- the child doing something some days and not others
- the child's performance changing when the environment changes
- the task demands changing substantially
- the child's performance being unexpectedly successful or better than usual on an occasion
- differences in the way each adult assists the child with the task

Child factors   Key aspects of children's performance to consider are their: (1) motivation to complete the task, (2) knowledge about how to do the task, and (3) ability to do the task (see Chapters 8 and 9 for further discussion on performance analysis in CO-OP and PRPP). Child motivation can be critical to successful performance and can be addressed more easily once motivation has been isolated as a barrier (e.g. by emphasising the benefits of completing the task or making the task more manageable for the child). Filling gaps in children's knowledge about what to do during performance can also facilitate performance. Often parents assume children know what to do because they have told them. However, discussion with children or observation of their performance frequently reveals they lack key information about what to do (Polatajko & Mandich, 2004). The first OPC session often results in an action plan to investigate the child's knowledge further. Discussion of the steps of performance may also reveal that the child does not currently have the ability to complete the task as the parent expects and alternative approaches to the task can be explored. Often the detailed discussion enables parents to reach this conclusion themselves. Alternatively, the therapist may guide the parent to observe the child more closely or share information about developmental stages related to performance of the task before exploring alternative ways to manage the task.

Task factors Consideration of the number or sequence of steps and the expected standard of the task can be barriers or bridges to enabling performance and are often amenable to change. As parents describe the child's current and preferred performance, the therapist listens for and may cue parents to identify additional steps or alternative sequences of steps of the task which could enable performance. For example, the parent may report that the child transitions from play to mealtimes more easily when given a 'warning' 2 min before changing tasks. The warning may become an added step in the mealtime routine.

Environment factors The proximal physical and social environments are most frequently adapted to facilitate performance when using OPC. Examples of changes to the physical environment that can improve performance include reducing background noise, using adaptive equipment or using visual communication aids. Examples of social environment changes include changes to parents' interaction style (e.g. from authoritative to collaborative) or changes to teaching/learning strategies. Social environment changes can be difficult for parents but are usually more acceptable when discussed in view of goal achievement and when alternative interactions are clearly described, modelled and rehearsed with coaching by the therapist.

Identify parents needs in implementing change

The final step of CPA is to determine parents' needs in implementing changes in the performance context. This step is critical to the success of many goals addressed with occupational therapists because of parents' influence on the performance context. Within OPC, enabling parent implementation of change is recognised as a complex aspect of the therapist's role in facilitating goal achievement. There are three key considerations when coaching parents' implementation of performance enabling change. These are attending to their: (1) interpretation of performance, (2) motivation for change, and (3) learning needs. Information regarding these areas is noted by the therapist throughout the session and addressed as necessary to support parent action.

Parents' interpretation   Parents' interpretation of performance guides their responses in the performance situation (Long, Gurka, & Blackman, 2008). Parents are more likely to be receptive to alternative interpretations when they feel that their own perspective is understood and respected. Hence, an understanding of their interpretation is critical to facilitating change in parents' actions. The intention is to support parents' implementation of change by conveying respect for parents' interpretation, and exploring the usefulness of interpretations in achieving the goal. By acknowledging and discussing parents' interpretation of their child's performance, the therapist essentially explores situations from the parents' world view rather than imposing the therapist's view. For example, the therapist may convey an understanding of parents' interpretations by saying:

● I can understand how you might think that.
● How do you manage to keep positive about the situation?
● So what have you tried to deal with his 'laziness' so he can get ready for school on time? How has that worked?

Without agreeing or disagreeing with parents, the therapist assists them to explore the usefulness of interpretations in facilitating children's perform-ance. Through a process of reframing, parents can shift their perspective to a position in which an alternative approach to the task is congruent with their beliefs. Achieving this requires the therapist to be aware of how the parent is interpreting the situation as well as being aware of one's own interpretations.

Parents' motivation   Parental motivation may vary throughout interactions since it is affected by numerous internal and external factors. It is usually high initially because goals have recently been established for parents' greatest concerns. However, as goal performance is explored, motivation can diminish or shift. Conflict in motivation can also arise (e.g. between the achievement of goals and implementation of actions). In later stages, parents' motivation is sustained by the obvious improvement they observe. Hence, proposed changes are designed with the expectation that an obvious improvement in performance occurs within a few days or, at most, 2-3 weeks. The improvement may be in the parents' experience of the task (e.g. the parent no longer gets a sore back when bathing the child) or in the child's success (e.g. mastery of bike riding). If performance does not obviously improve following parents' actions in the performance context, there is no expectation that the parent will continue these. The therapist can further support parents' motivation by:

● Offering parents a printed copy of their goals or keep a copy of them in view during sessions;
● Directing conversation to the best performance since the last session;
● Encouraging, praising and celebrating progress, change or learning.

When the therapist is alert to shifts and conflict in parents' motivation, these can be respectfully explored with parents in order to reach a point of action that is acceptable to the parent and anticipated to improve performance in the goal task. A revision of goals or an adjustment to the planned actions for the following week may be needed to address shifts in motivation. As discussion about parents' action plans becomes specific, conflicts in motivation can arise. These can be resolved when acknowledged and respectfully explored. For example, a mother may have a goal of extending her pre-school child's range of food. CPA may lead her and the therapist to the hypothesis that the child is protesting about the strangeness of new food (rather than about the sensory qualities of the food). Hence, a new strategy of persisting with one new food for several meals (despite a child's protest) may be proposed. The therapist may notice the parent hesitating when summarising planned actions for the following week. Exploring this with the parent may reveal a conflict between the parent's motivation to keep her child calm and motivation to extend the child's range of foods. Gentle acknowledgement and exploration of this motivation conflict enables the parent and therapist to identify adjustments to the plan that are still likely to lead to performance improvement (such as a supportive phone call from the therapist or conscious positive self-talk by the parent prior to mealtimes).

Parents' motivation cannot be assumed, even when goals have been selected by parents. Parents' motivation is particularly attended to at points when implementation of change to the performance context is being discussed and when performance improvement is being reviewed (i.e. clarifying parents' motivation to aim for further improvement). Addressing parents' motivation is a key factor in the success of parents' goal achievement.

Parents' learning needs When facilitating occupational performance, parents have particular learning needs which are critical to their ability to implement change. These three learning needs correlate with the three enabling domains of OPC, namely *emotional support*, *information* exchange and *a structured process*. The parent (as learner) may need: (1) emotional support such as encouragement to implement an idea, (2) information about alternative teaching strategies or techniques such as to reduce word use and break instructions into steps, or (3) cues to follow a structured process in trialling new ideas before exploring further options. This may be necessary if the parent is generating more ideas than she or he is able to implement. Learning needs are addressed by:

- Observing and responding to parents' needs for support, information or structure in implementing plans;
- Asking parents if they have any unmet learning needs in relation to implementation of plans and then working with parents to address these.

Typical development

The exchange of information between parent and therapist occurs within the boundaries of *what is necessary for both therapist and parent to know* in order to facilitate improved performance of the goal. With this in mind, it can be (but is not always) useful to consider and discuss what is typical or what is next in the developmental sequence in relation to performance of the goal. Parents' information about what the child is normally able to do, has done occasionally or could previously do is essential for the therapist to understand the current developmental stage of the child in relation to performance of the task. This information assists the therapist to guide the parent towards actions that are most likely to facilitate performance. Equally, therapists' knowledge about typical developmental stages and age-norms can be critical information in assisting parents' insights into identifying ways of matching performance contexts with the child's performance needs.

Health conditions and impairments

An exchange of information about specific health conditions and impairments can also be useful when enabling performance. As with all elements of information exchange, the therapist asks parents what they already know about their children's health condition or impairment before offering further information. In doing so, the therapist reinforces parents' existing knowledge and competence and ensures that the information offered is specific to parents' information needs.

The therapist only explores information about conditions and impairments with parents when the CPA indicates that this information could facilitate performance. For example, the therapist may notice a pattern indicating planning difficulties in a parent's description of the child's performance of the morning routine. If the parent's attempts to facilitate the child's performance have only accommodated the child's motivation issues, the therapist would share information regarding her or his hypothesis of planning skill difficulties. In this situation, the parent shares essential information about the child's participation in family life that illustrates the presence of health conditions and impairments (i.e. planning difficulties) as well as information about the successful ways in which the family has engaged in meaningful tasks despite these difficulties.

The therapist remains focused on how exchanged information relates to goal achievement and invites parents to consider how information relates to the preferred performance. The translation of information on health conditions and impairments into the unique performance context of the family is critical to implementation of change because it clarifies the steps towards acting on the information. The therapist promotes the development of parents' performance analysis skills by asking parents to describe how the information is relevant to their children's performance at home or in the community. For example, the therapist may ask:

- So given (what we have just discussed), what could be arranged differently to assist mealtimes with your child over this next week?
- Does that (information, e.g. the impact of arousal level on sensory tolerance) sound relevant to what you have observed with (your child) at your home?

Teaching and learning strategies

Teaching and learning strategies focus on structuring the performance situation in ways that promote mastery and facilitate occupational performance. Teaching/learning strategies are often useful in facilitating performance during OPC as they can bridge the differences between children's current abilities and task demands. Within OPC, the emphasis is on exploring teaching/learning strategies collaboratively with parents and selecting strategies which match parents' needs and abilities (as well as the child's) and are applicable in home or community contexts. Often simply reframing interactions as teaching/learning strategies draws parents' attention to children's *learning needs* rather than their *inabilities*, thereby facilitating parents' insight into alternative approaches to tasks.

Many authors have categorised different types of teaching/learning strategies and linked specific strategies with specific learner needs (e.g. Daniels, 2001; Greber, Ziviani, & Rodger, 2007; Meichenbaum & Biemiller, 1998). During OPC, the therapist and parent exchange information about which teaching and learning strategies are currently being used and which are

Case example – teaching learning strategies

The story of Maria and Jacob (7 years) illustrates how coaching Maria in teaching/learning strategies led to improved performance for Jacob. Jacob has an intellectual disability which affects his ability to learn many age-appropriate skills. One of Maria's goals for Jacob was that he learns to button shirts himself. Previously Maria had used the teaching/learning strategies of *demonstration and explanation*, for example, 'watch me Jacob, see, it goes through here'. CPA with Maria identified that Jacob did not know what most of Maria's explanation meant. He had difficulty attending to Maria at the speed and volume of instructions she was using. When Maria asked Jacob to show her what he knew about doing up buttons, he held each side of the shirt and pressed them together ineffectually. When Maria attempted to explain how to button to Jacob, he attended for about 5 s before looking away or asking social questions. The therapist discussed the 'hand-over-hand' and 'verbal script' teaching/learning strategies with Maria relating them to the performance challenges observed and described. The use of a verbal script cued Jacob to key actions and minimised language. Maria added a *visual cue* of a character face, drawn on the thumbnail of Jacob's pushing thumb.

Jacob's attention to the task improved as the teaching/learning strategies simplified the task into smaller steps with less language. His enjoyment of the thumbnail character also assisted Jacob to attend. Jacob and Maria practiced doing buttons more often as a result of practice being more structured and enjoyable. Jacob mastered buttons within a month.

known to work well for the child. The therapist may share information about alternative teaching/learning strategies that are anticipated to better match the child's learning needs and are perceived by parents as *doable* and *likely to work* in the performance context.

Specialised strategies

Specialised strategies are specific procedures for enabling performance under specific conditions, such as when a child has a particular impairment or for particular tasks. Specialised strategies include techniques such as Collaborative Problem Solving (Greene et al., 2004), the Rainbow Shoe Tie Method (instructions for shoelace tying that match finger placement with coloured marks on the laces) and Comic Strip Conversations (Gray, 1994). Rather than using these techniques directly with the child, the therapist teaches the parent to use them as situations arise in normal family routines. The therapist may use demonstration, discussion, diagrams, modelling and in vivo coaching to teach parents the strategies. As with teaching/learning techniques used within OPC, specialist strategies are selected when they are expected to make a direct impact on occupational performance and when parents perceive them as doable and likely to work with their children. Although usually proposed by the therapist, parents often know about strategies; hence, they may simply need encouragement to try them. Always, parents' knowledge and perceptions of how and when strategies could be used within normal family routines are critical information for developing a successful plan of action.

Community resources and entitlements

Community resources and entitlements are an important area of information exchange that can support goal achievement for parents. Community resources such as parenting and disability support groups, resource libraries, websites or workshops can be important sources of social support and information for parents that contribute to goal achievement. Information about entitlements such as discounted memberships, income support and eligibility for services can also lead to practical assistance that enables parents to maintain their role in supporting their children's development and maintaining their own well-being. By first asking parents what they already know, the therapist is able to focus information where it is needed (and often learns a lot more about what is available locally!).

In summary, *information exchange* is an essential enabling domain within OPC because it:

- Provides opportunities for parents to demonstrate their knowledge, skills and resourcefulness builds independent, competent problem-solving;
- Shares specific information with parents better equips parents to work effectively with children towards improved performance;
- Listens carefully to parents' information about their children and the performance context enables therapists to guide CPA accurately.

Structured problem-solving process

A structured process of (1) setting goals, (2) exploring options, (3) planning action, (4) carrying out plans, (5) checking performance and (6) generalising provides the broad format of OPC sessions and is similar to many problem-solving interventions (e.g. D'Zurilla & Nezu, 2007; Polatajko et al., 2001; Stiebel, 1999; Vuchinich, 2004; Wade, Michaud, & Brown, 2006).

The problem-solving process and the rationale for its use are described briefly to parents at the initial session. Parents are informed that together with the therapist they will explore ways to better match the child's ability with the activity demands and the performance context, illustrated using the Person-Environment–Occupation (PEO) model Venn diagram (Law et al., 1996) which is incorporated into Figure 10.2. The structured process is explained as a series of steps to guide this exploration. The PEO is used to emphasise enablement and de-emphasise a single origin to the problem situation.

The six steps of the structured process are used iteratively rather than linearly and may be re-visited at any time during the session. Reference to each step is guided by the therapist in response to parents' insights and readiness for action. Sessions generally shift from an initial phase of reported or observed performance to an exploration phase of future enabling changes, and finally to a phase of planning the next action and generalising. For many parents, this systematic process is the key to enabling their children's performance.

A range of techniques is used by the therapist to guide parents towards performance enabling actions. Some of the most frequently used techniques are described here; however, this list is not exhaustive. Most techniques used within OPC are consistent with other client-centred (Law, Baptiste, & Mills, 1995), solution-focused (De Jong & Kim Berg, 2008) and strengths-based interventions (Powell & Batsche, 1997), with the exception of CPA

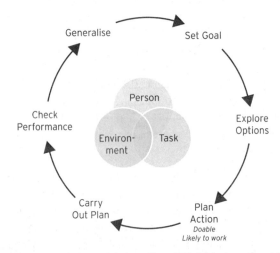

Figure 10.2 The structured process of Occupational Performance Coaching

which is unique to OPC but related to other occupation-centred perspectives (e.g. Fisher & Short-Degraff, 1993) and performance analysis methods (e.g. Chapparo & Ranka, 2006; Polatajko, Mandich, & Martini, 2000).

Set goal

Goal setting with parents is the first action within OPC sessions. Our experience suggests that parents often seek assistance for issues that are not of concern to the children whom the issue relates; therefore, OPC is designed to address the specific goals of parents. Parents are encouraged to collaborate with children when setting goals; however, the goals addressed in OPC reflect parents' priorities whether or not their goals are shared by other family members. It is important that children's concerns are acknowledged and other interventions are better suited to addressing children's goals (see Chapters 6 and 8) and can be used in conjunction with OPC. Goal setting frequently requires the whole first session of OPC and may need to be re-visited during the first few sessions as parents' priorities are clarified. It is imperative to revise goals if it appears they have lost their value to parents or have become unclear. Goal setting alone has an intervention effect (e.g. Locke & Latham, 1990); therefore, the time taken to establish clear, meaningful goals with families ultimately contributes to goal achievement.

OPC goals describe performance of occupations. For example, *Josh* plays quietly with his brother *for 10 minutes when at home*. Occupational goals usually make sense to parents because they reflect what their children want or need to do in everyday life. Occasionally parents describe goals of improvement in body structures and functions such as gross motor skills rather than occupations such as playing football with friends at the park. Goals describing improvement in body structures and functions (such as 'improving attention') are not suitable goals for OPC intervention because CPA cannot be applied (i.e. a specific task and context is required). However, the therapist can work with parents to isolate the occupational performance changes that will be observed when meaningful improvement in body structures and functions has occurred such as 'to follow instructions during the morning routine'. For example, the therapist can ask:

- What will you see is different at home (occupational performance) when Johnny's attention (performance component) has improved?
- What currently happens in the normal routine that has made you aware that attention is a problem for Johnny?

The performance context is a key source of solutions to performance difficulties and is used to make planned actions clearer. Although a child may have difficulty with attention in all contexts, focusing discussions on performance in one context (e.g. at home during dinner time) allows specific actions to be trialled and their effects to be clearly evaluated before attempting to generalise strategies to other contexts or abandoned them. Many of the solutions that assist a child's ability to attend sufficiently to eat a meal (e.g. eliminating distractions and ensuring supportive seating) will support attention to tasks in other contexts (e.g. at school). Other strategies will only work in specific contexts (e.g. to seat a parent next to the child rather than a sibling) and only become apparent when goals are context specific. Focusing on one task in one context at a time also makes it possible to explore other influences on performance (be they attentional, motoric, interpersonal or environmental) while remaining goal-focused.

Goals used within OPC are stated in the present tense and describe what children can do rather than what they will not or cannot do. For example, *Josh plays quietly* with his brother at home, rather *than Josh does not hit or throw things* at home. The former statement clearly describes the preferred performance rather than the absence of the current performance. This assists parents' visualisation of goal achievement and draws greater attention to the barriers and bridges to enabling performance. Goals are also time-limited. To date, the effectiveness of OPC has been examined using a maximum number of sessions (8 and 10) which essentially created a time frame for goal achievement from the outset of intervention (Graham, Rodger, & Ziviani, in review). When goals are achieved prior to the session limit, intervention is usually terminated.

Sub-goals

If the therapist feels sub-goals are needed, these describe steps of improvement in children's performance in the goal context in much the same way that Goal Attainment Scale (Kiresuk & Sherman, 1968) steps are described. Each step describes an observable difference in performance in the lived environment (see Chapter 6 for more detail). Sub-goals can be worded by:

(1) Describing single steps of improved performance (e.g. Johnny can sit on the toilet as a sub-goal towards toileting independently);
(2) Listing the amount of time or frequency of the performance of the goal statement (e.g. Johnny can play calmly with his brother for 2 min (step 1), for 5 min (step 2), etc.);
(3) Describing performance of the occupation in increasingly complex contexts (e.g. greets others at home (step 1), at pre-school (step 2) and in the community (step 3)).

Explore options

The *explore options* stage is largely guided by the CPA process described earlier. The emphasis is on an exploration of the performance situation and consideration of the options for enabling performance. Direct decision making about *planned actions* is deferred until options have been explored in depth.

While exploring options, therapists may trial techniques with children during performance of tasks and share their thinking with parents. For example, the therapist may talk aloud about what is being attempted, observed and considered while trialling a technique. When considering what techniques to trial, the therapist considers what will work to facilitate children's perform-ance as well as what parents feel is likely to work and that they are able to implement. The therapist's intention in working directly with children is to identify techniques that work and then coach parents' use of them.

As the session transitions to the stage of planning actions, a narrowing of ideas occurs in order to develop specific action plans for the following inter-val between sessions. The therapist guides parents to decide which of the discussed options they anticipate implementing and where, when and how they intend to do this.

Plan actions

The action planning stage involves summarising parents' intended actions over the following week. *Action plans* are checked with parents to ensure they are perceived as doable and likely to work in facilitating goal perform-ance at home or in the community. Doing so brings to light any parental motivation issues in implementing plans (refer to step 4 of CPA for further explanation). Parent-led decision making about the planned action is a critical step towards implementation of plans. The therapist pays close attention to parents' clarity in describing their plans and their optimism in the likeli-hood of success. Any ambiguity is clarified. Despondency (e.g. *I don't like my chances but I'll give it a go*) or detachment (e.g. *I'll try your idea if you like*) may reflect a low sense of self-efficacy or disagreement with the plan and needs to be addressed. Clarifying any hesitation, cynicism or anxious responses from the parent is essential. For example:

- You seem a little unsure about the plan. What is your concern?
- What would be more realistic?
- How confident are you that this plan will work on a scale from 1 to 10?

Emotional support or clarification of information may be needed before the parent is ready to implement changes within the performance context. Plans can be scaled down while still leading to valuable new information by:

- Deciding to observe the child's performance more closely, for example, to observe which parts of the task the child is able to do over the week;
- Asking the child what she or he knows about doing the task during performance;
- Encouraging parents to observe their internal reaction during performance;
- Extending time frames between sessions or choosing one part of the plan to implement.

When parents anticipate making changes with a clear sense of ownership of ideas and an expectation of success, they are far more likely to implement change and to achieve success.

Carry out plan

Carrying out the plan refers to parents' implementation of plans within normal family routines in which goal performance is required. At the initial session, the *carry out plan* stage is explained to parents briefly, but emphasising parent-implemented action. This raises both parents' anticipation of their own action and anticipation of a meaningful improvement in performance. Parents are advised that carrying out the plan refers to using it within the environment in which change is expected to occur and that this is important to find out if the plan actually works for this family.

At the first session, the therapist acknowledges to parents that no matter what happens when plans are implemented valuable information for understanding the performance situation will be gained. Difficulty in carrying out the plan at times is expected. Non-implementation of the plan in subsequent sessions informs the therapist that one of the CPA steps requires attention (e.g. the child's performance needs and the parents' motivation or learning needs). The therapist explores this with the parent by:

● Checking that the parent still thinks that the planned action is likely to work if it could be implemented;
● Listening for the specific difficulty in implementing the plan;
● Acknowledging that there were valid reasons why the plan was difficult to implement;
● Clarifying motivation conflict about implementing versus not implementing the plan;
● Inviting the parent to explore what she or he knows or suspects would make it easier to implement the plan.

Strategies to assist implementation of plans often relate to parents' management of their own self-regulation (e.g. anger at the child and anxiety about the child's response or their own competence). Pausing to take a breath before responding to the child, positive self-talk and reminding oneself of the goal are common strategies parents use to support their implementation of plans.

Check performance

Checking performance involves either observing the child's performance with the parent or asking the parent to report how performance of the task at home or in the community is going. This stage usually occurs at the beginning of subsequent sessions when the effects of previous plans are reviewed. Parents are also encouraged to check performance themselves during the week.

The intention of the therapist when checking performance is to highlight the link between parents' actions and children's more successful performance. Reflections focus on what was different or helpful in the performance context. For example, the therapist may ask how the child went at playing calmly during play dates at home, what was different in the sequence of events, arrangement of the context or parents' own thinking and action (or non-action). Identifying these differences usually requires probing by the therapist and careful listening to parents' narratives. During the first few OPC sessions, two responses from parents are common: first, that performance in goal situations is still 'awful', and second, that performance is better but it was just co-incidental.

When improvement has occurred, but parents are unsure about why, the therapist works from the assumption that the improvement was due to some alteration to the performance context made by the parent. The therapist works with the parent to identify what these differences might be by discussing:

- What was different about the performance and performance context this week?
- What they would make sure they do again next week?
- What they noticed helped, at least a small amount?
- What could they do more of that they suspect might help?

Where parents report no change in performance, the therapist continues the CPA based on a description of performance in which the parent attempted or carried out the plan. Children's response to parents' *attempts* to improve performance even when unsuccessful, provides important information in designing a plan for the following week. Probing and listening for examples of when performance was at its best, worst or even slightly different to normal are fruitful ways of developing a more effective action plan.

Generalise

From the first improvements in children's performance, the therapist prompts parents to consider other tasks, routines and situations (or other children if relevant) for which enabling solutions are applicable. This encourages parents' independent problem-solving and generalisation of strategies. For example, if adjusting child's seating led to improvement in eating at home, the therapist asks where else adjusting sitting position might improve eating. Generalisation prompts include asking parents about future situations in which previous action plans may be useful. Questions might include:

- What other task does your child do that you expect this strategy will be useful for?
- Where else have you noticed yourself automatically using this technique?
- When you think ahead to what life will be like in 6 months time, and you imagine that this situation is going well, what do you notice you/your child are doing?
- What would be the first sign you would notice that would remind you to adjust the situation to keep things going well?
- What would be the first action you would take to get things back on track, to keep the situation going well?

When assisting parents to generalise their current success to future situations, the therapist is mindful of conveying the expectation that parents will continue to be successful in supporting their children with the occupations they find challenging.

In summary, the *structured process* is an essential enabling domain because it:

- Assists the focus on goals;
- Prompts reflection on how specific actions affect goal achievement;
- Encourages parent self-competence by prompting autonomous decision making, action and judgement in relation to children's performance.

Conclusion

This chapter has described an intervention for working with parents of children with occupational performance challenges. We have situated OPC in the contemporary practice environment through an explanation of its theoretical background. Coaching processes were framed within three *enabling domains*, and illustrated through examples of dialogue and case study excerpts. The presented intervention integrates contemporary occupational therapy theory with behavioural, motivational and strengths-focused techniques to assist parents' creation of enabling contexts for children and themselves.

References

Bronfenbrenner, U. (1979). *The ecology of human development*. Cambridge, UK: Harvard University Press.

Chapparo, C., & Ranka, J. (2006). *Perceive Recall Plan Perform training manual*. Sydney, NSW: The University of Sydney.

D'Zurilla, T. J., & Nezu, A. M. (2007). *Problem-solving therapy: A positive approach to clinical intervention* (3rd ed.). New York, NY: Springer.

Daniels, H. (2001). *Vygotsky and pedagogy*. London, UK: Routledge Falmer.

De Jong, P., & Kim Berg, I. (2008). *Interviewing for solutions* (3rd ed.). Belmont, TN: Thomson Brooks/Cole.

Dunst, C., Trivette, C., & Deal, A. (1994). *Supporting and strengthening families: Methods, strategies and practices*. Cambridge, UK: Brookline Books.

Fisher, A., & Short-Degraff, M. (1993). Improving functional assessment in occupational therapy: Recommendations and philosophy for change. *American Journal of Occupational Therapy, 47*(3), 199-201.

Geldard, D., & Geldard, K. (2005). *Basic personal counselling. A training manual for counsellors* (5th ed.). Frenchs Forest, NSW: Pearson.

Graham, F., Rodger, S., & Ziviani, J. (2009). Coaching parents to enable children's participation: An approach to working with parents and their children. *Australian Occupational Therapy Journal, 56*(1), 16-23.

Graham, F., Rodger, S., & Ziviani, J. (in review). Enabling occupational performance of children through coaching parents: Three case reports. *Physical and Occupational Therapy in Pediatrics*.

Gray, C. (1994). *Comic strip conversations*. Arlington, TX: Future Horizons.

Gray, C., & Arnold, S. (2000). *The new social stories book*. Arlington, TX: Future Horizons.

Greber, C., Ziviani, J., & Rodger, S. (2007). The four quadrant model of facilitated learning. *Australian Occupational Therapy Journal, 54*, S31–S39.

Greene, R., Ablon, J., Goring, J., Raezer-Blakely, L., Markey, J., Monuteaux, M., et al. (2004). Effectiveness of Collaborative Problem Solving in affectively dysregulated children with oppositional-defiant disorder: Initial findings. *Journal of Consulting and Clinical Psychology, 72*(6), 1157–1164.

Kiresuk, T., & Sherman, R. (1968). Goal attainment scaling: A method for evaluating comprehensive community mental health programs. *Community Mental Health Journal, 4*(6), 443–453.

Knowles, M., Holton, E., & Swanson, R. (2005). *The adult learner: The definitive classic in adult education and human resource development* (6th ed.). Amsterdam: Elsevier Butterworth-Heinemann.

Law, M., Baptiste, S., & Mills, J. (1995). Client-centred practice: What does it mean and does it make a difference. *Canadian Journal of Occupational Therapy, 62*(5), 250–257.

Law, M., Cooper, B., Strong, B., Stewart, D., Rigby, P., & Letts, L. (1996). The person-environment occupation model: A transactive approach to occupational performance. *Canadian Journal of Occupational Therapy, 63*(1), 9–23.

Locke, E., & Latham, G. P. (1990). *A theory of goal setting and task performance*. Englewood Cliffs, NJ: Prentice-Hall.

Long, C. E., Gurka, M. J., & Blackman, J. A. (2008). Family stress and children's language and behaviour problems. *Topics in Early Childhood Special Education, 28*(3), 148–157.

McKenna, K., & Tooth, R. (2006). *Client education: A partnership approach for health practitioners*. Sydney, NSW: University of New South Wales Press.

Meichenbaum, D., & Biemiller, A. (1998). *Nurturing independent learners*. Cambridge, MA: Brookline.

Murphy, B. C., & Dillon, C. (2008). *Interviewing in action in a multicultural world*. Belmont, TN: Thomson.

Nezu, C., Palmatier, A., & Nezu, A. (2004). Problem-solving therapy for caregivers. In E. Chang, T. D'Zurilla, & L. Sanna (Eds.), *Social problem solving: Theory, research and training* (pp. 223–238). Washington, DC: American Psychological Association.

Polatajko, H. J., & Mandich, A. D. (2004). Enabling occupation in children: *The Cognitive Orientation to daily Occupational Performance (CO-OP) approach*. Ottawa, ON: CAOT Publications ACE.

Polatajko, H. J., Mandich, A. D., & Martini, R. (2000). Dynamic performance analysis: A framework for understanding occupational performance. *American Journal of Occupational Therapy, 54*(1), 65–72.

Polatajko, H., Mandich, A., Missiuna, C., Miller, L., Macnab, J., Malloy-Miller, T., et al. (2001). Cognitive Orientation to Daily Occupational Performance (CO-OP): Part III: The protocol in brief. *Physical & Occupational Therapy in Pediatrics, 20*(2/3), 107–123.

Powell, D., & Batsche, C. (1997). A strengths based approach in support of multi-risk families: Principles and issues. *Topics in Early Childhood Special Education, 17*(1), 1–26.

Rogers, C. R. (1951). *Client-centered therapy: Its current practice, implications and theory*. Boston, MA: Houghton Mifflin.

Stiebel, D. (1999). Promoting augmentive communication during daily routines: A parent problem-solving intervention. *Journal of Positive Behavior Interventions, 1*(3), 159–169.

Vuchinich, S. (2004). Problem-solving training for families. In E. Chang, T. D'Zurilla, & L. Sanna (Eds.), *Social problem solving: Theory, research and training* (pp. 209–222). Washington, DC: American Psychological Association.

Wade, S., Michaud, L., & Brown, T. (2006). Putting the pieces together: Preliminary efficacy of a family problem-solving intervention for children with traumatic brain injury. *Journal of Head Trauma Rehabilitation, 21*(1), 57–67.

World Health Organisation. (2001). *International classification of functioning, disability and health (ICF)* (Short version ed.). Geneva: World Health Organisation.

Chapter 11

Occupation-centred Intervention in the School Setting

Elizabeth A. Hinder and Jill Ashburner

Learning objectives

The objectives of this chapter are to:

- Provide insights into the occupations of the school student and those of the school-based occupational therapist.
- Illustrate the unique contribution of occupational therapy to the educational experience and outcomes of learners with special needs.
- Describe the central tenets of an education–ecological model.
- Highlight key influences of contemporary education and inclusive practice on occupation-centred practice in schools.
- Focus on the collaboration with the educational team that underpins occupation-centred information gathering and intervention.

Occupation in action: Timmy's tale

From the second-story staffroom the team can see disaster unfolding in the playground below.

Atop the climbing castle, just beside the slide sits Timmy – stiff, statue-like, suspended.

'How on earth did he make it up there?' 'Who is going to get him down?' 'Where is the duty-teacher hiding?'

Suddenly, Curtis, the King of the Castle, appears from behind, towering over Timmy's tiny frame.

'Oh no!' Curtis breaks the 'hands and feet to ourselves' rule. *'This is going to be ugly!'*

(Continued)

227

As if discovering your feet are off the ground isn't tough enough, to be violated by touch, pushed-and-shoved no less, sent hurtling down the slipperiest of slides, only to crash land in hideous sand ... this will surely be the bitter end.

Two of the disaster response team deploy immediately down the stairs. As they reach the playground they realise something is seriously wrong with the scene. There is no screaming to be heard. There is no duty-teacher racing to the castle.

'Has Timmy completely shut-down?' 'Is he injured?' 'Has Curtis gagged him in anticipation of the 'thinking corner'?'

The response team is stilled in its tracks ... Timmy is seen ascending once more, tentatively crossing the moat on the suspension bridge, edging to the slide. Timmy stops and stiffens.

Curtis suddenly booms 'Ready, Set, GO!'

Timmy shoves with all his might ... The Castle King is dethroned. Timmy's high-pitched squeals of delight can be heard throughout the kingdom. The ruckus continues. Round two, then three, then more. 'Grab the camera, Mum will want to see this'. The bell has gone, but not even the King can convince Timmy to leave the castle. The team could not be more thrilled with the tale's ending.

New goals abuzz already ... 'Managing activity transitions from play-ground to classroom may need some work?!'

Timmy is a player (although a little perseverative some may per-ceive), a participant.

'Was it all that targeted work on gravitational insecurity and sensory-motor experiences as part of the class's Be-Active program?', 'That turn-taking practice at morning greeting', 'Mum's diligence with family time in the park?', 'The school's new Friendship Program', 'Time at the messy play table?', 'The recommendations for sandpit time?', 'Ready-set-go drills in Physical Education class?', 'Perhaps the trained assistant last term for supported peer play time?'.

Or, has it been the team's unflinching focus on Timmy one day becoming a member of the royal kingdom?

Understanding the occupations of the school student

Participation in the occupations of schooling is a fundamental element of being a child in today's world and one which shapes the futures of young people and communities. School is recognised as having a major influence on children, and outside the family, purported to be the primary contributor to societal social, economic and psychological outcomes (Law, Petrenchik, Ziviani, & King, 2006).

Not all children benefit equally from the educational opportunities on offer, experience the same membership of a school community, successes in performance or readiness for transition to adult roles and occupations. Children challenged by disability and disadvantage may benefit from access to occupational therapy services, integrated within their education. Occupational therapists, working as team members, are optimally positioned to facilitate engagement in everyday school occupations and attainment of positive educational and meaningful life outcomes.

For occupational therapists, occupation is the lens through which experiences are viewed, the destination towards which opportunities are focused and the means through which goals are attained. For those working in school settings, the distinctive compass that guides this occupational journey is education, the business of teaching and learning. From the time the student enters the school grounds until the school bell signals day's end, the child is expected not only to participate in the education programme, but also to manage daily living and social tasks critical to school success (Pape & Ryba, 2004). The school-based occupational therapist must attend to student occupations in academic, social and self-help domains, as well as extracurricular and post-school life goals (Swinth, Spencer, & Jackson, 2007). In addition to the occupational roles of learner, player and classmate, possible student roles may include band member, sportsperson or debater. Appreciation of life roles held beyond the school yard is also important in understanding the child's unique occupational profile. These are addressed further in Chapter 12.

A child's occupational engagement leads to skill mastery, role identity and performance competence (Rodger & Ziviani, 2006). The child's occupational repertoire and achievements are shaped by his or her opportunities and challenges at school (Polichino, Frolek Clark, Swinth, & Muhlenhaupt, 2007), particularly as school may be viewed as the child's first workplace (Chapparo & Hooper, 2002). The occupational roles of a student are to some extent pre-determined by the expected daily education routines. Certain obligatory school occupations (which may not be seen as desirable by students) comprise the 'need to do' rather than 'want to do' activities of schooling, much like some aspects of the adult worker role.

Like others, children with disabilities have a strong need for belonging, acceptance and positive recognition. From a student's perspective, the social experience of school can be more important than academic success. Motivation, attitude and self-perception have a strong impact on learning (Jalongo, 2007), as highlighted in *Timmy's Tale*. Children are more likely to seek optimal challenges if they have experienced success and avoid challenging tasks if they have experienced failure, exclusion or criticism (Case-Smith, Richardson, & Schultz-Krohn, 2005).

Understanding specific occupational contexts and their impact on student role execution and participation is critical for the school-based occupational therapist. School-based occupational therapists can use their occupational lens to promote awareness of the child's and family's perspectives on learning and participation (Handley-More & Chandler, 2007) as seen in the following: Kate is a bubbly 'tweenager' who shares with her friends a passion for fashion, movies and Hollywood gossip. Break time at school is filled with 'model shoots', 'red carpet events' and 'personal training sessions'. Kate has a mild intellectual impairment. In this last year of primary school, she is having some difficulties keeping up in science and maths, despite the curriculum adjustments that have been made. The class teacher is looking to include Kate in the tutorial group with five other students, which runs each lunch-time for 20 min. The occupational therapist raises the team's awareness of the valued occupations and activities Kate currently engages in at break time, providing avenues for recreation, physical activity and restoration from the demands of the morning academic programme. Perhaps above all else, the occupational therapist helps the team appreciate Kate's participation and accomplishment in her occupational roles as a player and a friend. These areas have been a focus of the Individual Education Plan over the years. Staff members are keen to regroup with Kate and her family to re-examine learning goals and strategies. In the meantime, fractions will wait.

Educationally relevant occupational therapy in schools

Social, political and professional influences have steered the evolution of school-based therapy services, converging into three fundamental features of school-based practice (Whitmere, 2002):

(1) contextually based assessments
(2) educationally relevant intervention plans
(3) collaborative consultation

Occupational therapists working towards effective school-based practice must shift between education systems and occupational therapy frames of reference (Muhlenhaupt, 1993). Therapists must first seek to understand the unique culture, routines and philosophies of schools, legislative and policy frameworks, and the way these influence practice (Swinth et al., 2007). Appreciation of the implicit socio-cultural expectations of the education environment enables therapists to practice with cultural diplomacy and responsiveness (Simmons Carlsson, 2006).

The school system contrasts sharply with traditional occupational therapy practice areas (Muhlenhaupt, 1993). A paradigm shift in cultures, attitudes and practices from a dominant biomedical model to an education–ecological model is required (Simmons Carlsson, Hocking, & Wright-St Clair, 2007). This may involve re-framing the expectations of other team members, such as teachers and parents who have not experienced collaborative goal-directed therapy (Hanft & Shepherd, 2008). Some may experience uncertainties tran-sitioning from a family-centred early childhood to a school-focused model (Alliston, 2007). Taking time to clarify service parameters and understand others' expectations and roles is essential (Friend & Cook, 2007).

Educational relevance refers to therapy services which assist in explaining and enhancing a student's performance and participation at school (Hanft & Place, 1996). Interventions translocated from a biomedical model into a school context do not necessarily constitute educationally appropriate or responsive services. Occupational therapists must explicitly examine and address the student's occupational roles, abilities and performance within the education setting. Bundy (1993, 1995) referred to four key areas of student performance, to which occupational therapists can contribute:

(1) Acquiring information (e.g. accessible learning materials and compatible instructional methods);
(2) Expressing learning (e.g. handwriting, keyboarding, assistive technology and augmentative communication access);
(3) Assuming the student role (e.g. regulating behaviour, interacting with classmates and manipulating learning materials);
(4) Performing school self-care (e.g. toileting, eating lunch and dressing for swimming) and mobility activities (e.g. using wheelchair and maintaining sitting posture).

The occupational therapist working in schools cannot adopt an all-encompassing or rehabilitation role (Cantin, 2007), nor work towards occupational therapy-specific objectives. Endeavours must be targeted towards supporting the teaching and learning process, and enabling the student to achieve the educational goals agreed upon by the whole team (Dole, Arvidson, Byrne, Robbins, & Schasberger, 2003). School-based therapists need to delineate school-related needs from those that do not influence a child's education and empower families to access other community resources for issues that fall beyond the scope of practice of school-based occupational therapy (Dunn, 2000). For example, the occupational therapist might provide the team with information to enable the family to choose an appropriate home-visiting service for bathroom modifications.

Ways of working in schools

Collaborative practice is necessary for successful inclusive education (Bose & Hinojosa, 2008; Friend & Cook, 2007; Hines, 2008) and effective occupational therapy in schools (Hasselbusch & Penman, 2008). Collaborative consultation refers to the interactive process involving individuals with diverse expertise who work together, as equal partners, to enhance the academic achievement and functional performance of students (Hanft & Shepherd, 2008). Co-responsibility (Giangreco, Cloninger, & Iverson, 1998) and horizontal power-sharing (Townsend et al., 2007) are central tenets of team-centred practice. The development of collaborative relationships in schools requires conscious investment of time and effort (Hanft & Shepherd, 2008). Teachers and caregivers must be seen as equal team members, while students themselves remain the central focus of the collaborative partnership. In this chapter, 'education team' refers to the student, family, educational and related personnel who work together towards common educational goals.

Therapeutic interventions can inadvertently have negative collateral effects, such as compromised instruction time, schedule disruption, social segregation or stigmatisation. Service providers in schools are urged by Giangreco (2000) to consider if the service is only as specialised as is necessary, compared to that delivered to peers. The question is not whether the student may benefit from therapy (Bundy, 1993), but rather, from a less is more perspective, what is required for the student to benefit fully from education. Occupational therapists must therefore look for unobtrusive ways to support students within available routines, schedules and daily life situations, minimising occupational hindrance or educational disruption (Ziviani & Muhlenhaupt, 2006).

Planning educational programmes for diverse learners

For students with special needs, education practices have been profoundly influenced by the development of the *Salamanca Statement and Framework for Action on Special Needs Education* (United Nations Educational Scientific and Cultural Organization & Ministry of Education and Science Spain, 1994), which heralded unprecedented attention to the rights of all learners. The central tenets of this statement include:

- Every child has a basic right to education.
- Every child has unique characteristics, interests, abilities and learning needs.
- Education services should take into account these diverse characteristics and needs.
- Those with special educational needs must have access to regular schools.
- Regular schools with an inclusive ethos are the most effective way to combat discriminatory attitudes, create welcoming and inclusive communities and achieve education for all.

While not universal, many countries (e.g. Australia, Canada, New Zealand, the UK and the USA) have followed this lead in the development of inclusive policies, procedures and practices (Giangreco et al., 1998). The Salamanca Statement cites occupational therapists as one of the resource personnel who can play a lead role in supporting the educational needs of students. Giangreco (2001) asserted the education team should first consider expected learning outcomes for the student with a disability, before considering supports required. Supports may include those designed to cater for personal and physical needs, to educate others about the nature of the student's disability and its impact on learning, and accommodations to the environment or curriculum to enable the student to participate. Occupational therapists can form part of this support structure, using a unique understanding of the student's disability and school occupations to work towards desired learning outcomes.

Two key pedagogical practices underpinning inclusive education include differentiated instruction and 'Universal Design for Learning' (van Kraayenoord, 2007). Differentiated instruction involves modification to curriculum, teaching structures and practices to ensure instruction is relevant, flexible and responsive to student needs. Modifications may involve content simplification or reduction, use of different resources, additional instruction or assistance, re-teaching concepts or use of peer tutoring. Expectations may be changed by altering the expected output required or enabling the student to present work in a different way (Westwood, 1998).

For example, the occupational therapist recommends adaptive ruling and compass equipment (using different resources), and alteration of expected design scale (adjusting expected outcomes), to enable Chris, a student with hemiplegia, to achieve success in Technical Drawing classes.

'Universal Design for Learning' (Rose & Meyer, 2006) aims to ensure that products (e.g. curriculum) and environments (e.g. classrooms) are designed to be usable by as many people as possible. In contrast to differentiated instruction, it aims to address the diversity of learners at the point of curriculum development, rather than attempting to adapt or retrofit the curriculum. Multiple means of representation such as video, text, speech, Braille and images are made available to provide students various ways of acquiring and expressing learning. Advances in technology (e.g. textbooks in digital format) are enabling more students to use multiple means to demonstrate learning aptitude. School-based occupational therapists may use universal design principles when advising on programmes or environments that are accessible to students with diverse needs.

For example, the occupational therapist collaborates with the school technology committee and Principal, advocating for installation of assistive software on all school computers to suit the variety of learners on campus who experience challenges with reading on-screen text (including those with disabilities, learning difficulties and students from different linguistic backgrounds).

van Kraayenoord (2007) maintains that a combination of differentiated instruction and universal design principles is usually required to effectively meet the needs of students with diverse learning needs. Curricula and teaching strategies should be developed using 'Universal Design for Learning' principles; however, further modification may still be necessary to meet the needs of all learners.

Occupation-centred information gathering in educational settings

The team's priority education goals and desired outcomes need to be identified at the outset. The process must begin with identifying occupations the student needs and wants to do, from the perspective of all team members (Swinth et al., 2007). The intervention that follows should have this same outcomes focus. In other words, start where you mean to finish (Molineux, 2004).

Contemporary school-based occupational therapy requires an occupation-centred approach to assessment as described in Chapter 7. The focus is on occupational engagement at school, rather than underlying performance components (e.g. capacity to produce an assignment rather than visual-motor skills for handwriting). Improvements in performance components have not been found to translate automatically to gains in occupational performance (Mathiowetz & Haugen, 1995). Component skills are only evaluated when the cause of the occupational issue is not apparent and there is a need to clarify the nature of the performance difficulty in order to support success (Dunbar, 2007; Hocking, 2001). The student's capacity to complete a task under optimal conditions may not always equate to daily school performance. Attention must also be paid to the student's intrinsic habits and motivations (Keilhofner, 2002). There may also be extrinsic environmental barriers, such as under-estimation or unrealistic expectations of the student or school routines, environments or staff attitudes that are not conducive to optimal performance. Therefore, an ecological assessment approach, focused on uncovering obstacles to occupational engagement and success, is essential (Quake-Rapp, Miller, Ananthan, & Chiu, 2008).

In order to examine the 'fit' between the student and the school environment, the therapist evaluates contextual factors (Hanft & Shepherd, 2008), including the:

- Physical environment (e.g. accessibility of classroom, bathroom, playground, sporting facilities, etc.);
- Social environment (e.g. playground observations may reveal bullying issues that underlie a student's maladaptive behaviour);
- Cultural environment (e.g. differences between schools and classrooms in structure, permissiveness, standards of behaviour, flexibility and tolerance of diversity) (Stoll, 2000);
- Sensory environment (e.g. levels of background noise, visual clutter, crowding, etc.);
- 'Virtual' environment, as digital technologies have an increasing role in students' occupations (Hanft & Shepherd, 2008) (e.g. conducting research, accessing information electronically, completing assignments, communicating, social networking and engaging in 'virtual' realities and communities).

The temporal aspects of school participation also warrant assiduous consideration (Hanft & Shepherd, 2008) such as the:

- Daily schedule (e.g. of a student with arthritis who experiences fatigue);
- School routine and break schedule (e.g. for a student with spina bifida required to manage self-catheterisation and wishing to join her friends at recess);

- School calendar (e.g. a significant curriculum adjustment proposed for the new school year with a new teacher, rather than at the end of a school year);
- Transitions (e.g. from an early childhood setting to school or elementary to high school). These are critical periods for occupational therapy evaluation, to determine needs in preparation for transition and predict adjustments required in new settings (Myers, 2008).

School-based occupational therapists also need to gather information on the instructional approaches used in the classroom and contribute to discussions on their suitability to particular students. For example, 'active learning' principles (Bonwell & Eison, 1991) that are used to cognitively engage students with the learning material may be advantageous for students who have difficulty remaining still or focused; however, increased sensory challenges may overwhelm other learners (Anderson, 2001). 'Cooperative learning' (Gillies, 2007) where small groups of students work together may challenge those who have difficulties with social interaction (Macintosh & Dissanayake, 2006). 'Constructivist learning' (Liu & Matthews, 2005) which focuses on student-guided 'construction' of knowledge may challenge individuals with limitations in cognition and memory. These students may benefit from direct or explicit instruction, such as the provision of a worked example to guide their learning (Kroesbergen & Van Luit, 2005).

The assessment process in schools may include a combination of: record reviews (e.g. school file, previous education, therapy or health service reports and referral information); interviews with education team members (including the student and parents) about the student's history, concerns, priorities and preferences; narratives, structured and unstructured observations; and the use of informal and formal assessment tools. The occupational therapist can be pivotal in advocating that student voice, irrespective of communication competencies, be captured and truly reflected in the education planning process. Children as young as 5 years are able to rate their own competence, and select and prioritise goals (Missiuna & Pollock, 2000). The occupational therapist, wherever possible, involves the student in assessment, in order to foster engagement and self-determination from the commencement of the collaborative partnership (Dunbar, 2007).

Skilled observation may be used to determine the student's ability to perform aspects of the student role, habits and routines. Observations of the student may be naturalistic (without a pre-determined behaviour in mind) or systematic (specific behaviours elicited by a pre-determined set of environmental stimuli) (Hintze & Matthews, 2004). It is especially important to observe the occupations and environments that have been identified as most challenging for the student. The *Observation of the School Environment* (Hanft & Shepherd, 2008) is designed to assist in structuring observations of the classroom environment.

Standardised, norm-referenced assessments measuring performance and component skills were used almost exclusively in school settings.

However, contemporary tools and methods are now needed to facilitate occupation-centred goal setting and outcome measurement of significance to the student and team. These tools enable:

(1) Self- or caregiver-report that tap the meaning of the occupation to the child and/or his or her family;
(2) Examination of not only the child's perception of their skill, but also how important the occupation is to them;
(3) Empowerment of the child and/or his or her family to set their own goals.

Table 11.1 describes examples of student self-assessments tools, team goal setting and planning tools, and measures that can be used to determine capacity of the child to assume the student role, express learning and perform the self-care and mobility activities required at school. Assessment must not be viewed in isolation, or an end in itself, but rather interwoven throughout the entire therapy process (Laver Fawcett, 2007). Systematic data collection should be used to determine the impact of intervention on educationally important occupational domains, such as student accomplishment of learning tasks and participation in the education context (Swinth et al., 2007).

Occupation-centred programme planning and intervention in schools

Information gathered regarding valued occupations and priorities is used to steer a top-down, occupation-centred approach to intervention, integrated into the education programme (Polatajko, Davis, Stewart, Cantin, & Amoroso, 2007). Intervention aims to maximise the fit between the student's abilities and the demands of school occupations, curriculum and classroom activities, expectations of teachers, and the school's physical, social and cultural environments (Moyers, 2005). The focus must be on successful participation in needed and valued school occupations (Dunbar, 2007), functional outcomes (Law, 2006) and development of a positive student identity (Simmons Carlsson et al., 2007).

Intervention in schools to address occupational challenges may focus on:

● Provision of advice regarding modifications or adjustments to the environment, to lessen the discrepancy between setting demands and the student's ability to learn (Rourk, 1996);
● Changing the expectations, skills or behaviours of others, to facilitate the student's participation in education (Dunn, 2000);
● Specific interventions to develop performance capacities into the functional skills required for access and participation in the education programme.

Research indicates clearly that an intervention focus on component abilities often fails to improve function and participation at school (Denton, Cope, & Moser, 2006). Therefore, the focus must remain on access to and participation

Table 11.1   Assessment tools for education settings

Assessment focus			Tool examples
Goal setting and planning	Student self-assessment/interview		• Student Interview Questionnaire (Sage, 2008) • Child Occupation Self-Assessment (Keller, Kafkes, Basu, Federico, & Kielhofner, 2005) • *School Setting Interview* (Hemmingson, Egilson, Hoffman, & Keilhofner, 2005) • *Canadian Occupational Performance Measure* (Law et al., 2005) • *Perceived Efficacy and Goal Setting* (Missiuna, Pollock, & Law, 2004)
	Student-centred team goal setting and planning		• Making Action Plans (Falvey, Forest, Pearpoint, & Rosenbury, 2004) • *Choosing Outcomes and Accommodations for Children: A Guide to Planning for Students with Disabilities* (Giangreco et al., 1998) • *Vermont Interdependent Services Team Approach* (Giangreco, 1996) • *Goal Attainment Scaling* (Kiresuk, Smith, & Cardillo, 1994)
Performance of occupational role of student	Ability to assume student role	Role of 'learner' (e.g. classroom behaviour regulation, following directions and rules, manipulation of classroom objects)	• *School Function Assessment* (Coster, Deeney, Haltiwanger, & Haley, 1998)
		Role of 'player' (e.g. social skills, play and recreational skills)	• *School Function Assessment* (Coster et al., 1998) • See play and leisure assessments listed in Chapter 7

(Continued)

Table 11.1 (Continued)

Assessment focus			Tool examples
	Ability to express learning	Handwriting speed and legibility	• *The McMaster Handwriting Assessment Protocol* (Pollock et al., 2008) • *Developmental Assessment of Speed of Handwriting* (Barnett, Henderson, Scheib, & Schulz, 2007) • *Evaluation Tool of Children's Handwriting* (Amundsen, 1995)
		Use of keyboarding devices, computers, communication output devices, etc.	• The *School Function Assessment Assistive Technology Supplement* (Silverman, Stratman, Grogan, & Smith, 2003) • *Lifespace Access Profile* (Williams, Stemach, Wolfe, & Stanger, 1994)
	Ability to perform self-care and mobility tasks		• *Pediatric Evaluation of Disability Inventory* (Haley, Coster, Ludlow, Haltiwanger, & Andrellos, 1992)
Assessment of school environment	Observations of the physical, sensory, cultural, social, virtual environments Student's assessment of support at school		• Observation of the School Environment (Hanft & Shepherd, 2008) • Student Perceptions of Classroom Support Scale (O'Rourke & Houghton, 2008)

in education and removal of obstacles to occupational engagement, rather than remediation. A multifaceted intervention using a combination of compatible approaches is often effective (Muhlenhaupt, 2003).

Using an ecological intervention approach, the school becomes the therapeutic context (Hasselbusch & Penman, 2008). The occupational therapist, wherever possible, uses the natural situations, routines, curriculum and resources within the school environment to collaboratively design education programmes and interventions. Occupational therapy interventions need to be grounded in curriculum content and in the classroom and schoolyard (Ziviani & Muhlenhaupt, 2006). Attention must be given to not only the curriculum, teaching and learning processes, but also the non-academic and extracurricular activities that form part of the student's full school experience (Ziviani & Muhlenhaupt, 2006). Intervention should involve selection and custom-design of activities that are meaningful and appealing to the student and allow him or her to experience success (Heah, Case, McGuire, & Law, 2007).

Collaboration in service delivery

As with assessment, best practice programme planning and intervention must reflect the agreed priorities of the education team. Options can be negotiated in a collaborative partnership that recognises the rights of individuals to consider alternatives, choose or decline interventions, and take risks and responsibility for decisions (Townsend et al., 2007). Attitudes communicated and supports provided at school can be crucial to development of positive life pathways for individuals with disabilities (King, Willoughby, Specht, & Brown, 2006).

Intervention in the school context requires the therapist to adopt interactive clinical-reasoning processes and work alongside team members at their pace to arrive at shared understandings and mutually owned solutions (Hasselbusch & Penman, 2008). Attention to adult-learning preferences, tolerance for change and awareness of the individual needs of parents and other adult team members are required (Handley-More & Chandler, 2007). Soliciting information on a teacher's philosophy of classroom management and past experiences enables the therapist to tailor suggestions to suit specific situations (Hasselbusch & Penman, 2008). Teachers value interventions they consider feasible and appropriate for their students and that are accompanied by materials and professional development support as needed (Wehrmann, Chiu, Reid, & Sinclair, 2006).

In accordance with evidence-informed practice, occupational therapists have a responsibility to provide meaningful information regarding the effectiveness of potential interventions, and the pros, cons and possible consequences of each option available (King et al., 2007). The optimal solution, based on theory and quantitative evidence, may prove impractical in the circumstances or not acceptable to the team. Therefore, by providing alternate strategies and different approaches to address the identified issues, the occupational therapist enables students and their teams to select an approach considered the best match for their specific school situation (Dunbar, 2007). See Chapter 15 for a further discussion of balancing evidence, experience and pragmatic issues in professional decision making. Effective collaboration requires blending of direct occupational therapy services with the team and system supports for students, families, educators and the school system. Hanft and Shepherd (2008) have contended collaboration should not be viewed as a type of service delivery model, but rather as the interactive team process underpinning practice including direct student, team and system supports.

Direct or 'hands-on' occupational therapy services must be explicitly related to current curriculum content or school task priorities. Wherever possible, these supports should be delivered within the context of typical lessons or natural school activities and routines (Hanft & Shepherd, 2008). To achieve positive outcomes, direct supports should be delivered in confluence with team and/or system supports (Hanft & Shepherd, 2008).

Frances, the school-based OT, was asked to review Angie's toileting needs and provide advice for placement of rails in the proposed amenities block. Angie was a convivial, self-assured student aged 10 years. On initial interview, Angie's skills and aspirations highlighted her future capacity to live and work independently. In-home support to assist with dressing, bathing and meal preparation would be likely to be required throughout Angie's life. However, Frances felt Angie's inability to use the toilet independently may limit her future participation in social, community and work environments. Rather than restricting intervention to rail prescription, Frances explored with the team ideas for developing Angie's toileting skills. They realised that this would require some changes to Angie's school day for a period, and to the OT timetable, but all agreed that independent toileting was important for Angie to achieve the fullest participation in her desired future.

Frances completed observational assessment and task analysis which revealed that Angie was able to transfer from her power wheelchair to the toilet independently using a rail in an accessible bathroom; however, she required assistance to manage her underpants. She could maintain a standing position while holding a rail, but she lacked the ability to reach and reposition her underpants. Grasping the fabric of her garments was also challenging. Frances provided information to Angie's mother who adapted several pairs of Angie's underpants. Loops sewn on both sides using a rigid cloth tape formed openings through which Angie could place her thumb to help pull her underpants up and down.

Frances, Angie and Mrs. Brown, the teaching assistant, worked together in the bathroom once a day for the following week, practicing and refining the new components of the task. Mrs. Brown worked with Angie on all other toileting occasions that week and was asked by Frances to allow Angie to persist for 5 min before stepping in to help if needed. By the end of the third week, Angie had mastered the task, albeit slowly. Angie's investment at age 10 years, and that of her team, afforded her independence and dignity as she progressed through school and college to her full-time work as a medical receptionist.

Team supports are those strategies used to enhance the competency of another to support a student's participation and achievement, by increasing the knowledge and skills of key people in the student's day (Hanft & Shepherd, 2008). The focus is on equipping personnel to enable occupational success at school (Hasselbusch & Penman, 2008). This may involve collaborative consultation, co-teaching, monitoring progress, educating others, supporting individual education planning processes or re-framing the understandings of others. Re-framing may either lay the foundation for agreed curriculum adjustments or make adjustments unnecessary by altering team perspectives (Hasselbusch & Penman, 2008). In addition, peer coaching and modelling are powerful team support strategies (Van Meter & Stevens, 2000).

Lunchtime participation was proving a challenge for Joel, and those around him. 'Intervention' involved the occupational therapist, speech-therapist and class teacher working with Joel's classmates. In a series of lessons, Joel's peers learned specific friendship skills to support his successful participation in the hustle and bustle of snack time. They were provided with personal communication resources that could help them get the message across to their friends more effectively if things were not going to plan (visual symbols reinforcing what needed to happen, e.g. 'Scraps go in the bin'). In science, they learned about the senses and identified their class-mates' preferences. They decided that 'smelly' snacks might best be left for home time. The class designed a digital Social Story™ using PowerPoint® entitled 'Lunchtime and Playtime at Eastville Primary'. The teacher decided this would be a great resource to share with the students in the Prep entry class. The speech-therapist thought this would be a useful tool for her work with the new students in the English as Second Language group. The grounds person painted bright new lines on the long benches to define sit-ting spaces. Two buddies nominated to take turns to remind Joel to 'finish eating'. Everyone wanted to have plenty of time to play together, as Joel is Eastville's soccer legend ... and always has to kick-off!

Hanft and Shepherd (2008) describe system supports as the formal and informal initiatives and communications that support schools to respond to diverse learner needs. These serve to benefit students beyond those directly receiving occupational therapy services.

The local school authority is building a new super-campus that will merge the existing primary and secondary facilities. The occupational therapist works with the district planning taskforce to address two particular areas of identi-fied need. She provides information to the parents and citizens' association on universal design for learning principles and successfully advocates for the purchase of school furniture that is ergonomically sound and multi-adjustable. She contributes to the design of a new playground that will be accessible and appealing to a wide range of students, from those with disabilities to active able-bodied students seeking physical challenges. During the planning process, the occupational therapist uses available opportunities to provide education about children's occupations, physical activity, play and development to the wider community, including the increasingly well-versed construction company.

A contemporary occupational therapy framework used in educational settings, known as the Match the Activity to the Child (MATCH) strategy (Lockhart & Missiuna, 2007), is illustrated in the case of Adam below and in Table 11.2.

Adam is a 9-year-old boy, in a 4th grade class, who has an impressive ability to produce elaborate illustrations of dinosaurs. He has a diagnosis of Asperger's syndrome. Adam was referred because his teacher and parents shared concerns about his increasing emotional regulation difficulties in the classroom. A class behaviour management plan using a star chart was ineffective, as Adam rarely accrued the 10 stars required for a reward. When asked about things he would like to change about school, Adam replied: 'shut the loud kids up when I'm trying to think'. The teacher reported Adam often complained that other students had 'hit' him when they inadvertently brushed past. The occupational therapist noticed that Adam became visibly distressed during a noisy co-operative learning task. He walked to the back of the room, began to twist his hair and hum. When the teacher tried to re-direct

Table 11.2 MATCH strategies to assist Adam

MATCH strategy	Examples for Adam
Modify the task	• Teaming Adam with quiet self-directed student for cooperative learning tasks as alternative to group work
Altering expectations	• Reducing number of stickers required for reward and expanding target behaviours to be rewarded
Teach: using a different teaching approach	• Increasing use of visual instructions, rather than relying on auditory instruction • Capitalising on Adam's strengths and interests in learning tasks, appointing him as illustrator for group projects • Developing *Sensory Story* (Marr, Mika, Miralgia, Roerig, & Simmott, 2007) to teach Adam to manage situations with excessive noise by using Apple® iPod with calming music
Changing the environment	• Re-positioning Adam's desk and grouping with a quiet cohort of classmates • Providing classroom retreat corner with self-selected cushions and calming music on headsets
Helping by understanding	• Educating team about functional significance of sensory processing issues for Adam • Assisting teacher to recognise signs of escalating sensory reactions, reducing 'overload' events and supporting participation • Teaching Adam to alert teacher of stress by using 'I need a break' card

him to the learning task, he cried and threw his pencil across the room. The Sensory Profile School Companion (Dunn, 2006) revealed high levels of sensitivity to noise and touch. Systematically recorded observations confirmed the team's suspicions that Adam's emotional and behavioural difficulties were often precipitated by group activities in which Adam was exposed to high levels of noise and unexpected touch.

Regardless of the supports delivered, intervention needs to be dynamically interrelated with ongoing assessment as a means to evaluate responses and make adjustments as required (Youngstrom, 2005). A student's occupational needs, contexts and roles are not static throughout schooling. Evaluation of the outcomes of occupational therapy intervention needs to focus on changes in occupational performance (e.g. ability to perform, enhanced ability to perform or prevention of potential performance problems), and participation in life situations, along with addressing subjective experiences (e.g. perceptions of change, satisfaction with performance or life quality) (Youngstrom, 2005). The ultimate goal of any occupational therapy intervention is collaboration to promote students' academic achievement and engagement in school-related occupations, as part of a full and fulfilling schooling experience (Hanft & Shepherd, 2008).

Conclusion

The stories shared in this chapter illuminate implementation of contemporary occupational therapy practice in the school environment. An occupation-centred approach to information gathering and intervention in schools means services are embedded within routines and rhythms of the school day to support the occupational engagement and success of the school student.

References

Alliston, L. (2007). Principles and practices in early intervention: A literature review for the Ministry of Education, New Zealand. *Education Counts*. Retrieved 15 March 2009 from http://www.educationcounts.govt.nz/publications/special_education/22575.

Amundsen, S. J. (1995). *Evaluation tool of children's handwriting*. Homer, AK: OT Kids Inc.

Anderson, K. L. (2001). Voicing concerns about noisy classrooms. *Educational Leadership, 4*, 77–79.

Barnett, A., Henderson, S. E., Scheib, B., & Schulz, J. (2007). *Developmental assessment of speed of handwriting*. Bloomington, MN: Pearson.

Bonwell, C., & Eison, J. (1991). *Active learning: Creating excitement in the class-room*. Washington, DC: Jossey-Bass.

Bose, P., & Hinojosa, J. (2008). Reported experiences from occupational therapists interacting with teachers in inclusive early childhood classrooms. *American Journal of Occupational Therapy, 62*(3), 289–297.

Bundy, A. (1993). 'Will I see you in September?' A question of educational relevance. *American Journal of Occupational Therapy, 47*(9), 848–850.

Bundy, A. C. (1995). Assessment and intervention in school-based practice: Answering questions and minimizing discrepancies. *Physical & Occupational Therapy in Pediatrics, 15*(2), 69–88.

Cantin, N. (2007). Occupation-based enablement: A practice mosaic: Practice exemplar 7.1. In E. A. Townsend, & H. J. Polatajko (Eds.), *Enabling occupation II: Advancing an occupational therapy vision for health, well-being & justice through occupation* (pp. 191–193). Ottawa, ON: CAOT Publications.

Case-Smith, J., Richardson, P., & Schultz-Krohn, W. (2005). An overview of occupational therapy for children. In J. Case-Smith (Ed.), *Occupational therapy for children* (5th ed., pp. 2–30). St. Louis, MO: Elsevier Mosby.

Chapparo, C., & Hooper, E. (2002). Self-care at school: Perceptions of 6 year old children. *American Journal of Occupational Therapy, 59*(1), 67–77.

Coster, W., Deeney, T., Haltiwanger, L., & Haley, S. (1998). *School Function Assessment*. San Antonio, TX: Psychological Corporation.

Denton, P. L., Cope, S., & Moser, C. (2006). The effects of sensorimotor-based intervention versus therapeutic practice in improving handwriting performance in 6- to 11-year-old children. *American Journal of Occupational Therapy, 60*(1), 1627.

Dole, R. L., Arvidson, K., Byrne, E., Robbins, J., & Schasberger, B. (2003). Consensus among experts in pediatric occupational and physical therapy on elements of Individualized Education Programs. *Pediatric Physical Therapy, 15*(3), 159–166.

Dunbar, S. B. (2007). *Occupational therapy models for intervention with children and families*. Thorofare, NJ: SLACK Inc.

Dunn, W. (2000). *Best practice occupational therapy: In community services with children and families*. Thorofare, NJ: SLACK Inc.

Dunn, W. (2006). *Sensory profile school companion*. San Antonio, TX: Psychological Corporation.

Falvey, M., Forest, J., Pearpoint, J., & Rosenbury, R. (2004). *All my life's a circle: Using the tools: Circles, MAPS and PATHS*. Toronto, ON: Inclusion Press.

Friend, M., & Cook, L. (2007). *Interactions: Collaboration skills for school professionals* (5th ed.). Upper Saddle River, NJ: Pearson Education.

Giangreco, M. F. (1996). *Vermont interdependent services team approach: A guide to coordinating educational support services*. Baltimore, MD: Paul H. Brookes.

Giangreco, M. F. (2000). Related services research for students with low incidence disabilities: Implications for speech language pathologists in inclusive classrooms. *Language, Speech and Hearing Services in the Schools, 31*, 230-239.

Giangreco, M. F. (2001). Interactions among the program, placement and services in educational planning for students with disabilities. *Mental Retardation, 39*(5), 341-350.

Giangreco, M. F., Cloninger, C. J., & Iverson, V. S. (1998). *Choosing outcomes and accommodations for children: A guide to educational planning for students with disabilities*. Baltimore, MD: Brookes.

Gillies, R. M. (2007). *Cooperative learning: Integrating theory and practice*. Thousand Oaks, CA: Sage Publications.

Haley, S. M., Coster, W. J., Ludlow, L. H., Haltiwanger, J. T., & Andrellos, P. J. (1992). *Pediatric evaluation of disability inventory*. Boston, MA: New England Medical Centers Hospital Inc.

Handley-More, D., & Chandler, B. E. (2007). Occupational therapy decision-making process. In L. L. Jackson (Ed.), *Occupational therapy services for children and youth under IDEA* (pp. 59-87). Bethesda, MD: AOTA Press.

Hanft, B., & Shepherd, J. (Eds.). (2008). *Collaborating for student success: A guide for school-based occupational therapy*. Bethesda, MD: AOTA Press.

Hanft, B. E., & Place, P. A. (1996). *The consulting therapist: A guide for OTs and PTs in schools*. San Antonio, CA: Therapy Skill Builders.

Hasselbusch, A., & Penman, M. (2008). Working together: An occupational therapy perspective on collaborative consultation. *Kairaranga, 9*(1), 24-31.

Heah, T., Case, T., McGuire, B., & Law, M. (2007). Successful participation: The lived experience among children with disabilities. *Canadian Journal of Occupational Therapy, 74*(1), 38-47.

Hemmingson, H., Egilson, S., Hoffman, O., & Keilhofner, G. (2005). *School setting interview*. Chicago: Model of Human Occupation, Department of Occupational Therapy, College of Applied Health Sciences, University of Illinois.

Hines, J. T. (2008). Making collaboration work in inclusive high school classrooms: Recommendations for principals. *Intervention in School and Clinic, 43*(5), 277-282.

Hintze, J. M., & Matthews, W. J. (2004). The generalizability of systematic direct observation across time and setting: A preliminary investigation of the psychometrics of behavioural observation. *School Psychology Review, 33*, 258-270.

Hocking, C. (2001). Implementing occupation-based assessment. *American Journal of Occupational Therapy, 55*(4), 463-469.

Jalongo, M. R. (2007). Beyond benchmarks and scores: Reasserting the role of motivation and interest in children's academic achievement. *Childhood Education, 83*(6), 395-407.

Keilhofner, G. (2002). *A model of human occupation: Theory and application* (3rd ed.). Philadelphia, PA: Lippincott Williams & Wilkins.

Keller, J., Kafkes, A., Basu, S., Federico, J., & Kielhofner, G. (2005). *Child Occupational Self Assessment (COSA)*. Chicago: Model of Human Occupation Clearinghouse, Department of Occupational Therapy, College of Applied Health Sciences, University of Illinois.

King, G., Currie, M., Bartlett, D. J., Gilpin, M., Willoughby, C., & Tucker, E. A. (2007). The development of expertise in pediatric rehabilitation therapists: Changes in approach, self-knowledge and use of enabling and customizing strategies. *Developmental Neurorehabilitation, 10*(3), 223–240.

King, G., Willoughby, C., Specht, J. A., & Brown, E. (2006). Social support processes and the adaptation of individuals with chronic disabilities. *Qualitative Health Research, 16*(7), 902–925.

Kiresuk, T. J., Smith, A., & Cardillo, J. E. (1994). *Goal Attainment Scaling: Applications, theory, and measurement*. Philadelphia, PA: Lawrence Erlbaum Associates.

Kroesbergen, E. H., & Van Luit, J. E. H. (2005). Constructivist mathematics education for students with mild mental retardation. *European Journal of Special Needs Education, 20*(1), 107–116.

Laver Fawcett, A. J. (2007) *Principles of assessment and outcome measurement for occupational therapists and physiotherapists: Theory, skills and application*. Chichester, UK: John Wiley & Sons.

Law, M. (2006). *Autism spectrum disorders and occupational therapy, briefing to the Senate Standing Committee on Social Affairs, Science and Technology*. Canadian Association of Occupational Therapists, 9 November 2006, Ottawa, ON. Retrieved 13 April, 2009 from http://canchild.icreate3.esolutionsgroup.ca/en/childrenfamilies/resources/Autism_Brief_Nov_06.pdf.

Law, M., Baptiste, S., Carswell, A., McColl, M. A., Polatajko, H., & Pollock, N. (2005). *Canadian Occupational Performance Measure* (4th ed.). Ottawa, ON: CAOT Press.

Law, M., Petrenchik, T., Ziviani, J., & King, G. (2006). Participation of children in school and community. In S. Rodger, & J. Ziviani (Eds.), *Occupational therapy with children: Understanding children's occupations and enabling participation* (pp. 67–90). Oxford, UK: Blackwell Publishing Ltd.

Liu, C. H., & Matthews, R. (2005). Vygotsky's philosophy: Constructivism and its criticisms examined. *International Education Journal, 6*(3), 386–399.

Lockhart, J., & Missiuna, C. (2007). *Adolescents with motor difficulties: A resource for educators*. Retrieved 15 March 2009 from http://www.canchild.ca/Portals/0/education_materials/pdf/MATCH_Adolescent.pdf.

Macintosh, K., & Dissanayake, C. (2006). Social skills and problem behaviours in school aged children with high functioning autism and Asperger's syndrome. *Journal of Autism and Developmental Disorders, 36*, 1065–1076.

Marr, D., Mika, H., Miralgia, J., Roerig, M., & Simmott, R. (2007). The effect of sensory stories on targeted behaviours in preschool children with autism. *Physical & Occupational Therapy in Pediatrics, 27*(1), 63–69.

Mathiowetz, V., & Haugen, J. B. (1995). Evaluation of motor behavior: Traditional and contemporary views. In C. E. Trombly (Ed.), *Occupational therapy for physical dysfunction* (4th ed., pp. 157–185). Baltimore, MD: Williams & Wilkins.

Missiuna, C., & Pollock, N. (2000). Perceived efficacy and goal setting in young children. *Canadian Journal of Occupational Therapy, 67*(2), 101–109.

Missiuna, C., Pollock, N., & Law, M. (2004). *The Perceived Efficacy and Goal Setting system*. San Antonio, TX: PsychCorp.

Molineux, M. (Ed.). (2004). *Occupation for occupational therapists*. Oxford, UK: Blackwell Publishing.

Moyers, P. (2005). Introduction to occupation-based practice. In C. H. Christiansen, C. M. Baum, & J. B. Bass-Haugen (Eds.), *Occupational therapy performance participation and well-being* (3rd ed., pp. 221–240). Thorofare, NJ: SLACK Inc.

Muhlenhaupt, M. (1993). Frames of reference for pediatric occupational therapy. In P. Kramer, & J. Hinojosa (Eds.), *Influence of settings on the application of frames of references* (pp. 445–473). Baltimore, MD: Williams & Wilkins.

Muhlenhaupt, M. (2003). Enabling student participation through occupational therapy services in schools. In L. Letts, P. Rigby, & D. Stewart (Eds.), *Using environment to enable occupational performance*. Thorofare, NJ: SLACK Inc.

Myers, C. T. (2008). Descriptive study of occupational therapists' participation in early childhood settings. *American Journal of Occupational Therapy, 62*(2), 212–220.

O'Rourke, J., & Houghton, S. (2008). Perceptions of secondary school students with mild disabilities to the academic and social support mechanisms implemented in regular classrooms. *International Journal of Disability, Development and Education, 55*(3), 227–237.

Pape, L., & Ryba, K. (2004). *Practical considerations for school-based occupational therapists*. Bethesda, MD: AOTA Press.

Polatajko, H. J., Davis, J., Stewart, D., Cantin, N., & Amoroso, B. (2007). Specifying the domain of concern: Occupation as core. In E. A. Townsend, & H. J. Polatajko (Eds.), *Enabling occupation II: Advancing an occupational therapy vision for health, well-being & justice through occupation* (pp. 13–36). Ottawa, ON: CAOT Publications.

Polichino, J. E., Frolek Clark, G., Swinth, Y., & Muhlenhaupt, M. (2007). Evaluating occupational performance in schools and early childhood settings. In L. L. Jackson (Ed.), *Occupational therapy services for children and youth under IDEA* (3rd ed.). Bethesda, MD: AOTA Press.

Pollock, N., Lockhart, J., Farhat, L., Jacobson, J., Bradley, J., & Brunetti, S. (2008). *The McMaster handwriting assessment protocol*. Retrieved 15 March 2009 from http://www.canchild.ca/Default.aspx?tabid=2140.

Quake-Rapp, C., Miller, B., Ananthan, G., & Chiu, E. (2008). Direct observation as a means of assessing frequency of maladaptive behaviour in youths with severe emotional and behavioural disorders. *American Journal of Occupational Therapy, 62*(2), 206–211.

Rodger, S., & Ziviani, J. (2006). *Occupational therapy with children: Understanding children's occupations and enabling participation*. Oxford, UK: Blackwell Publishing.

Rose, D. H., & Meyer, A. (Eds.). (2006). *A practical reader in universal design for learning*. Cambridge, MA: Harvard Education Press.

Rourk, J. D. (1996). Nationally speaking: Roles of school-based occupational therapists: Past, present, future. *American Journal of Occupational Therapy, 50*(9), 698–700.

Sage, J. (2008). Student Interview Questionnaire. In B. Hanft, & J. Shepherd (Eds.), *Collaborating for student success: A guide for school-based occupational therapy* (p. 39). Bethesda, MD: AOTA Press.

Silverman, M., Stratman, K., Grogan, K., & Smith, R. O. (2003). *School Function Assessment Assistive Technology Supplement (SFA-AT)*. Milwaukee, WI: University of Wisconsin-Milwaukee.

Simmons Carlsson, C. (2006). *The "culture of practice" of Ministry of Education, special education occupational therapists and physiotherapists*. Auckland University of Technology, Auckland: Unpublished master's thesis.

Simmons Carlsson, C., Hocking, C., & Wright-St Clair, V. (2007). The 'why' of who we are: Exploring the culture of practice of Ministry of Education, special education occupational therapists and physiotherapists. *Kairaranga, 8*(2), 6-12.

Stoll, L. (2000). *School culture*. Retrieved 15 March 2009 from http://www.leadspace.govt.nz/leadership/articles/school-culture.php.

Swinth, Y., Spencer, K. J., & Jackson, L. L. (2007). *Occupational therapy: Effective school-based practices within a policy context*, Document OP-3. Centre on Personnel Studies in Special Education, University of Florida. Retrieved 13 April 2008 from www.coe.ufl.edu/copsse/docs/OT_CP_081307/1/OT_CP_081307.pdf.

Townsend, E. A., Beagan, B., Kumas-Tan, Z., Versnel, J., Iwama, M., & Landry, J. (2007). Enabling occupation II: Occupational therapy's core competency. In E. A. Townsend, & H. J. Polatajko (Eds.), *Enabling occupation II: Advancing an occupational therapy vision for health, well-being & justice through occupation* (pp. 87-133). Ottawa: CAOT Publications.

United Nations Educational Scientific and Cultural Organization, & Ministry of Education and Science Spain. (1994). *The Salamanca Statement and Framework for Action on Special Needs Education*. Retrieved 15 March 2009 from http://www.unesco.org/education/pdf/SALAMA_E.PDF.

van Kraayenoord, C. E. (2007). School and classroom practices in inclusive education in Australia. *Childhood Education, 83*(6), 390-394.

Van Meter, P., & Stevens, R. J. (2000). The role of theory in the study of peer collaboration. *Journal of Experimental Education, 69*(1), 113-127.

Wehrmann, S., Chiu, T., Reid, D., & Sinclair, G. (2006). Evaluation of occupational therapy school-based consultation service for students with fine motor difficulties. *Canadian Journal of Occupational Therapy, 73*(4), 225-235.

Westwood, P. (1998). Reducing classroom failure. *Australian Journal of Learning Disabilities, 3*(3), 4-12.

Whitmere, K. (2002). The evolution of school-based speech-language services: A half century of change and a new century of practice. *Communication Disorders Quarterly, 23*(2), 68-76.

Williams, W. B., Stemach, G., Wolfe, S., & Stanger, S. (1994). *Lifespace access profile for individuals with severe and multiple disabilities: Revised edition*. Sebastopol, CA: Lifespace Access Profile.

Youngstrom, M. J. (2005). Categories and principles of intervention. In C. H. Christiansen, C. M. Baum, & J. B. Bass-Haugen (Eds.), *Occupational therapy performance participation and well-being* (pp. 396-419). Thorofare, NJ: SLACK Inc.

Ziviani, J., & Muhlenhaupt, M. (2006). Student participation in the classroom. In S. Rodger, & J. Ziviani (Eds.), *Occupational therapy with children: Understanding children's occupations and enabling participation* (pp. 241-260). Oxford, UK: Blackwell Publishing.

Chapter 12

Enablement of Children's Leisure Participation

Anne Poulsen and Jenny Ziviani

Learning objectives

The aims of this chapter are to:

- Present the Engaging and Coaching for Health (EACH)-Child concept as a way to think about evaluation, intervention and facilitation of active leisure participation for children aged 6–12 years.
- Provide an overview of leisure evaluations and methodological approaches currently available for appraising children's leisure participation.
- Describe a practical approach towards building a leisure portfolio for children that is viable and sustainable within their communities, considering social, economic and individual circumstances.
- Propose a system for enabling healthy leisure participation and for evaluating and modifying ongoing engagement.
- Provide a clinical example of the EACH-Child leisure-coaching approach when planning future interventions.

Introduction

Leisure is a term most frequently used to describe older children's use of free time. In free time, there are choices and there is fun! With all these choices, as Robert Louis Stevenson assures us, 'we should all be as happy as kings'. Thus, leisure is associated with positive affect – the hallmark of subjective well-being. Enabling healthy engagement in leisure pursuits is a key concern of occupation-centred practice for children of all ages. Leisure activities can be a creative therapeutic tool, or a targeted component of a holistic occupational performance plan. Advocacy for healthy and inclusive leisure participation for all children regardless of economic, individual or social circumstances is consistent with an occupational justice agenda.

A primary focus of this chapter will be on how occupation-centred practitioners facilitate children's engagement in discretionary leisure pursuits during out-of-school hours. To this end, the leisure experiences of children aged 6–12 years will be explored. Play of preschool-aged children and leisure are complementary and overlapping occupational performance areas; however, preschoolers are not the focus of this chapter. Fun, enjoyment and happiness are positive affective experiences associated with satisfying engagement in both areas.

Children's leisure predominantly occurs during out-of-school hours and as such occupies over half a child's waking hours each week. In Western nations, holidays and vacation time occupy an additional 10–12 weeks a year. Hence, the potential impact of leisure time for offering productive and satisfying occupational engagement with attendant physical and mental health benefits is substantial. From a time-use perspective alone, it is logical to consider leisure-time behaviour as a window of opportunity for the promotion of health and well-being.

Importantly, pleasurable leisure activities can serve as vehicles to directly or indirectly assist goal achievement. Positive leisure engagements can improve subjective well-being, including short-term mood enhancement and longer lasting thoughts about life satisfaction in general. This occurs through fulfilment of three basic psychological needs identified by Deci and Ryan (2000) in their theory of self-determination. To strengthen a child's self-perceptions of general life satisfaction, two basic psychological needs must be fulfilled – choice or autonomy and competence or mastery. Both of these can be afforded in leisure situations. For example, self-selected and discretionary leisure engagement fulfils the psychological need for autonomy. Skill acquisition across physical, social, cognitive and psychological domains fulfils the need for competence or mastery. Relatedness or a sense of belonging or connection with others is the third element. These socialisation and friendship-building aspects can be attended to in leisure when planning interventions to promote socially oriented objectives.

Researchers argue that the strongest benefit of extracurricular activities for primary school-aged children is fostering relationships with peers (Schneider, Richard, Younger, & Freeman, 2000). Children are exposed to differing socialisation experiences with adults, inter- and cross-generational family members and neighbourhood peers. Diverse social interactions during leisure time provide socialisation experiences where social networks are created and a range of rules and scripts learned. Out-of-school hours provide an opportunity for social capital (through partnerships, friendships and community contacts) to be acquired (Larson, 2001).

Outcomes of healthy leisure engagement

By its very nature, leisure is often associated with high levels of intrinsically motivated activity. Intrinsic motivation is the desire to do something simply for its own sake, because it is interesting and enjoyable (Deci & Ryan, 2000). When children are intrinsically motivated to engage in activities, a range of adaptive outcomes are seen. These include positive affect, high levels of persistence and on-task behaviour. Utilisation of positive coping strategies at times of increased pressure and high personal effort during activity engagement are also evident.

Creating opportunities for intrinsically motivated leisure has multiple benefits and represents a powerful tool to facilitate a child's personal growth and flourishing. Specific competencies are acquired in an atmosphere of intense absorption. High interest in personally valued pursuits is associated with time transformation, a state where time seems to stand still or pass by without conscious awareness. These are components of the state of flow, as well as high levels of enjoyment, involvement, control and a merging of action and awareness (Csikszentmihalyi, 1990).

Levels of intrinsic motivation change, however, when leisure becomes structured and externally controlled. When an external locus of causality is perceived by the child, interest levels may fall and extrinsic sources regulate the child's behaviour. Coercion, bribery and elaborate reward schemes offer little potential for encouraging self-determined activity participation. Disadvantages of these external regulators include decreasing participants' intrinsic interest and can impact on a child's inherent enjoyment in an activity; heightened anxiety and concerns about the outcomes of activity engagement; and a low likelihood for long-term enjoyment and ongoing participation. While intrinsically motivated activities require no external inducement to be repeated, extrinsically motivated activity engagement is dependent on the presence of outside agents for ongoing performance. A reduction in the amount of child self-direction and a low internal locus of causality engenders a more work-like atmosphere.

Experienced practitioners recognise the importance of offering choice and fostering an autonomy-supportive environment when facilitating a child's personal growth. This is particularly important at the outset of an intervention when personal goals are child-determined rather than adult-determined. Collaboration and agreement on goal selection, prioritisation and management requires careful negotiation, particularly when invested parties disagree. Discrepancies between child-determined goals and those selected by parents, teachers and referring agents are common. The benefits of collaboration to achieve positive outcomes and reduce goal conflict are clearly seen in successful goal achievement (see Chapter 6).

Personally salient goals improve a child's subjective quality of life, and inclusion of leisure-focused goals selected by the child improves psychological well-being. When children set their own goals, and particularly when a leisure-oriented goal is included in the overall plan, the level of persistence is stronger and challenges are tackled with greater enthusiasm. As will be seen later in this chapter, therapist support requires a skilful blend of coaching qualities and intervention practices on the part of the therapist to achieve the aim of self-determined, self-actualised occupation-centred participation.

Practitioners, who are occupation-focused, carefully observe and listen to their clients when matching child characteristics according to affordances within their environment. The adoption of models such as the *Synthesis between Child, Occupational Performance and Environment in Time* (SCOPE-IT; Poulsen & Ziviani, 2004) assists practitioners to visualise the contributing factors to promote optimal outcomes for each individual. Operationalising these principles to enable children to actively participate in leisure pursuits within the community is the purpose of this chapter. The Engaging and Coaching for Health (EACH)-Child concept will be presented to assist practitioners to collaboratively advise clients about factors contributing to a match between children's leisure requirements, needs and abilities within their social and physical environments.

EACH-Child: model of leisure coaching

EACH-Child (Ziviani, Poulsen, & Hansen, 2008) was conceived as a way of describing a child-focused, family- and community-based way in which occupational therapists can support children in attaining their leisure participation goals. It promotes attending to a child's strengths and interests in leisure activities, and evaluating them alongside a background of information about environmental supports and barriers for these pursuits. Included in this appraisal is a detailed analysis of the leisure activity requirements, including information about leisure demands and sustainability of leisure participation for that child and family. EACH-Child is diagrammatically presented in Figure 12.1 and comprises a sequence of steps that need to be considered when scaffolding leisure opportunities for children.

Engagement

The first step in scaffolding leisure-oriented community participation involves 'engagement'. Examining current leisure opportunities and identifying leisure interests of personal relevance affords individual children the freedom to explore what is possible. Therapists can use assessments to guide this process or can employ a structured interview to determine the type of activities which might appeal. This process can be empowering for some children who may have only been presented with traditional (usually competitive) team sports which can challenge their sense of competence, if they are not highly skilled. To support this exploratory process, therapists should equip themselves with information about what is offered in their local communities.

Once activity options have been identified, the individual contextual situation of the child and family needs to be considered. This involves evaluating the social and physical environments which can act as facilitators or barriers to participation. Specifically, the therapist discusses costs related to activity participation, availability within the child's school or community

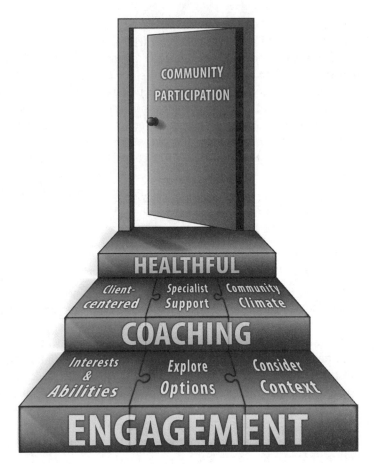

Figure 12.1 EACH-Child. Reproduced with permission

context, social and/or peer supports for involvement and seasonal fluctuations in activity availability. Additionally, as family infrastructure is one of the most salient facilitators of children's ongoing participation, therapists discuss family leisure profile interests, time availability and transport considerations.

Coaching

The second step involves finding the right match or fit between the child, activity and environment. Therapeutic expertise is required in making decisions about leisure pursuits that will match the child's abilities and interests and meet the family's needs and resources. An appreciation of leisure experiences and the factors contributing to or preventing healthy participation will enhance professional input into family-centred decisions about withdrawal from or persistence with ongoing leisure pursuits. Therapists utilise their skills in activity analysis, as well as teaching and learning, to help improve specific task performance. Hand in hand with this, the therapist needs to be alert to the motivational climate in which the activity is being acquired. An environment which involves mastery rather than competition is more likely to prevent children from 'dropping out'.

The interface with sporting or activity coaches who can supplement the therapist's interventions with more specialised knowledge of what is needed for specific activities is a critical but underutilised component of many intervention plans. By utilising specialist knowledge and embedding the intervention in a community context, the child is well positioned for skill acquisition to enable full participation.

Community participation

The third step of community participation is by no means final. Changes in the child and/or environment can mean that parents need to be vigilant to signs of avoidance or displeasure. All children experiment with a range of leisure pursuits in the process of finding some that may have long-term sustainability. Observing children undertaking these pursuits and listening to their reports of their experiences will help ensure that the activity is meeting their leisure, and personal and social needs. If not, the activity and the child's motivation, the context and/or the child's skill levels need to be reviewed.

Step one: creating successful engagements

Engaging children and families in a leisure dialogue requires a child-centred approach where the aim is finding an optimal match or fit between child, activity and environment characteristics. During the first step of the EACH-Child process, the child's interests and abilities are explored, and then leisure options and participation experiences investigated. Finally, the leisure context is evaluated. The overriding concern is identification of the best fit between these factors to promote a successful engagement.

Table 12.1 provides clinicians with a practical reference for selecting evaluation tools and methodologies to begin the matching process or to inform proposed child, activity and environment partnerships. Although a limited range of evaluation tools is currently available for children aged 6–13 years, occupational therapists continue to provide substantive contributions to this body of knowledge, alongside the disciplines of therapeutic recreation, ecological and positive psychology.

Documentation of leisure-time participation using population-based tools has been possible with surveys developed by social scientists and economists as a means of quantifying objective patterns of time use. An informative review of time-use approaches is presented by Juster, Ono, and Stafford (2003). The Canadian Occupational Performance Measure (COPM; Law et al., 1998) provides a user-friendly semi-structured interview of occupational performance where

Table 12.1 Assessment of interests, participation and contexts relevant to children's leisure

Assessment	Target group	Purpose	Psychometric properties
Pediatric Interest Profiles: Survey of Play for Children and Adolescents (Henry, 1998)	Children and adolescents between 6 and 21 years with and without disability	To obtain a profile of play/leisure interests	Internal consistency Cronbach's alpha range 0.59–0.80 (subscales), 0.93 for total scores. Test–retest variously reported 0.45–0.85. Content and construct validity reported
Assessment of Ludic Behaviours (parent interview portion) (Ferland, 1997)	Preschool-aged children with disability	Profile of attitude and interests	Limited
Paediatric Activity Card Sort (PACS; Mandich, Polatajko, Miller, & Baum, 2004)	Children between 6 and 12 years with various disabilities	Level of engagement in a range of activities including play	Content validity reported through various studies
Preferences for Activities of Children (PAC; King et al., 2004)	Children and youth 6–21 years of age	Determine activity preference of children and youth	Internal consistency ranges from 0.67 to 0.84. Items drawn from literature, expert panel and pilot study. Construct validity is based on longitudinal outcome data and factor analytical studies which have identified five factors accounting for around 30% of the variance over two studies
Children's Assessment of Participation and Enjoyment (CAPE; King et al., 2004)	Children and youth 6–21 years of age	To identify participation in and enjoyment of activities outside of school	Test–retest reliability range from 0.67 to 0.86 for participation, and 0.12 to 0.73 for enjoyment. Items drawn from literature, expert panel and pilot study. Construct validity is based on longitudinal study outcome data and comparisons with PAC, discriminate analyses on the basis of gender and presence of disability

Instrument	Purpose	Psychometric properties
Leisure Diagnostic Battery (LDB; Witt & Ellis, 1984) Developed for youth with disability	Assess perceived freedom in leisure as well as perceived barriers to participation	Test-retest reliability coefficient 0.72. Alpha coefficients range from 0.83 to 0.96 depending on individual scales. Validity has been addressed through factor analysis
Assessment of Life Habits for Children (LIFE-H; Fougeyrollas et al., 1998) Developed for children with disability	Determine the disruption in the accomplishment of life habits, defined as behaviours that ensure survival and development of a person. Accomplishment, assistance required and satisfaction for part of the recreation, arts and culture subcomponents	Adapted from adult version and consultation with expert panel. Strong association between PEDI, WeeFim and IFE-H education/recreation 0.79–0.91 Internal consistency of categories 0.73–0.90 except for interpersonal relations
Child & Adolescent Scale of Participation (CASP; Bedell, 2004; Bedell & Dumas, 2004) Developed for young people 3 years and upwards with and without acquired brain injury	Designed to examine participation in activities related to home, school and community. Of relevance are items related to social, play or leisure activities in neighbourhood and community	Test-retest reliability for total score of short form 0.67 and long form 0.73. Inter-rater reliability: participation 0.70, task supports 0.68 and performance 0.73 Items developed from life domains identified from the literature, the ICF, consumers and professionals. The CASP has a high test-retest intraclass correlation (0.90) and high internal consistency (0.98). Factor and Rasch analyses suggest the CASP functions as a unidimensional scale
Time-use Diaries (Juster et al., 2003; Juster & Stafford, 1985) Self-report for children over the age of 11 years or proxy report	Various forms: stylised estimates, recall time diary, self-report diary and experience sampling method (ESM)	Stylised estimates – less reliable than recall time budgets and time diary methods (Plewis, Cresser, & Mooney, 1990) Recall time diaries have moderate reliability achieved with multiple diaries. Validity demonstrated through comparison with other approaches (e.g. ESM) (Plewis et al., 1990) Self-report diaries have moderate reliability and validity – may provide slightly more valid data than recall time budgets (Juster & Stafford, 1985) Experience sampling method has low reliability (due to small sample sizes) (Juster et al., 2003); however, comparison with results from time diaries shows strong convergence (Larson & Verma, 1999)

(Continued)

Table 12.1 (Continued)

Assessment	Target group	Purpose	Psychometric properties
The Canadian Occupational Performance Measure (COPM; Law et al., 1998)	All ages and client groups	Provides a measure of occupational performance (including leisure)	Internal consistency has been reported as 0.56 for performance and 0.71 for satisfaction (Law et al., 1998). Test-retest reliability around 0.80 (Carswell et al., 2004)
Home Observation for Measurement of the Environment (HOME; Bradley, 1994, 2000; Bradley et al., 2000)	Infants to adolescents 15 years	Quantity and quality of stimulation support and structure in home environment of which play is a component	Internal consistency above 0.80. Test-retest early childhood scale 0.05–0.70. Inter-rater reliability variously over 85% Construct validity literature based. Construct validity supported in research
Test of Environmental Supportiveness (TOES; Bundy, 1999)	18 months to 15 years	Observational measure developed as a companion measure for the Test of Playfulness with the aim of determining the level of supportiveness of an environment for play	The measure is in early stages of development. Preliminary evidence suggests high levels of internal consistency and Rasch analysis indicates that items conform to expectations of measurement model. Details should be accessed from author
Children's Perception of Physical Activity Environment (Hume et al., 2006)	Preadolescents (10–11 years)	Children's report on perceptions of physical and social environments at home and in the neighbourhood that inform involvement in physical activity	Items drawn from literature Preliminary findings support test-retest percentage agreement between 68% and 100%. ICC values between 0.72 and 0.92 reported for continuous items

participants can reflect on the things that they do in a day. Because of the seasonal variation in leisure-time behaviour, selective probing to provide a full picture of out-of-school time-use trends over the past year or so is necessary to supplement the COPM. See Chapter 6 for other goal-setting tools and Chapter 7 regarding occupation-centred assessments.

During Step one of the EACH-Child process, the emphasis is on understanding leisure-time occupational performance from the child's perspective. The initial consultation includes baseline data collection using formal and informal evaluation tools to build a picture of the match between current strengths, abilities and interests, and environmental characteristics. A series of interactive discussions informs goal formation.

These discussions can be facilitated through leisure mapping (Figure 12.2). A circle, representing the child, is first drawn in the centre of a page. To commence the first level of mapping, the child generates a list of current leisure pursuits. The instructions are as follows: 'Think about how you spend your time out of school. What will you do today, tomorrow, this week or next? What sorts of things did you do last week? Tell me about some of these things you do or want to do'.

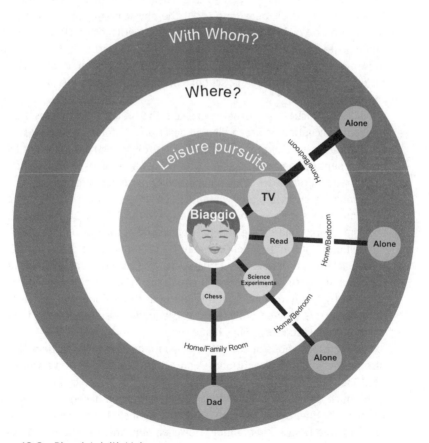

Figure 12.2 Biaggio's initial leisure map

The activities are then written in a series of circles spaced around the child's circle. Even if only one or two leisure interests are suggested, this is sufficient to start a leisure map. Connector lines between the child and the identified leisure interests are drawn with variation in the positioning, size and choice of colours to highlight factors such as the strength of a current leisure interest. For example, solid black lines might represent current leisure interests while future leisure interests might be represented by dotted lines. Consistent ways of representing data are recommended to allow for follow-up reflection. Leisure mapping is an enjoyable idiographic technique that can generate a considerable amount of discussion about current and future leisure pursuits.

A web of information about affective experiences, social support networks, time commitments and other ecological information can be collected and added to the leisure map. It is recommended that this information is added in concentric circles surrounding the initial drawing. This helps the child consider the ecological aspects surrounding leisure participation. This information is organised during an initial brainstorming session when key questions about where an activity takes place (the physical environment level), and with whom an activity is pursued (the social environment level), are asked. For younger children, questions about the physical environment are limited to: 'Where do you do this activity - at home (write down H) or away from home (write down A)?' Questions about the social environment are limited to, 'How many people do you do this activity with?' If more information is given, for example, whether siblings, school mates or neighbours are involved, then this can be added.

While the leisure map is being created, the practitioner acts as a sounding board accepting and recording all descriptive information and discussing the clearest means of presenting this. The pros and cons of different leisure engagement options can be listed with pluses and minuses beside the item. In this way, information concerning viability of selected leisure options can be graphically evaluated on a whiteboard or large sheet of paper. Commercial mind-mapping software can also be utilised to facilitate the generation of leisure maps, and children are able to keep a copy of their own map.

Additional information sources may be required to complete the leisure map. Background details about the social and physical environment, activity demands, costs and seasonal fluctuations in activity availability may be supplied by family members or through utilisation of internet or hard copy databases. This may be provided in subsequent sessions, or collected after children have taken their maps home.

Further explorations of subjective evaluations of activity participation can also be investigated. Practitioners can ask the child to assign a value from 1 to 10 for each activity on a dimension such as level of enjoyment, by asking 'How much do you enjoy doing this activity? Imagine giving it a mark out of 10 for fun'. Other subjective appraisals can be included according to area of focus for the leisure intervention. However, enjoyment is the first aspect to rate. For example, self-concept perceptions of level of ability might be probed at a later date with a question on competence, 'How do you rate the way you do this activity?' This approach requires participants to analyse activities on a series of affective or cognitive dimensions.

At the same time as the leisure map is constructed, an activity analysis of child-identified leisure pursuits occurs. Child-identified leisure pursuits include those listed in a child's goal list as being a desired future option, a problematic current activity or an intensely pleasurable and satisfying pursuit. Obtaining this information will ensure a close match between the child's current ability levels and entry level into the leisure pursuit. Instances where there is a mismatch between the child's current abilities, activity demands and environmental characteristics can be pinpointed to inform interventions. Practitioners then decide whether a specialised intervention is required to change child or environmental capacity and will step up to the second phase of EACH-Child.

Before moving on from Step one, both the child and his/her family will have a clear picture of leisure possibilities and probabilities that have been considered taking into account interests, abilities, contextual supports and barriers. This process represents a leisure FIT-ID, focusing on the current levels of fit or matching between child, activity and environment. In Step two, the child is coached in areas where talent or capacity can be developed. Areas where personal growth might be nurtured in current or future leisure environments are highlighted and then a plan for intervention is developed during the second step of the EACH-Child process.

Step two: coaching to promote personal growth

First and foremost, client-centred leisure coaching is an empowering intervention for the consumer. Throughout the second step of EACH-Child, the child's needs, interests and abilities are constantly monitored. Concurrently, there is observation and appraisal of physical and social aspects of the leisure environment. Three key principles underpin the coaching step of the EACH-Child process: (1) maintaining a client-centred approach, (2) including specialised interventions founded on self-determination theory principles of psychological need fulfilment for autonomy, competence and relatedness, and (3) looking towards the future to evaluate sustainability within a supportive community climate.

A client-centred approach

Client-centred coaching requires active listening and reflection on child reports and integration of information from parental observations and feedback about the child's current leisure experiences. Enjoyment of the leisure activity is essential to document initially. Asking the child about positive affective experiences during the leisure activity is a transparent, revealing indicator of sustainability and future retention of the leisure experience. Encouraging children and parents to evaluate leisure participation through self-appraisals of fun or enjoyment is an important part of the coach's role. Asking a direct, but closed question, such as 'Did you enjoy ... leisure activity ...?', can tap this affective element. Alternatively, open-ended questions such as 'How was ... leisure activity ... today?', with a probe about levels of enjoyment, can gauge this aspect of the leisure experience.

Further questions aimed at exploring the child's perceptions of the social environment and the psychological and/or physical demands of the activity can also be framed as open-ended questions; for example, 'Who came along today?', 'What things did you try today?', 'Could you tell me more about ...?', 'What new things happened during ...?', 'What was the best part about ...?', 'What's your opinion about ...?' and 'What was it like when ...?' are open-ended facilitators where probing will almost certainly need to follow. Process-oriented rather than outcome-oriented discussions may need to be actively modelled to parents to facilitate discussions about the leisure experience. In this way, a decreased emphasis on outcomes such as results, win–lose scenarios, social comparisons and competitive statements can be engendered, while an increased focus on reasons for participation and the experiences that occur during the leisure activity can be discussed (see Table 12.2).

A supplementary evaluative strategy to explore the strength of children's self-perceptions of affective (e.g. fun), cognitive (e.g. learning), motivational and active experiences during leisure includes using visual analogue scales. Graduated circle and facial expression scales are favourably received by children with limited reading skills. However, all self-reporting methods are sensitive to social desirability and reactivity to administrators, as well as being influenced by the variable verbal, reading or writing skills of each child. Nevertheless, self-report scales remain an important means of evaluating leisure engagement experiences.

Self-report scales have improved reliability and reproducibility when used with older children (from 7 years upwards), with developmental status and mental age being an additional consideration (Chambers & Johnston, 2002). Numbered Likert-type scales are suitable for children aged 10 years and older with the number of response choices being a less important consideration than complexity of items' description and cognitive capacity of the child. Dichotomous thinking of young children represents the greatest barrier to use of these techniques. Therefore, responses that are clustered at extreme endpoints of a scale indicate that this is a difficult and, perhaps, inappropriate task for a particular child.

Older children and parents can be educated to recognise growth-enhancing characteristics of positive leisure experiences. For example, the deep absorption and time transcendence associated with high levels of intrinsically motivated activity pursuit can be highlighted as parts of flow, and identified as a state of optimal activity engagement. Almost without knowing it, a child who is engaged in flow activities continues to acquire further skills and to attain personal growth. Affective experiences of fun time are clear indicators of ongoing engagement and whether that experience is likely to be voluntarily re-visited. Multiple methods are required to monitor a child's engagement in leisure

Table 12.2 Leisure questions

Leisure Questions	Rating scale
Enjoy	How much do you *enjoy* doing it?
	0 1 2 3 4 5 6 7 8 9 10
	Don't enjoy Enjoy a lot
Interest	How *interested* are you in doing it?
	0 1 2 3 4 5 6 7 8 9 10
	Not interested Very interested
Concentration	How much do you *concentrate* while you do it?
	0 1 2 3 4 5 6 7 8 9 10
	Don't concentrate Really concentrate
Stress	How *stressful* is it?
	0 1 2 3 4 5 6 7 8 9 10
	Not stressful Very stressful
How well	*How well* do you do it? (How do you rate your success so far?)
	0 1 2 3 4 5 6 7 8 9 10
	Not well Very well
Difficult	How *difficult* is it?
	0 1 2 3 4 5 6 7 8 9 10
	Not difficult Very difficult
Your idea	How often is it *your idea* to do it?
	0 1 2 3 4 5 6 7 8 9 10
	Not often All the time
Somebody else's idea	How often is it *somebody else's idea* to do it? (You feel you have to do it)
	0 1 2 3 4 5 6 7 8 9 10
	Not often All the time
Force yourself	How often do you have to *force yourself* to do it?
	0 1 2 3 4 5 6 7 8 9 10
	Not often All the time
Want	How much do you *want* to do it?
	0 1 2 3 4 5 6 7 8 9 10
	Not much A lot
Learn	How often do you do it to *learn* something or improve your skills?
	0 1 2 3 4 5 6 7 8 9 10
	Not often All the time
Competition	How often do you do it to *win*?
	0 1 2 3 4 5 6 7 8 9 10
	Not often All the time

pursuits: structured and semi-structured interviews, child self-reports and ratings which supplement information from other reports and observations.

Specialised interventions

In the EACH-Child model of leisure coaching, all interventions are based on meeting children's basic psychological needs for autonomy, relatedness and competence (ARC). Self-determination theory assumes that individuals are naturally curious about the world and intrinsically motivated to explore, pursue innate interests, build competencies and repeatedly engage in enjoyable and satisfying pursuits (Deci & Ryan, 2000). As one experienced clinician (Henderson, personal communication, 23 March 2008) commented, 'Specialised interventions provide an ARC of discovery on the journey to MARS (Mastery, Autonomy, Relatedness and Self-determination)'.

The ARC of psychological need fulfilment provides a theoretical foundation to help practitioners develop, evaluate and re-frame specialised interventions aimed at increasing a child's fulfilment of these needs and helps the child move from little or no intrinsic motivation ('*I don't want* to do it') to a stage where there are high levels of intrinsic motivation ('*I want* to do it'). Deci and Ryan (2000) identified three additional types of motivation. High levels of externally regulated motivation exist for the state of extrinsic motivation ('*I have* to do it'). Progressively more internalisations are seen in children who have introjected motivation ('I do it because *I should* do it'), and then identified motivation ('*I choose* to do it because it will be good for me').

Practitioners can plot a child's level of motivation for activity engagement using the Rocket Model of Motivation (Figure 12.3). This model provides a useful framework for envisaging a child's journey to self-determined activity engagement.

A: autonomy principles to promote personally meaningful choice

Autonomy can be evaluated by looking at how meaningful choices are facilitated through adoption of child-directed versus adult-directed information exchange. The use of autonomy-focused language that allows freedom of choice encourages personal decision-making and self-corrections when progress is impeded or obstacles recognised can be observed and fostered throughout the intervention. Adult conversational control is minimised and programme adaptations occur following child-identified detection. Provision of a supportive environment allows free exchange of information and a climate where the ongoing needs of the children and changing environmental circumstances are collaboratively addressed.

One technique that supports client-centred practice and autonomous personal growth is motivational interviewing (MI; Markland, Ryan, Tobin, & Rollnick, 2005). A core group of MI techniques, called OARS, is central to adopting a MI style. These include O for open-ended listening, A for using affirmative statements, R for reflective listening and S where summaries that promote self-efficacy are provided throughout each session.

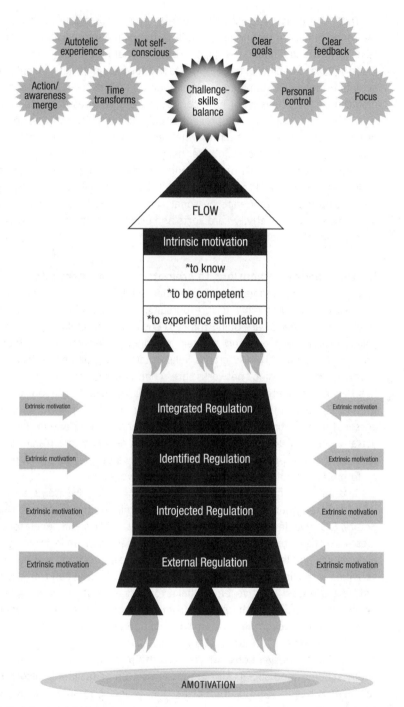

Figure 12.3 Rocket Motivation Model (adapted from self-determination continuum (Deci & Ryan, 2000), nine principles of flow (Jackson & Csikszentmihalyi, 2000) and Vallerand's (1997) hierarchical model of intrinsic and extrinsic motivation)

Practical means of facilitating interests and encouraging learning about the range of leisure resources available in the community include working on leisure maps and filling in the gaps through utilisation of multimedia sources. Electronic resources providing up-to-date information about current leisure activity options can supplement other sources such as local newspapers and magazines. The provision of hard copy resources requires dedicated time to collect, regularly update and present in child-friendly format. Consideration of leisure characteristics such as whether the activity is seasonal/non-seasonal, competitive/non-competitive, flexible, costly or dependent on a specialised/inexpensive environment and specialised equipment demands, gender-specific/neutral, age-specific/multi-age inclusive and socially evaluative/accepting will influence personal choice. Choice instruction sessions using choice books, activity card sorts and practice in deciding 'what is right for me' can inform leisure mapping.

R: relatedness interventions to promote social connectivity

To ensure that relatedness needs are addressed, coaches may need to take a broad view of the child's leisure pursuits, using a social lens to evaluate whether social needs are being fulfilled. Ensuring that children have opportunities to develop bridging as well as bonding networks is part of this process. Bridging networks create links outside familiar people in a child's everyday life. Bonding networks are characterised by strong personal ties between affiliated members of the family or neighbourhood and close friends. Bridging networks offer a means for expanding opportunities for personal growth, broader identity formation and 'getting ahead'. They also act as a buffer in times of need when bonding networks are fragile or have fallen apart. The provision of a social support safety network is dependent on formation of both bonding and bridging networks.

Children's engagement in occupations such as family rituals and festivals can strengthen bonding links between family members (Fiese, Hooker, Kotary, & Schwagler, 1993). Holidays and outings, picnics and spectator activities have the potential to increase social connectivity, while offering novel experiences and learning opportunities. Mealtimes, afternoon tea, eating out activities with friends or relatives and transportation time can frame leisure-time experiences. Positive emotional experiences that occur in heterogeneous leisure groups with children from different cultural, educational and socioeconomic backgrounds offers socialisation and personal growth opportunities through the formation of bridging networks.

Specialised interventions where friendship programmes, mentorships, buddy schemes and social skills groups are set up or facilitated also address relatedness needs. Identification of barriers to inclusive social participation, such as ego-oriented or competitive, and socially evaluative motivational climates in external leisure pursuits are important to recognise. Networking and parent training in recognition of adverse leisure environments, inclusive and exclusive social settings, dense and disparate network groups and personal interest-driven as opposed to parent or external source-driven leisure groups are additional aspects of the coaching support role.

C: competence interventions to promote mastery

Occupation-focused practitioners are experienced in the design and grading of intervention programmes to increase children's competencies to participate in leisure pursuits of their own choosing. Task breakdown through identification of component skills and appropriate sequences of component skills is a foundation component of occupational performance analysis. Practitioners' experiences and leisure skill knowledge will vary; therefore, collaboration with the child, family and other experienced adults or activity leaders will aid the task analysis of prerequisite component skills for the desired leisure pursuit. Enlisting the aid of community members (e.g. retirees with specialised skills such as making adapted equipment and availability to mentor children in specialist hobbies) requires time, effort and dedicated nurturing, but promotes social connectivity and enriches outcomes.

Activity modifications such as adaptations in time (e.g. breaks and session length), area (e.g. decreasing the size of a playing field and expanding team size to decrease distances covered) and equipment (e.g. larger, softer balls, fixed striking platforms, lowered hoops and auditory cues for participants with visual impairment) can be considered. Other factors that might be altered to promote mastery and ensure positive outcomes include the different endpoints (e.g. competitive versus non-competitive outcomes) and altering participant roles (e.g. having buddies for running and water carrier positions). The presentation of instructions and verbal feedback offer possibilities for increasing compliance, enjoyment and skill enhancement (e.g. using brief, repeated instructions, sending descriptions of activity home beforehand to promote practice in privacy of own home, providing demonstrations, using gestural and language prompts, modelling, breaking activities into manageable portions and grading skill progression).

Pragmatic concerns regarding mastery of skill-based interventions include making decisions about frequency of learning sessions, types of instructions and feedback. The length of sessions can be optimally tailored for age, level of difficulty, attention span and tolerance. Timing of sessions also varies with content, and provision of opportunities that vary in time, place, instructor and social settings, thus ensuring transferability and sustainability.

The basic principles supporting occupational performance mastery translate across clinical and non-clinical settings. In all leisure interventions aimed at increasing competence in a skill area, the ratio between the challenge of the activity and skills required for the activity needs to be balanced. A challenge/skill imbalance creates negative affect and maladaptive behavioural responses. For example, highly challenging activities can induce anxiety when skills are perceived to be inadequate. Alternatively, boredom may occur when skills are too advanced for an easy task. Optimal balance between challenge and skill creates the necessary conditions for experiencing flow, with its attendant benefits of enjoyment and personal growth (Csikszentmihalyi, 1990).

MI techniques can be incorporated in specialist interventions aimed at developing competencies and confidence. Promoting self-efficacy through adult-initiated positive affirmations during skill-building activities is an MI technique. In Cognitive Orientation to daily Occupational Performance (CO-OP), child-checking using questioning about competence behaviour is one of the four central components of the intervention (Missiuna, Mandich, Polatajko, & Malloy-Miller, 2001). The concept of child-detected efficacy rather than other-referenced evaluations is emphasised. Examples of questions related to progress, effort and goal achievement include, 'How did you go this time compared to last time?' or 'How would you rate your plan/effort?'

Strategies to satisfy the basic psychological need for competency in targeted, therapeutic interventions abound. Frequently, this wealth of knowledge is restricted to provision of services in artificial, clinical settings. Creating opportunities for mastery through collaboration with community partners is underutilised because it means working outside clinical environments and embedding practice in non-clinical environments. Limited budgets and disease-focused models prevent full development of this essential aspect of occupational performance interventions.

Community climate

There is a need for collaboration with community partners to embed the leisure intervention in an ecologically sensitive framework. The community climate supporting the intervention requires understanding to gauge the possibilities for ongoing engagement and sustainability. Therapists can expand each child's social and leisure capital through community opportunities and explore kinship, neighbourhood and leisure-specific networks.

In addition, families' strengths and weaknesses, relationships and interactions, priorities and lifestyles will impact on sustainability of children's leisure pursuits. It is necessary to consider whether the leisure activity will meet a family's needs and be viable in stressed family environments, and whether the family supports the child's leisure goals. Ongoing supports and barriers, such as financial considerations, transport arrangements, family approval and disapproval of the leisure participation, need to be taken into account when evaluating ongoing participation. The level of family satisfaction with the leisure activity will substantially predict ongoing child engagement.

A site visit to conduct a needs assessment to gather local and cultural information to ensure community leisure options are feasible, acceptable, effective and equitable for each child is important. Affordances and barriers to participation must be considered. Alongside this is the need to investigate and facilitate supportive partnerships and collaboration. Assessments of the motivational climate can be incorporated in these site visits where not only the climate is appraised, but other leader characteristics are also observed (e.g. instructional processes, problem-solving, communication, socialising and interactions before, during and after activity sessions).

Motivational climates can be broadly divided into *ego-oriented/competitive* environments that emphasise social achievement and other-referenced performance, or task-oriented mastery climates that emphasise learning and *self-referenced skill acquisition* (Nicholls, 1989). Ego-oriented climates may deter potential participants when the children's knowledge, skills and perceptions of their abilities are low. In these motivational climates, achievement is measured in comparison to others or to a normative reference point, and stigma may be associated with poor performance. There is increased social comparison during competitive group activities where performance is publicly appraised. Organised sports can operate in an exclusive manner with less competent individuals withdrawing from these activities. Barriers can exist to prevent or limit full participation, because of ego-oriented motivational climates where the emphasis is on social comparison and performance outcomes. De-emphasising a 'win at all costs' mentality while focusing on process outcomes (e.g. mastery-oriented coaching strategies) is recommended.

While leisure can enhance social participation, adverse experiences can negatively impact social development, particularly in ego-oriented motivational climates. It is therefore important to consider the level of support and the characteristics of the motivational climate in each activity so as to maximise social development, and ensure healthy, growth-enhancing participation. The practitioner is therefore required to seek out underutilised options and non-competitive activities for children who may be particularly vulnerable in competitive leisure pursuits, such as children with poor motor skills who wish to participate in structured physical activities and sports. There is a need to address parental and child concerns/fears about having low motor ability, lost opportunities, wasted effort, fears of letting others down and embarrassing self-representational failure.

Advocacy for physical activity participation of all community members rather than the physically elite promotes social inclusiveness and provides opportunities for improving self-confidence. Non-competitive, life-long physical activities offer a vehicle for healthy, physically active leisure. Identification and removal of barriers to participation requires interdisciplinary collaborative efforts within the community. Advocacy for more community support for inclusive leisure means actions must be considered at the policy level as well as community organisation level. Needs assessment to gather local and cultural information to ensure that interventions are feasible, acceptable, effective and equitable has the potential to inform standards development, current and future fiscal and legislation/changes and information campaigns. The over-arching principle of service provision aimed at ensuring that all children have positive leisure experiences is critical for increasing perceptions of efficacy, skill development and enjoyment that will lead to life-long adoption of positive attitudes to community participation.

A case study using EACH-Child

Biaggio was 10 years and 5 months old when his mother consulted a private occupational therapist about his poor gross motor skills which she saw as contributing to his current social and emotional difficulties. From an early age, Biaggio achieved motor developmental milestones later than his older sister and brother, as well as his numerous cousins. He was a solitary child at preschool, standing on the sidelines rather than actively joining in other children's games. During his school years, Biaggio was stigmatised by peers who derided his weight, poor physical coordination and friendships with girls rather than boys.

During out-of-school hours, Biaggio spent long periods of time in front of his own television set located in his bedroom. Leisure mapping revealed a strong focus on sedentary, screen-based activities that were largely solitary and indoors. He also enjoyed reading non-fiction historical and scientific texts and conducting science experiments in the privacy of his bedroom. Occasionally he would play a masterful game of chess or checkers with his father.

Information gained from the short form of the Leisure Diagnostic Battery (Witt & Ellis, 1989) revealed low perceived leisure competence and low perceived control of events and outcomes during his leisure experiences. Biaggio described past experiences in the local soccer team where he was assigned to be a goal keeper because of his large size. However, his slow reaction time and poor eye-hand coordination skills had contributed to low self-concept perceptions of physical ability which were reinforced whenever he let a ball slide through his legs or hands. The public humiliation and feelings of pressure to perform in this competitive environment contributed to increased levels of anxiety. He eventually refused to participate in this activity and avoided team sports and organised physical activities during and after school.

During the first sessions with Biaggio, the therapist explored his abilities, interests and options. Concurrently, information was collected on the social and physical context of past, current and future leisure options. This represented the first stage of the EACH-Child process. In addition to completing the Leisure Diagnostic Battery and starting a leisure map (see Figure 12.2), a picture of current strengths was compiled. The results of the Movement Assessment Battery for Children (M-ABC: Henderson & Sugden, 1992) showed stronger performance on Balance sub-tests than Ball Skills or Manual Dexterity items. Static Balance was superior to Dynamic Balance with Biaggio demonstrating ability to focus well and hold a posture, such as standing on a balance board, even when unexpected external distractions provided an additional level of unanticipated difficulty. The Children's Perception of Physical

Activity Environment Scale (Hume, Ball, & Salmon, 2006) provided information about home and neighbourhood leisure environments. Biaggio reported
an impoverished leisure environment at home, but described a rich array of
potential social and physical activity opportunities in the neighbourhood.
Within close proximity to his home was a man-made lake where canoes, kay-
aks and sailing boats could be hired. Bike paths surrounded the lake connecting the natural bushland outer areas of the suburb with built-up areas.

To start the matching process, the collected data were summarised and
Biaggio began to consider current leisure engagement and identify future
activities that might be ecologically sustainable. Using the leisure mapping process, Biaggio added a new circle for each potential leisure project.
He identified three activities of high personal interest: kayaking, cycling and
rollerblading. Although he was unable to ride a bike or rollerblade, and had
never been in a kayak, his strong intrinsic motivation to attempt these activities, coupled with his innate strengths on the M-ABC for static (although not
dynamic) balance, meant that a potential match could be evaluated. In addition, the environmental affordances of his neighbourhood supported engagement in these leisure pursuits.

Potential barriers to activity engagement were identified in the second
phase of the EACH-Child approach. Specialist support was necessary to promote skill acquisition for each leisure pursuit. CO-OP (Missiuna et al., 2001)
was selected as the specialist intervention to provide this level of child-centred support. Biaggio's demonstrated capacity for learning and problem-
solving suited this task-oriented approach based on cognitive principles and
motor learning theory. Biaggio's parents were unable to afford the hire fees
for kayaking or cycling. A cousin's discarded rollerblades were found for the
rollerblading sessions; however, they were a size too large.

It seemed as though Biaggio's leisure interests could not be sustained. In
fact, at one point the barriers to future participation seemed insurmount-
able. His own resourcefulness provided the impetus for finding solutions to
these difficulties. During an internet search, he located an on-line resource
where rollerblades could be purchased for an affordable price. Encouraged
by this early success, Biaggio and his leisure coach explored vacation and
after-school options that were either free or strongly subsidised. He was
reluctant to attend these sessions without a peer or adult mentor. Hence, the
identification of potential leisure buddies was a new focus of the coaching
process.

While waiting for coaching options to 'click' into place, CO-OP focused on
skill acquisition to achieve Biaggio's personal goals of rollerblading and riding a bicycle. A borrowed bike provided opportunities for graded practice in
a safe location away from the gaze of onlookers. Rollerblading proved to be
a short-lived interest, while bicycling became a pursuit that occupied large
amounts of time. Biaggio traded the rollerblades for a bicycle and began
exploring his neighbourhood in the company of cousins and two boys who
attended his local school. Friendships were forged and Biaggio introduced

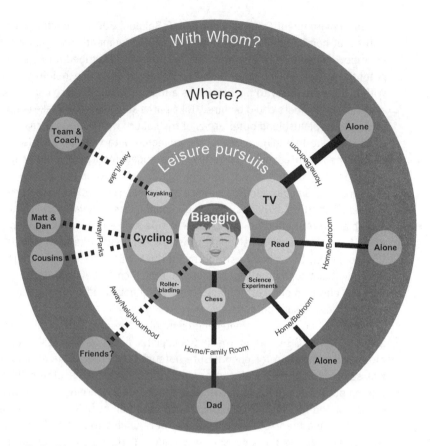

Figure 12.4 Biaggio's subsequent leisure map

his new companions to the somewhat dubious pastime of making tennis ball bombs, using scrapings from sparklers.

Community participation was achieved through informal and ongoing leisure-time engagement experiences with neighbourhood companions. Biaggio became involved in social physical activities and was involved in more outdoor activities following the EACH-Child intervention. An imbalance between time spent in structured and unstructured leisure-time pursuits was observed. On discharge, a final leisure map was drawn where Biaggio was able to identify future leisure pursuits of interest. Two more circles were added. One involved pursuing the kayaking option as a high school activity or moving on to rowing when this option became available. See Figure 12.4. Both options were structured physical activities which offered socialisation opportunities with team members and adult leaders which would have improved the balance between 'grow and learn time' and 'chill out time' during the out-of-school hours.

Conclusion

The centrality of leisure in the daily lives of children has been emphasised. Enablement of children's leisure participation represents an important and growing area of practice. The EACH-Child process is a theoretically grounded, practical means of facilitating children's growth utilising leisure interventions that are creative, stimulating and sustainable. This collaborative approach is consistent with adoption of a strong client-centred approach, where children are encouraged and supported in their pursuit of self-determined goals. A case study demonstrating utilisation of the EACH-Child approach in daily practice has been described.

References

Bedell, G. M. (2004). Developing a follow-up survey focused on participation of children and youth with acquired brain injuries after discharge from impatient rehabilitation. *NeuroRehabilitation, 19*, 191-205.

Bedell, G. M., & Dumas, H. (2004). Social participation of children and youth with acquired brain injuries discharged from inpatient rehabilitation: A follow-up study. *Brain Injury, 18*, 65-82.

Bradley, R. H. (1994). The HOME Inventory: Review and reflections. In H. Reese (Ed.), *Advances in child development and behavior* (pp. 241-288). San Diego, CA: Academic.

Bradley, R. H. (2000). Deceived by omission: The difficulty of matching measurement and theory when assessing the home environment. *Journal of Research on Adolescence, 10*, 307-314.

Bradley, R. H., Corwyn, R. F., Caldwell, B. M., Whiteside-Mansell, L., Wasserman, G. A., & Mink, I. T. (2000). Measuring the home environments of children in early adolescence. *Journal of Research on Adolescence, 10*, 247-288.

Bundy, A. (1999). *Test of Environmental Supportiveness*. Fort Collins, CO: Colorado State University.

Carswell, A., McColl, M. A., Baptiste, S., Law, M., Polatajko, H., & Pollock, N. (2004). The COPM: A research and clinical review. *Canadian Journal of Occupational Therapy, 71*, 210-222.

Chambers, C. T., & Johnston, C. (2002). Developmental differences in children's use of rating scales. *Journal of Pediatric Psychology, 27*, 27-36.

Csikszentmihalyi, M. (1990). *Flow: The psychology of optimal experience*. New York, NY: Harper & Row.

Deci, E. L., & Ryan, R. M. (2000). The "what" and "why" of goal pursuits: Human needs and the self-determination of behavior. *Psychological Inquiry, 11*, 227-268.

Ferland, F. (1997). *Play, children and physical disabilities and occupational therapy*. Ottawa, ON: University of Ottawa.

Fiese, B., Hooker, K., Kotary, L., & Schwagler, J. (1993). Family rituals in the early stages of parenthood. *Journal of Marriage and the Family, 55*, 633-642.

Fougeyrollas, P., Noreau, L., Bergeron, H., Cloutier, R., Dion, S., & St-Michel. G. (1998). Social consequences of long term impairments and disabilities: Conceptual approach and assessment of handicap. *International Journal of Rehabilitation Research, 21*, 127-141.

Henderson, S. E., & Sugden, D. A. (1992). *Movement Assessment Battery for Children*. Kent, UK: The Psychological Corporation.

Henry, A. D. (1998). Development of a measure of adolescent leisure interests. *American Journal of Occupational Therapy, 52*, 531–539.

Hume, C., Ball, K., & Salmon, J. (2006). Development and reliability of a self report questionnaire to examine children's perceptions of the physical environment at home and in the neighbourhood. *International Journal of Behavioral Nutrition and Physical Activity, 3*, 3–16.

Jackson, S. A. (2000). Joy, fun and flow state in sport. In Y. L. Hanin (Ed.), *Emotions in sport*. Champaign, IL: Human Kinetics.

Juster, F. T., Ono, H., & Stafford, F. P. (2003). An assessment of alternative measures of time use. *Sociological Methodology, 33*, 19–54.

Juster, F., & Stafford, F. P. (1985). *Time, goods and well-being*. University of Michigan, Ann Arbor: Institute for Social Research.

King, G., King, S., Rosenbaum, P., Kertoy, M., Law, M., Hurley, P., et al. (2004). *Children's Assessment of Participation and Enjoyment & Preferences for Activities of Children*. San Antonio, TX: PsychCorp Harcourt.

Larson, R., & Verma, S. (1999). How children and adolescents spend time across the world: Work, play, and developmental opportunities. *Psychological Bulletin, 125*, 701–736.

Larson, R. W. (2001). How U.S. children and adolescents spend time: What it does (and doesn't) tell us about their development. *Current Directions in Psychological Science, 10*, 160–164.

Law, M., Baptiste, S., Carswell, A., McColl, M. A., Polatajko, H., & Pollock, M. A. (Eds.). (1998). *Canadian Occupational Performance Measure* (2nd ed., Rev.). Ottawa, ON: CAOT Publications ACE.

Mandich, A. D., Polatajko, H. J., Miller, L. T., & Baum, C. (2004). *Paediatric Activity Card Sort*. Ottawa, ON: CAOT Publications ACE.

Markland, D., Ryan, R. M., Tobin, V. J., & Rollnick, S. (2005). Motivational interviewing and self-determination theory. *Journal of Social & Clinical Psychology, 24*(6), 811–831.

Missiuna, C., Mandich, A. D., Polatajko, H. J., & Malloy-Miller, T. (2001). Cognitive orientation to daily occupational performance (CO-OP): Part I – Theoretical foundations. *Physical and Occupational Therapy in Pediatrics, 20*, 69–81.

Nicholls, J. G. (1989). *The competitive ethos and democratic education*. Cambridge, MA: Harvard University Press.

Plewis, I., Creeser, R., & Mooney, A. (1990). Reliability and validity of time budget data: Children's activities outside school. *Journal of Official Statistics, 6*, 411–419.

Poulsen, A. A., & Ziviani, J. M. (2004). Can I play too? Physical activity engagement patterns of children with developmental coordination disorders. *Canadian Journal of Occupational Therapy, 71*, 100–107.

Schneider, B. H., Richard, J. F., Younger, A. J., & Freeman, P. (2000). A longitudinal exploration of the continuity of children's social participation and social withdrawal across socioeconomic status levels and social settings. *European Journal of Social Psychology, 30*, 497–519.

Vallerand, R. J. (1997). Toward a hierarchical model of intrinsic and extrinsic motivation. In M. P. Zanna (Ed.), *Advances in experimental social psychology* (Vol. 29, pp. 271–360). New York: Academic Press.

Witt, P. A., & Ellis, G. D. (1984). The Leisure Diagnostic Battery: Measuring perceived freedom in leisure. *Society and Leisure, 7*, 109–124.

Witt, P. A., & Ellis, G. D. (1989). The Leisure Diagnostic Battery. State College, PA: Venture Publ Inc.

Ziviani, J. & Poulsen, A. A. & Hansen, C. (2009). Movement skills proficiency and physical activity: A case for Engaging And Coaching for Health (EACH – Child). *Australian Occupational Therapy Journal*, 56, 259-265, doi: 10.111/j.1440-1630.2008.00758.

Chapter 13

Acute Hospitals: A Challenging Context for Occupation-centred Practice with Children

Sylvia Rodger and Rebecca Banks

Learning objectives

Specifically this chapter aims to:

- Identify therapists' perspectives on being occupation-centred in children's hospitals and the obstacles encountered.
- Provide some strategies to assist occupational therapists working in hospitals to be more occupation-centred.
- Demonstrate the application of occupation-centred practice by describing two case studies from a children's burns unit and a feeding therapy service for infants and children with complex medical conditions.

Introduction

Molineux (2004) described the translation of an occupational focus from theory into practice as being simultaneously simple and difficult. This difficulty is rooted, he suggested, in the very nature of most modern work environments and particularly reductionist medical settings. Acute medical settings pose specific challenges to occupational therapists who aspire to occupation-centred practice (Baum, Berg, Seaton, & White, 2002; Pollard & Walsh, 2000). Yet there appears to be limited information available to guide and support therapists in reconciling an occupation-centred practice paradigm with the (often incongruous) acute orientation of hospitals, especially with children. This chapter aims to explore how occupational therapists in children's hospitals describe, justify and implement occupation-centred practice despite the inherent challenges of their working environment. Given the paucity of literature on this topic, we conducted several focus groups with 19 paediatric occupational therapists based in hospitals in Queensland, Australia, to explore the nature of their occupation-centred practice, how this was challenged by hospital settings and specific strategies employed to counter these workplace pressures. An occupational therapy (OT) manager from an adult hospital in Victoria, Australia, who had recently championed her department's transition towards a more occupation-centred model of service provision, was also consulted to provide a perspective on how this process may be operationalised from a management level.

We hope that this chapter will encourage readers to consider that the key to occupation-centred practice in acute hospital contexts may lie in re-evaluating and re-framing our reasons for intervention, so that occupation becomes our fundamental focus.

Occupation-centred practice in hospital settings: lessons from the literature

Does occupation-centred practice 'fit' in acute hospitals?

Molineux (2001) has argued that if we wish to claim occupation as the defining characteristic of our profession, we must re-frame our practice and clearly demonstrate our 'own commitment to occupational research, occupational education and occupational practice' (p. 94), in spite of workplace constraints. Thus, all clinical practice, even within acute settings, should be occupationally focused and articulated in the language of occupation. Whilst a seemingly straightforward direction, there is some evidence which suggests that not only is this difficult to do, but there also exists some ambivalence amongst members of the profession about whether occupation *is* our core concern. This professional uncertainty is exemplified by the varying accounts from occupational therapists of their roles within acute hospitals. Reportedly, descriptions range from enabling clients' functional skills development (Molineux, 2004) to 'gap filling' or behaving 'chameleon like' so that tasks which serve the interests of the clients' health and well-being but are not prioritised by other members of the health care team are addressed (Fortune, 2000). Additionally, some therapists focus on client capacity to perform basic functional movements and tasks that are not necessarily immediately relevant to or consistent with their usual context (Persson, Erlandsson, Eklund, & Iwarsson, 2001). In accord with the focus of this book, we propose in this chapter that it is not just worthwhile but essential that OT practice, regardless of clinical setting, remains theoretically and philosophically aligned with the profession's ethos of facilitating people's engagement in meaningful occupations which enables participation in important life roles.

Why is occupational therapy practice in acute hospital settings inherently challenging?

Although this question has not been the specific target of research in children's hospitals, challenges have been described in some accounts (Crooks & Wavrek, 2005). Research from Australian metropolitan adult hospital settings (Wilding & Whiteford, 2007, 2008) provides some further insight into this issue.

Wilding and Whiteford (2007, 2008) employed participatory action research (PAR) methodology to explore the everyday practice of occupational therapists in acute adult hospital settings. It became evident that in these settings there was a strong focus on:

- remediating illness and injury
- improving health by treating disease
- the primacy of the medical profession in terms of medico-legal requirements, management of patient care and initiating referrals to other health professions (Wilding & Whiteford, 2007)

Wilding and Whiteford (2007) interviewed 10 occupational therapists with 3–10 years experience and another with more than 10 years experience to examine how they explained and justified their practice and the application of occupation-focused theory and evidence which informed their practice. Participants described their role as 'enhanc[ing] their patients' health through doing, and [acting] as experts in doing ...' (p. 189). However, their explanations of OT to others (i.e. clients, colleagues and administrators) were purposefully devoid of professional jargon (e.g. 'occupation' and other occupational language). Instead they used terms such as 'activities' and 'function', and drew parallels with other professions such as physiotherapy. These explanations typically included simplified descriptions of OT processes and philosophical beliefs (e.g. empowerment, motivation and enablement) and highlighted the relationship between environment and activity participation. Although these graded explanations and analogies were purported to be more easily understood by colleagues, the occupational therapists felt this was a 'double-edged sword'. By representing OT in basic, uncomplicated terms, it could be misconstrued as relatively straightforward and therefore meriting less respect.

The participants also reported epistemological tensions in acute hospitals. They felt there was a mismatch between the philosophy, theory and practice of OT and medicine (Wilding & Whiteford, 2007). Occupational therapists were frequently frustrated by the constraints of the hospital environment on their practice, highlighting particularly the tensions between antagonistic reasoning processes (i.e. top-down versus bottom-up). The hospital context forced them to engage in bottom-up reasoning, where medical conditions are fore-grounded as the primary cause of occupational dysfunction and therefore should be the focus of intervention. This was clearly demonstrated by the nature of referrals to OT, which were determined by biomechanical problems and contained directions from medical staff about the nature of OT intervention required. Feelings of being misunderstood and overlooked by other health professions were compounded by different understandings of 'occupation', health and well-being.

These findings concurred with Fortune's (2000) interviews with six British occupational therapists in child and youth mental health practice. Similarly, these therapists avoided any philosophical reference to 'occupation' in their explanations of their role, opting instead to describe their intervention in terms of what needed to be done. Fortune (2000) described this as *paradigm-independent practice* – where context, clients' and/or colleagues' needs dictate OT services rather than our own professional paradigms/service models. She hypothesised that in the absence of a sound framework to guide their practice, occupational therapists risk losing their identity. Therefore, she advocated for 'occupationally informed therapy' (p. 229) and recommended that occupational therapists define their roles in line with sound theoretical underpinnings of occupation. These views have received support from subsequent literature (Molineux, 2004).

Occupation-centred practice in hospitals: lessons from the frontline

Considering the limited literature in this area, we undertook two focus groups with occupational therapists working in Queensland children's hospitals to: (1) ascertain the perspectives of therapists with first-hand knowledge of working with children in acute hospitals and (2) compare their experiences to their counterparts in adult hospitals as described in the literature. Details of the participants, hospital settings and procedures of the focus groups are provided in box below.

Background to focus groups

Participants
Nineteen occupational therapists with experience ranging from less than 12 months to over 25 years working with children and families in children's hospitals participated in two focus groups. Eighteen were female. Caseloads included developmental, mental health, surgical, orthopaedic, medical, oncology, burns/plastics/wound care, infants and neonates, feeding therapy, neurological, rehabilitation, intensive care, cystic fibrosis and diabetes.

The settings
Brisbane, an Australian capital city with just under 2 million people, has two large tertiary-level acute children's and women's hospitals which provide services for children from birth to 14 years of age. These hospitals

(Continued)

are major referral centres that comprise 24 h emergency departments, neonatal and paediatric intensive care units, theatres, and inpatient and outpatient services. Attached to each is a large allied health department with services including OT, physiotherapy, music therapy, speech pathology, audiology, social work, psychology and dietetics. Thus, these hospitals exemplify settings commonly described in the literature (e.g. Crooks & Wavrek, 2005). One participant worked in the children's wards of a smaller regional general hospital, located approximately 80 km from Brisbane.

Focus groups procedure

Ethical clearance was obtained to conduct two focus groups. Occupational therapists provided written consent agreeing to participate in and digital recording of the discussions. Each of the major children's hospitals hosted one focus group, with 12 and 7 therapists attending each of the groups, respectively. Each discussion was facilitated by at least one of the authors. The focus groups were of 1.5–2 h duration and followed a purposefully designed schedule of open-ended questions with probes to explore issues further as they were raised in discussions. The following key questions were asked:

● How familiar are you with the term 'occupation-centred practice'?
● What does 'occupation-centred practice' mean in a children's hospital context?
● Describe the OT process in this context.
● What are the barriers to occupation-centred practice at the hospital?
● What strategies can help overcome these barriers?

Summaries and key themes from each of the focus groups were distributed to all participants within 2 weeks for member checking (Patton, 2002). The authors independently read the written transcripts and summaries and coded the data based on standard content analysis techniques. Discussions between the authors enabled identification of key themes. Quotes from participants are reported in the following text.

What does 'occupation-centred practice' mean in acute children's hospital?

> We pride ourselves on trying to use our occupational focus in everything we do. So … looking holistically at our work, particularly a child's occupational roles, and how [being in hospital] will impact upon that, then working to help the children do the things that they need and want to do as part of their occupation, despite being in a different environment (hospital) or despite their illness or disability.

As illustrated in the above quote, our participants indicated that despite their apparent focus on biomechanical performance and specific performance components in practice with children in acute settings, the underpinning philosophy and framework guiding their clinical reasoning was essentially occupation-centred. Being occupation-centred was described as part of the 'core business' of OT – an approach shared by all therapists, influenced by client-centredness, a holistic perspective and occupation-focused principles including valued life roles and occupations. From the individual practitioner's perspective, occupation-centred practice was described as 'a framework for how you prioritise and work and intervene with the child'. From a management perspective, it was described as 'a fundamental concept that underpins a lot of what we do ... and certainly underpins anything that we present or plan'. When presented with the core features of occupation-centred practice described in Chapter 2, participants identified three features which consistently characterised their practice within acute children's hospital settings: (1) a client-centred orientation, (2) individualised intervention, and (3) interventions that were contextually relevant to the child's circumstances (i.e. being hospitalised).

Occupational therapists justified their acutely focused interventions minimising later occupational dysfunction or disruption for the child and his/ her family.

One participant elaborated on this with an example from the 'hands caseload'. Referral to OT for a splint is common after an acute hand injury. The requested OT intervention was primarily medically oriented (i.e. to remediate physical injury) and presented limited opportunities for engagement with the child and family members, in terms of participating in decision making and goal setting. In this instance, clinical reasoning is guided predominantly by the medical condition, the therapist's knowledge of wrist anatomy and the goal of supporting the wrist and associated structures to promote healing and proper joint alignment. Although the primary reason for OT involvement with the child is the acute injury, intervention will not necessarily cease at this point. The occupational therapist employs a complex thinking process which enables him/her to look beyond the immediate injury to longer term goals and implications, such as supporting the child to use his/her hand appropriately for daily tasks and to cope at home and school whilst the injury is healing. This 'future-thinking' perspective, that is, considering the implications of the hand injury for participation in meaningful occupational and role performance, distinguishes OT input from that of other health professions.

These accounts mirror the findings of Mattingly and Fleming (1994) who described the 'underground practice' of occupational therapists working in medical or hospital settings. This concept of a 'hidden' practice conveys the discrepancy between what occupational therapists perceive as their role and what is observed and interpreted from their interventions by others. Although our participants did not use the term 'underground practice', it was evident that their seemingly biomechanical focus was driven by a reasoning process clearly grounded in occupation. Similar to the therapists from Mattingly and Fleming's (1994) study, the occupational therapists in Brisbane children's hospitals believed that an overtly holistic approach to practice would mitigate their credibility within the medical culture of their workplace. Thus, occupationally driven interventions would be 'hidden' by redefining problems and treatment goals in biomedical terms.

How is occupation-centred practice discussed?

Although an occupational focus was considered integral to their practice, participants generally did not document this (e.g. in reports or progress notes) or otherwise communicate this explicitly. The term 'occupation-centred practice' was not a part of their daily hospital vernacular. They preferred to couch their descriptions of OT roles and services in medical terms such as 'function' and language which was meaningful, specific and relevant to the child and family, such as 'play skills', 'school participation', 'feeding', 'functional skills' or 'everyday tasks'. Adapting their descriptions during communication with client/s, other health professionals and hospital administrators was a strategic decision.

> When you think about working in an acute hospital, other professions and funding sources don't regard occupation-centred practice as something that they are going to acknowledge and back financially and regard as an important hospital service ....
> I don't think [occupation] is something that means a lot to anybody outside the profession, to be honest.

These findings reflect the literature described earlier relevant to adult hospital settings (e.g. Mattingly & Fleming, 1994; Wilding & Whiteford, 2007, 2008), in that occupational therapists find our professional language and jargon to be very different to that of other health professions and therefore problematic. Whilst being poorly understood is hardly unique to the acute setting, it seems more pronounced within the acute environment since other disciplines have more clearly defined roles and share a biomechanical focus.

What does occupation-centred practice look like in the hospital setting?

Giving meaning to hospitalisation

An important and distinguishing feature of the OT role in acute hospital settings was perceived to be in providing meaning to the hospitalisation experience within the context of the child's and family's life. Assisting the child and his/her family to understand, prepare for and cope with potentially frightening and painful medical procedures and treatments such as diagnostic and intervention procedures exemplifies this role. Occupational therapists would explain their treatments and outcomes in terms of the impact on the child, his/her ability to engage in typical and valued roles and occupations, and the family members and their meaningful occupations and roles. To assist with coping, for example, meaningful, age-appropriate occupations could be used to distract and/or reward the child during and after painful dressing changes. This role will be further illustrated in the burns case study presented later in this chapter.

Participants felt that their occupational focus was more valued and more readily accepted by other health professionals and clients when working with children with chronic conditions requiring regular and/or prolonged hospitalisation. Since the child would be admitted for extended period/s of time, the hospital context was recognised as an occupational environment for the child and therefore there was less resistance to focusing on engaging in and performing meaningful activities. Since the child would have long-term medical requirements, it was believed that other health professionals could better appreciate OT contributions (e.g. assisting child and family to adjust, facilitating participation in occupations and roles such as play and school, and enabling meaningful social engagement and interactions).

Education of child and family: enabling understanding and informed participation

A strong theme which emerged from both focus groups was the key role occupational therapists play in educating the child and family to help them make sense of and deal with the child's admission to hospital, and to facilitate appropriate, timely and informed participation of children and their parent/s in decision making. As described by one participant, 'I think a lot of what we do is a lot just talking, and explaining and educating, not just around what our role is, but helping [the child and family] understand the process'. Thus, within the overall approach of the health care team, the OT contribution includes: (1) providing individualised and age-appropriate explanations to children and their families regarding medical procedures and outcomes; (2) facilitating clients' informed participation in goal setting and interventions; and (3) helping them to understand how interventions may impact on the child's future coping, psychosocial development and occupational performance. Occupational therapists achieve this by drawing on their unique blend of skills including a holistic approach, varied communication styles and techniques, knowledge of medical conditions and typical childhood development, and the impact of environment on occupational performance.

> We educate because we understand those caregivers are important to that child and without [the caregivers] understanding and being educated, they're not available to that child to give the support that they [children] necessarily need.

Although the child's health condition was the reason for hospital admission and therefore the dominant focus for the medical staff and dictated the health care services provided, our participants also described a unique feature of their role in supporting parenting occupations and roles (e.g. care-giving and meaningful interactions with their child). This intervention was considered more critical for particular caseloads (e.g. infants, feeding and mental health). Since other health professionals, the child and his/her family tend to focus on the medical condition, appreciation of the potential role of OT is not immediately apparent. Therefore, the onus is on occupational therapists to advocate for their interventions and enabling parental occupations and co-occupations (e.g. feeding and play). The role of occupational therapists in supporting parents will be demonstrated in one of the feeding case studies later in this chapter.

Challenges to occupation-centred practice in hospitals

The nature of hospital environments

Acute hospitals are notoriously unpredictable work environments for health professionals. Similar to other studies (Crooks & Wavrek, 2005; Wilding & Whiteford, 2007), our participants described a range of challenges impacting on their ability to be occupation-centred practitioners in children's hospitals. It seems that the most significant barrier to occupation-centred practice is the acute medical orientation which dominates hospital culture and influences all aspects of the work environment:

- Prioritisation of medical interventions and procedures to address the child's acute health needs;
- Hierarchy of referrals according to medical expertise and medical requirements;
- Co-ordination of the health care team by medical professionals (which compounds the two previous points);
- Availability and capacity of the child and parents to participate and engage in interventions (depending on factors such as grief and coping, physical illness and competing family responsibilities such as work and care for other children/dependents).

Children admitted to hospital are usually in acute stages of illness, and require multiple diagnostic and/or surgical interventions to manage life-threatening conditions. Thus, contact with medical professionals is understandably prioritised over contact with occupational therapists, whose input may be perceived to be less immediately relevant. It is very difficult to persevere with a focus on occupational issues, when colleagues, children, families and hospital administration are much more concerned with immediate health issues. As one participant put it, it is extremely challenging to be 'proactive rather than reactive' when the rest of the health care team is focused on responding to changes in medical status and biomechanical issues.

There exists significant pressure on occupational therapists to be consistent with the priorities of their colleagues and child and family by focusing on acute health issues and care pathways (e.g. positioning, splinting and wound care). Since referrals to OT are initiated by medical professionals whose focus is on acute issues, it is challenging to remain occupation-centred:

> On days when you're just running and chasing and responding [to the pager] all day, it is easy to become task-focused rather than remaining focused on the overarching occupational focus.

These comments are reinforced by findings from Mattingly and Fleming (1994), who indicated that the hospital context restricts OT practice by limiting it to biomedical approaches which makes it difficult to address the 'lived body' and disability as it affects the person's occupations, roles and relationships. Most health professions follow standardised protocols based on a medical diagnosis/classification of illness which does not always align with our desire to be individual-focused.

On admission to hospital, a child's typical participation in occupations and roles is brought to a sudden halt and thus problems in these areas are less evident. Hospitalisation is often perceived as a discrete and unpleasant episode within a child's life during which they are removed from valued activities, environments and social interactions. It is difficult for an occupational therapist to assess and/or anticipate occupational dysfunction when their only knowledge of the child is outside of his/her own context. Hospital policies (e.g. related to home visits) may also make it difficult for therapists to access home or school environments in preparation for discharge. As one participant commented:

> I find that a huge challenge to assess performance and participation in this environment when the kids aren't feeling well and the tools that we use do not match the kid's [context].

Finally, the intrinsic pressures of working in a hospital such as rapidly changing medical status, pressure for quick discharge once acute crisis has resolved, bed shortages and large caseloads make it very difficult for an occupational therapist to be creative and think beyond the immediate point of time.

Difficulty in engaging in the entire occupational therapy process

We asked the focus group participants to comment on the OT process as depicted in Chapter 2 with relation to their own working experiences. They indicated that whilst ideal, in reality this process would be very difficult to follow in its entirety and identified several factors militating against the provision of this optimal input. Rather than being continuously involved in the child's care throughout admission, the therapist is typically referred to during discrete points for a specific purpose, such as conducting a developmental assessment to aid diagnosis of a medical condition or assistance in discharge planning. As such, OT intervention is often a 'disjointed' service rather than a comprehensive, integrated progression from admission to discharge.

There were several concerns also raised with the feasibility of goal setting consistent with an occupation-centred focus in an acute medical environment. The priority given to medical issues tends to dictate immediate goals, whereas occupational goals may be more appropriate once acute medical issues have been resolved or managed.

Collaborative goal setting was also noted to not always be appropriate or realistic. For example, infants in Neonatal Intensive Care Units (NICUs) are often seen without parents in attendance and so the onus is on the health care team to determine the most appropriate goals for the infant (e.g. positioning, environmental modifications to decrease physiological distress or increase tolerance of handling). Furthermore, the associated trauma of the event leading to hospitalisation (e.g. burn injury) may impact on the child's and family's capacity to participate in planning and goal setting. As explained by one therapist:

> Can you expect them to sit down and think about their goals when they're ... still struggling with the fact that their child almost died? But we still need to get on with our work and set our own goals.

Similarly, another participant noted that:

> When they're in hospital to address something, it's ... life threatening ... they will just disregard everything, they just block it out, other than stuff that is immediately relevant to the recovery.

It is recognised that particularly in the early stages of admission, the child and family are dealing with significant and overwhelming emotional issues. As such their ability not only to participate in the goal-setting process, but also to be of mind to take on board information so that they can make appropriate decisions may be diminished. Hence, our participants emphasised the importance of providing the child and parent/s with information to enable appropriate and *timely* involvement in planning and implementation of health care interventions. Goal setting was described as an iterative rather than a linear process. OT referral originates from a specific medical issue (e.g. feeding difficulties), which tends to influence initial goals. An occupational focus, however, enables therapists to 'peel back the layers' and identify other goals requiring attention in order to best serve the client and family. This will be illustrated in the feeding case study later in the chapter.

A predominantly occupational focus during assessment, intervention and evaluation was also noted to not always be appropriate. For example, for a child feeling acutely unwell, it may be more client-centred to evaluate discrete performance components and then anticipate occupational disturbances, rather than expect the child to complete actual tasks. The nature of the presenting condition was often a key determinant in how appropriate an occupational focus was. One participant described this as needing to focus on both immediate issues (consistent with the acute medical issue) whilst remaining cognisant of potential longer term issues and outcomes. Consider a teenager who has a lesion to forearm flexor tendons from falling on a broken bottle; he/she is unlikely to have persistent issues once the injury has healed. Thus, it is more appropriate to focus at the physical body structure and activities level (ICF; WHO, 2001) in fabricating the splint, and educating the teen about its use and how it may impact performance in certain activities whilst worn. In contrast, for a child with a brain injury, whilst the initial referral for OT may be similar in that it is for splinting (during coma to prevent contractures due to hypertonicity), the child is much more likely to have persistent physical and cognitive issues impacting on daily occupations and life roles; therefore, an occupational focus is far more appropriate and able to be implemented over time.

Strategies to foster occupation-centred practice in children's hospitals

Despite these hurdles, participants from both focus groups were able to identify a number of strategies which facilitated their implementation of occupation-centred practice.

Communication and education

The most significant strategy was the need for communication and education of fellow health workers about their role. In efforts to advocate for and educate others about the OT role, several participants (although they were in the minority) deliberately used and defined the term 'occupation' when reporting to other health professionals via progress notes and other documentation. One participant described trying to use occupational language to explain the assessments used and interventions provided to the child in terms of the impact on the occupations of play, self-care and schoolwork.

This strategy is consistent with Molineux's (2004) call for therapists to 'use the language of occupation' (p. 94), and therapists in Wilding and Whiteford's study (2007) who introduced headings such as 'occupational performance, occupational history, occupational engagement' and other occupational language into their reports. These changes in language were noted to improve therapists' levels of confidence, strengthen professional identities and heighten organisational feelings of empowerment (Wilding & Whiteford, 2007). Even relatively simple changes in language appeared to be transformative, leading to enhanced personal and professional identities as occupational therapists and an enhanced professional profile within the organisation (Wilding & Whiteford, 2008). Our participants recommended regular and clear communication of the purpose and contributions of OT to multiple audiences (i.e. clients, health care team and administrators) via multiple channels (e.g. verbal discussions, written reports and progress notes).

Demonstrating outcomes

Participants also found it beneficial to communicate explicitly the links between OT interventions which positively impacted on medical procedures and outcomes. This was particularly highlighted for psychosocial interventions. For example, a child may be resistant to certain interventions or using a specific piece of equipment which has implications for their treatment, progress and ultimate medical outcomes. Therefore, it is important to make the team aware of the need to address psychosocial issues to help the child adjust to and accept the equipment/device (e.g. walker and wheelchair) or cope with medical procedures (e.g. distraction activities during painful procedures or preparation for medical interventions). In such circumstances, our participants believed it was easier for other health professionals to recognise and appreciate the potential input of occupationally focused interventions. When other staff were aware of the links between OT and improved outcomes (e.g. reduced intervention times since the child was more receptive/relaxed), they were likely to refer to OT more regularly and initiate such referrals earlier.

Visibility and advocacy

Occupational therapists also highlighted the importance of being visible within the multi-disciplinary team by attending all ward rounds, team meetings and case conferences, visiting the ward regularly and checking admissions lists. This enabled practitioners to be proactive rather than reactive in acquiring referrals. However, it is important to ensure that implementation of this strategy does not overburden an already pressured workload.

Since OT is not always clearly understood by medically focused professions, it is important for therapists to act as advocates for themselves as well as for children's access to OT services. Individual therapists felt that support and promotion of occupation-centred practice within the OT team was critical to maintaining their approach. One stated:

> It's really easy in a busy, traumatic acute setting to become caught up in things and losing [sic] sight of your ultimate goal and what your professional role is. So I think having support within OT and ... keeping in touch with the professional core skills is a really useful thing to do.

This statement reflects the value of having departmental strategies in place to support occupation-centred practice. With this in mind, we consulted with a manager of an OT department from an acute adult hospital setting in Victoria, Australia, who had recently managed a process of change within her service to ensure that it was more occupationally oriented. Presented in below box are her suggestions for supporting occupation-centred practice from a management perspective.

Strategies to enhance occupation-centred practice in hospital settings (Ralda Bourne, personal communication, St. Vincent's Hospital, Melbourne, Australia, 2009)

Develop a consistent OT profile across the hospital

- Develop and agree to an OT profile within the OT department which is consistently adopted by all individual therapists. Details could include recommendations for use of language/terminology in documentation, encouraging explicit reports of clinical reasoning, establishing and attending reflective practice groups, etc.
- Negotiate how OT language should be used in practice and particularly when communicating with clients, health professionals and hospital administrators (in all verbal and written reporting media).
- Consistently make explicit links to occupational issues in referrals, thereby promoting continuity of care and occupational focus through different services.
- Identify the challenges to occupation-centred practice from multiple perspectives (e.g. clients, other health professionals, organisational and personal). Then, as a department, develop local strategies and identify ways of supporting one another to remain occupation-centred.

Institute in-service workshops/sessions to support changes in practice

Topics might include:

- Linking theory and practice - reinforcing our occupation origins by reviewing OT models.
- How to emphasise and make explicit our focus on occupation during OT assessment, intervention and service.
- A consistent approach to and language for documenting OT practice in charts, for example, creating templates for progress notes and reports. Headings could include: pre-admission occupational performance, performance components, current occupational performance, short-term and long-term implications for occupational performance, and recommendations.

The published literature to date indicates that acute care settings can challenge our professional identity and epistemological underpinnings. This was confirmed by our focus group participants, who have provided a grass-roots level perspective on OT practice in children's hospitals and also identified strategies to persevere with an occupation-centred focus despite the inherent challenges of their working environment. Strategies for promoting occupation-centredness within an OT department have also been provided from a management perspective. The strategies outlined above are generic and we recommend that therapists seeking to become more occupation-centred tailor such strategies to their local context.

Examples of occupation-centred practice in children's hospital settings

This section describes occupation-centred practice within two different caseloads in acute children's hospital settings. These scenarios are presented to highlight particular principles of occupation-centred practice in action, rather than to provide a detailed account of OT services in each instance.

Occupation-centred practice with children with burn injuries: James

This case study outlines the occupational therapist's role with a child with an acute burn injury from the initial acute phase of wound management and healing to rehabilitation and community re-integration. The occupation-centred approach is particularly useful in assisting James and his family to cope with hospitalisation, medical treatments and long-term implications associated with the burn injury. Seven-year-old James presented to the Emergency Department with flame burns covering 20% of his body. Burn depth ranged from superficial to full thickness and involved his face, axilla, chest and both upper limbs.

Information gathering
First, the occupational therapist needed to collect relevant information relating to James's pre-injury roles, activities and interests, alongside injury-related information including current coping, adjustment to injury/hospitalisation, total body surface area of burn (TBSA), depth of burn and possible acute care plans. This initial process identified meaningful occupations and roles for James and his family, which could be used to guide goal setting, enhance James's motivation for and participation in his treatment and develop his resources for coping.

Days 1–4 post-injury
Initial interviews with James and his parents described James's pre-morbid development, abilities, interests and roles. His interests include playing soccer on Saturdays and helping his mother cook pancakes or

cupcakes. He shared a close relationship with his older sister (aged 9 years) who reportedly became very anxious whenever James was hurt. James enjoyed school and had many friends; his teachers described him as an active participant at school and valued classroom member. James had expressed concerns to his mother that his friends might forget him or laugh at him when he returned to school. This interview also explored James's experiences with acute hospital environments and coping with injuries and pain. His parents described James as a child who hid his true feelings and preferred to put on a brave front when upset or scared. James had no prior experience with hospitals; his minor injuries had been attended to at home by his family.

Medical and occupational therapy interventions

For the first week of acute treatment, James's dressings were changed on the ward every 3 days. The injuries to his chest and upper arms injuries required skin grafting, which was followed by 3 weeks of dressing changes every 3 days. James's left axilla and elbow were splinted during the immediate course of healing, with a stretching regime initiated post-healing to mini-mise contracture. James found that wearing the splint full time impacted on his participation in self-care and other valued activities. The occupational therapist negotiated a compromise with James: if he co-operated with the splint wearing regime he could remove the splints twice daily, which would enable him to practise dressing himself and play balloon volleyball with his sister during her visits. This latter activity was not only meaningful, but also afforded James the opportunity to actively use his upper limbs above shoulder level and thus elicit extended range movements. To encourage his increasing participation in activities and endurance, James was also engaged regularly in physically-based therapy sessions.

Psychosocial adjustment and procedural preparation

For James, consideration of psychosocial issues was important in order to reduce the impact of the trauma, pain and hospitalisation on his potential engagement in occupational roles, both short- and long-term. The occupa-tional therapist performed a critical role in assisting James to cope with medical procedures and adjust to the hospital environment and his injury. The therapist understood that James might be reluctant to share his feelings and fears about certain treatments with the staff and therefore adopted the 'anticipate, prepare and distract' approach. Anticipating that James may be fearful of the dressing procedures, the therapist began preparing him well in advance of the procedure. This preparation included age-appropriate, specific and truthful information regarding the medication and dressing changes, and the operating theatre procedures and grafting. James's fears were assuaged by visiting the dressing room and seeing the surgical instruments ahead of the procedure, and by hearing information which *he* considered important: what his 'jobs' during treatment were, how much pain to expect and how the burn might look.

James's parents and sister also participated in this activity with the occupational therapist. The inclusion of his family not only relieved James's initial anxieties, but was also valuable in providing an avenue for the family to learn how they could help James cope. James, his family, nursing staff and the occupational therapist collaboratively developed a distraction plan for the dressing changes. Though this plan was periodically revised during the course of treatment, it always included interaction between James and his parents/family with a meaningful activity such as a game, book or video. The occupational therapist utilised James's interest in cooking (identified during initial assessment) as a motivator throughout his admission, to re-engage him in activities and as a reward for more physically-based therapy sessions.

Whilst wearing splints and unable to use his arms extensively, he was able to watch TV, videos and engage in touch screen-based computer activities.

Planning return to school

Once James's medical condition stabilised, the occupational therapist introduced James to the hospital teacher. This served two main purposes: (1) to give James the opportunity to re-engage in his valued student role and (2) to facilitate and increase contact with his school and classmates in preparation for his transition back to school. James established regular email contact with his friends and peers. This was valuable for not only resuming typical social interactions, but also allowing him to explain and describe his accident, subsequent hospitalisation and progress to his peers. In preparing James to return to school, the main aims were to anticipate potential difficulties with the transition and help James (and his classmates) to cope with support from James's family, teacher and occupational therapist. The occupational therapist and James discussed his concerns and fears, and anticipated reactions and questions he might receive from other children. Allowing James the opportunity to admit and express these feelings enabled him to develop appropriate coping strategies and rehearse answers to difficult questions, before attempting his return to the classroom. Another important strategy for facilitating return to school was scheduling a school visit at which James, his parents, the hospital school teacher and the occupational therapist met with his fellow students. Prepared and supported by the occupational therapist, James was able to explain his changed appearance and the purpose of wearing pressure garments to his classmates. Furthermore, his teacher was recruited as an additional channel for support and communication with James and his family.

Evaluation prior to discharge

Assessment of James's ADL performance and mobility prior to discharge was needed to ensure that appropriate supports were available to him at home. James was functioning independently and appropriately for his age, and accepted assistance with donning pressure garments. Since James's generalised adjustment to his burn injury experience and coping with scarring and wearing pressure garments would be an ongoing process, he was invited to attend the annual camp organised by the hospital burns centre. His interest in attending was enhanced not just by the scheduled camp activities, but also by the chance to re-engage with friends he had made during his hospitalisation.

Follow up

By age 11 years, James found that his reduced ROM restricted his engagement in sporting, school and self-care activities (e.g. dressing) and was re-admitted for contracture release surgery on his right elbow. Otherwise, James successfully returned to his pre-injury level of engagement in self-care, school activities and soccer.

In this case, there were a number of psychosocial issues surrounding his injury, treatment and recovery which if not properly addressed would have had significant implications for James's physical, emotional, social and cognitive development and life trajectory. By identifying James's valued occupations and roles and remaining occupation-focused, the occupational therapist was able to implement strategies which helped James to accept and cope with medical treatments, adjust to the long-term effects of his injury and resume participation in meaningful activities.

Feeding therapy services case study: Brayden and Fiona

In this second case study of feeding services in the special care nursery, the role of OT in supporting parent occupations is highlighted. Although the referral to OT services originates from the infant's feeding capabilities, the therapist peels back the layers utilising an occupation-centred approach to identify other issues which warrant intervention in order to effectively address the feeding difficulties and support infant occupations.

Fiona, mother to four children aged 3–14 years, gave birth to her fifth child Brayden at 35 weeks gestation. Small for gestational age, Brayden was also diagnosed with a complex condition known as tracheo-oesophageal fistula and oesophageal atresia shortly after birth. Brayden's tracheo-oesophageal fistula was surgically repaired within 24 h after birth but the resulting large central chest incision meant that he was restricted to supine lying with minimal handling and position changes. A jujenostomy tube delivered continuous feeds which met Brayden's nutritional requirements. This meant that Brayden was unable to establish oral feeding during his neonatal period, which necessitated a lengthy admission in the special care nursery. When Brayden had reached a chronological gestational age of 37 weeks, he was referred to the OT and speech pathology feeding team, to initiate an early intervention oral stimulation programme and support his developmental progression in preparation for future oral feeding.

Fiona and Brayden meet the Feeding Therapy Team

One of the occupational therapist's first priorities was to establish a supportive relationship with Fiona during her initial visits to the nursery to help her cope with her anxieties surrounding Brayden's medical condition and feeding difficulties. Fiona had successfully breastfed her other children and had looked forward to also sharing this experience with Brayden. The inability to engage with her son at this level was a source of emotional distress. Until Brayden's admission to the nursery, Fiona's primary contact with her son involved occasional Kangaroo care (i.e. skin-to-skin contact). Fiona could only visit Brayden every 2–3 days since she depended on volunteer hospital-provided transportation and also needed to care for her other children. Thus, Fiona's opportunities to bond with Brayden had been minimal. The occupational therapist needed to increase Fiona's confidence with handling, and support and enable meaningful interactions between Fiona and her medically fragile infant. Strategies included teaching Fiona alternative sensory-based activities, such as infant massage and sensory stimulation techniques (e.g. face-to-face social interactions and introducing appropriate toys over time) whilst Brayden was restricted to supine lying. Utilisation of such strategies enabled Fiona to overcome her fears regarding the seriousness of Brayden's condition and the stressful medical nursery environment and focus on a nurturing relationship with her son. Whilst supporting Fiona's developing parental occupations and interactions with Brayden, the occupational therapist also collaborated with the speech pathologist in applying strategies and techniques for early oral stimulation to promote non-nutritive sucking.

Graduation to babies' ward

Thirteen weeks after birth, Brayden was transferred to the babies' unit of the adjoining children's hospital for ongoing medical and surgical intervention. His hospitalisation continued for a further 6 months due to the complexity of managing his condition and awaiting surgical repair to his oesophageal atresia. Brayden remained unable to feed orally during this time. Fiona however remained hopeful that she would one day be able to breastfeed Brayden and therefore continued to express breast milk.

The collaborative focus for OT and speech pathology became facilitating Brayden's eventual readiness for oral feeding and future mealtime participation. Therefore, the occupational therapist provided direct developmental intervention to optimise Brayden's developmental progress and providing developmentally encouraging activities for Brayden to engage in with Fiona during her visits (see Figure 13.1). Since he was isolated from his natural home and family environments, it was imperative to provide Brayden with opportunities to master his physical, social and emotional developmental milestones. Typically, prone lying affords the infant sensory experiences which enable the development of head and oral control (which are needed for later co-occupations such as feeding, play, social interaction, etc.; see Figure 13.2). The occupational therapist compensated for Brayden's limited prone lying ability with alternate positioning strategies (see Figure 13.3).

Brayden and Fiona also attended a weekly infant massage and development group with two other mothers and their babies who had complex medical conditions. Whilst addressing Brayden's physical and sensory

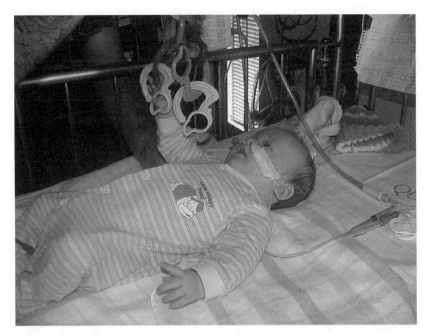

Figure 13.1 Learning to play in different positions (supine lying in hospital cot post-surgery). Reproduced with permission

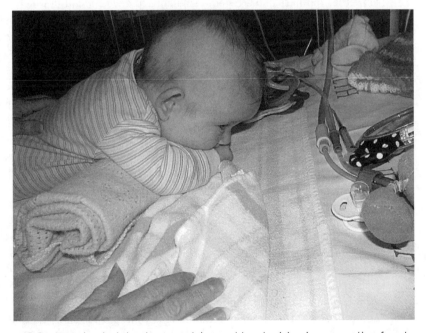

Figure 13.2 Learning to tolerate prone lying and head raising in preparation for play with toys post-surgery. Reproduced with permission

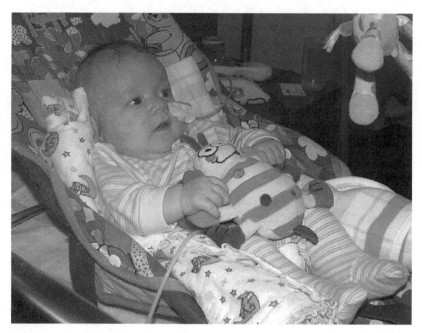

Figure 13.3 Sitting supported in chair for social interaction and play. Reproduced with permission

developmental needs, this intervention also provided Fiona with support from other mothers and created a small group environment in which these mothers and their babies could enjoy social interaction (an experience that they had missed due to hospitalisation). Brayden had been receiving massages regularly since birth and was observed to readily anticipate and consistently enjoy this experience within the group and consequently did not demonstrate any of the sensory defensive behaviours typically observed in infants with his complex condition. These interventions and early experiences facilitated by the occupational therapist enhanced Brayden's self-regulation capacity. Self-regulation is an important foundation for higher level skills such as learning to feed, coping with the environment and social interaction.

Brayden had surgical repair of the oesophageal atresia at 7 months of age and shortly afterwards a small amount of oral feeding was introduced. He was eventually discharged at 8 months with nasogastric tube feeding and small amounts of oral feeding. Developmentally, Brayden was achieving age-appropriate milestones in most aspects of his development. However, due to the complexity of his post-surgical status, he was unable to establish breastfeeding. Despite the preparatory activities and interventions, Brayden's ability to suck from a bottle was limited and he was transitioned to a sipper cup with thickened liquid and introduced to pureed solids (see Figure 13.4). The majority of his nutritional requirements were supported by nasogastric tube feeding. The therapists supported Fiona in accepting her disappointment about Brayden's inability to breastfeed.

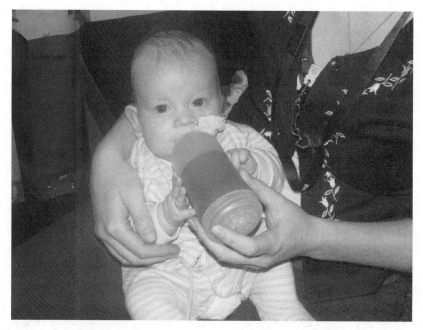

Figure 13.4 Learning to drink from a bottle. Reproduced with permission

Outpatient care

At 12 months, Brayden continued attendance at outpatient feeding therapy to support his ongoing development of oral feeding skills, interest in food and motivation to participate in mealtime experiences. During mealtimes at home with his family, Brayden sat in a high chair and readily enjoyed oral feeding experiences, albeit restricted in the quantity that he could physically manage. The outpatient feeding therapy sessions were also attended by some of his siblings, which afforded them opportunities to learn about Brayden's feeding limitations (e.g. that there are certain foods that are not safe to offer him). Fiona appreciated the ongoing support from the therapy team to help her adjust to the long-term nature of Brayden's feeding difficulties. It was anticipated that he will require long-term intervention and support to progress his eating skills development. Brayden's therapy would likely transition to a community-based therapy service in the future.

In this case study, although OT services were initiated due to feeding difficulties, the occupational therapist identified a number of other issues critical to Brayden's development and required attention. Specifically, she recognised that Brayden's progress, in the immediate and particularly the longer term, was dependent on enabling and supporting Fiona's parenting occupations. Based on this insight, a significant feature of the OT intervention was consequently to foster attachment between Brayden and Fiona, and recruit Fiona as an active intervention partner so that she could learn how to best support her son in reaching developmental milestones and engaging with his family.

Conclusion

This chapter has provided an overview of the challenges of occupation-centred practice in children's hospital settings from the perspectives of both the literature and therapists themselves. We have highlighted strategies to overcome these challenges as discussed by our informants and a hospital OT services manager. Three case studies were presented to illustrate how therapists can re-frame what they do and be explicit about how they practice in an occupation-centred manner. In the absence of significant literature in this area, it is hoped that this chapter provides a preliminary discussion about the 'how to' of being occupation-centred in children's hospital settings. Particularly we would like to emphasise that regardless of practice setting, OT practice with children focuses first and foremost on the occupations of children and their families.

Acknowledgements

Many thanks to Ms Kate Miller and Ms Belinda Kipping for their contribution of the burns case study and to Ms Lyndal Franklin for the feeding services case study. Thanks are also extended to the occupational therapists who attended the focus groups and contributed their thoughts and perspectives that informed the writing of this chapter. Their collaboration is greatly appreciated.

References

Baum, C., Berg, C., Seaton, M. K., & White, L. (2002). Fostering occupational performance and participation. In M. Law, C. M. Baum., & S. Baptiste (Eds.), *Occupation-cased practice: Fostering performance and participation* (pp. 27-36). Thorofare, NJ: SLACK Inc.

Crooks, L., & Wavrek, B. M. (2005). Hospital services. In J. Case-Smith (Ed.), *Occupational therapy for children* (5th ed., pp. 868-889). St. Louis, MO: Elsevier Mosby.

Fortune, T. (2000). Occupational therapists: Is our therapy truly occupational or are we merely filling gaps? *British Journal of Occupational Therapy, 63,* 225-230.

Mattingly, C., & Fleming, M. H. (1994). *Clinical reasoning: Forms of inquiry in a therapeutic practice.* Philadelphia, PA: F.A. Davis Company.

Molineux, M. (2001). Occupation: The two sides of popularity. *Australian Occupational Therapy Journal, 48,* 92-95.

Molineux, M. (2004). Occupation in occupational therapy: A labour in vain? In M. Molineux (Ed.), *Occupation for occupational therapists* (pp. 1-16). Oxford, UK: Blackwell Science.

Patton, M. Q. (2002). *Qualitative research & evaluation methods* (3rd ed.). Thousand Oaks, CA: Sage Publications.

Persson, D., Erlandsson, L. K., Eklund, M., & Iwarsson, S. (2001). Value dimensions, meaning and complexity in human occupation: A tentative structure for analysis. *Scandinavian Journal of Occupational Therapy, 8,* 7-18.

Pollard, N., & Walsh, S. (2000). Occupational therapy, gender and mental health: An inclusive perspective? *British Journal of Occupational Therapy, 55,* 425-431.

Wilding, C., & Whiteford, G. (2007). Occupation and occupational therapy: Knowledge paradigms and everyday practice. *Australian Occupational Therapy Journal, 54,* 185-193.

Wilding, C., & Whiteford, G. (2008). Language, identity and representation: Occupation and occupational therapy in acute settings. *Australian Occupational Therapy Journal, 55,* 180-187.

World Health Organisation (WHO). (2001). *International Classification of Functioning, Disability and Health (ICF).* Geneva, Switzerland: WHO.

Chapter 14

Enabling Children's Occupations and Participation using Assistive Technology

Desleigh de Jonge and Rachel McDonald

Learning objectives

The objectives of this chapter are to:

- Define assistive technologies and describe their benefits in enabling children with disabilities to acquire new skills and enable their participation in valued life roles.
- Describe one theoretical model, the Human Activity Assistive Technology (HAAT) model (Cook, Polgar, & Hussey, 2008), that can be used to inform the use of assistive technology (AT) for occupational engagement.
- Outline an occupation-centred practice process consistent with the HAAT model that can guide the use of AT with children and their families.
- Describe some assistive technologies that support children's engagement in play/leisure, productive and everyday occupations.

Introduction

This chapter addresses the use of assistive technology (AT) as a means of enhancing the participation of children with a range of impairments. Children typically engage in a range of play/leisure, school and self-care occupations, but when children have a physical, cognitive and/or social communicative impairment, their mastery of these occupations is often impacted. The role of occupational therapists is to enable children to engage in their occupational and social roles. Therapists promote engagement using a range of strategies such as helping children to acquire the skills to actively participate, modifying or adapting activities and the environment or selecting and supporting the use of AT.

What is assistive technology?

The World Health Organisation (WHO) defines AT as '... an umbrella term for any device or system that allows individuals to perform tasks they would otherwise be unable to do or increases the ease and safety with which tasks can be performed' (2004, p. 10). In this definition, the term 'AT' refers to both the physical device and the systems which enable a person to use that technology. This is also known as 'hard' *and* 'soft' *technology* (Cook et al., 2008; Waldron & Layton, 2008). Devices themselves which include equipment such as communication devices, wheelchairs and environmental control systems are known as 'hard' technologies. Supports or 'soft' technologies include the customising of the device to suit the individual, training to enable the person to use the device and providing advice regarding the device or maintenance of the device. AT ranges from simple low-tech options to sophisticated, 'high'-tech devices (Cook & Hussey, 2002). In essence, 'low' technologies are simple, inexpensive devices that are easy to make, such as a communication board. By contrast, 'high' technologies are expensive, sophisticated, dedicated technologies such as speech-generating devices or wheelchairs (Cook et al., 2008).

What can assistive technology offer children and families?

Children with disabilities often have impairments that limit their ability to participate in their life roles (Henderson, Skelton, & Rosenbaum, 2008). Most people use devices or technologies to assist them in their daily lives, for example, using a pen or computer to write or a remote control to turn the television on and off. Similarly, children with disabilities can benefit from AT in a number of ways.

First, technology is used to accommodate for lost function. For example, wheelchairs are provided to children who are unable to walk and speech-generating devices are provided to children who are unable to talk. Second, technologies are used to *assist* children to perform tasks or *augment* their performance. For example, children with dysarthria who are not able to communicate clearly can communicate more effectively with their peers and unfamiliar people using a speech-generating device. Children who find it difficult or effortful to walk long distances may find an electric wheelchair useful at school and in the community even though they may be able to walk a few steps. Figure 14.1 demonstrates how a mobile arm support and supportive seating can assist a high school student to manage home economics tasks. Third, technology can be used to assist families and carers to manage daily caretaking responsibilities. For example, when children cannot transfer in and out of bed or the bath/shower independently, a hoist or bath/shower chair can assist them to complete these tasks safely.

Technologies are not only useful in accommodating lost function, but can also enable skill acquisition and mastery and optimise occupational engagement and participation. For example, within the context of childhood development,

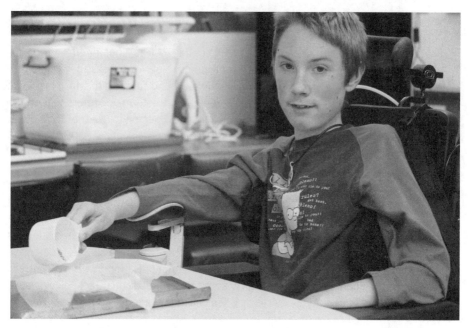

Figure 14.1 Participating in high school home economics using mobile arm support and supportive seating. Reproduced with permission

mobility is recognised as being essential for the development of an under-standing of the world through exploration as well as enhancing self-efficacy. Consequently, mobility devices have been developed for children in their first year of life to enable them to experience movement, explore and interact with the environment, leading to skill acquisition. In addition, technology allows children to enjoy a sense of control over where they go and where they can escape from, facilitating mastery and self-efficacy. It also provides a foun-dation for the development of skills to control more sophisticated mobility devices which these children will continue to need into the future. Similarly, the early use of communication technology provides children with many oppor-tunities to interact with people in their daily environments. In particular, it allows children to learn that the environment can be responsive to them, enabling them to link actions and outcomes.

AT can be used to enable the child to engage in activities that are mean-ingful to them. For example, a remote scanning device provides a child with limited dexterity with the capacity to change channels on the television. A joystick can be used to control a remote control car. A computer keyboard with large keys can enable a child with motor control difficulties to write. Text-to-speech software will allow a child with a vision impairment to access a story in the classroom or at home.

As members of families, classrooms and communities, children are often reliant on other people to assist them to actively participate in family, school and community occupations. Technologies can be used to facilitate this participation. For example, a switch-operated kitchen appliance allows

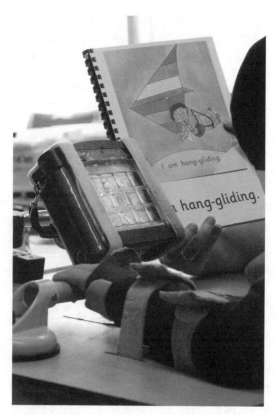

Figure 14.2 Using communication book and aid while stabilising other hand using a bar. Reproduced with permission

a child with limited physical function to participate in cooking patty cakes with siblings for a special family celebration. A range of computer-based programs can assist teachers in tailoring education for children with motor impairments to enable them to participate more fully in classroom learning activities. Figure 14.2 illustrates a boy using a communication book and aid to support his development of literacy skills. A lightweight stroller or wheelchair might enable the family to use public transport, allowing family participation in family-oriented community activities. A communication system can improve interaction, which is critical for promoting current and future relationships with other children, siblings, parents and other community members enabling social engagement.

A theoretical model for understanding assistive technology

Occupation-centred practitioners use theoretical models focusing on occupational performance and participation to underpin their practice. Occupation-centred models such as the Canadian Model of Occupational Performance and Engagement (CMOP-E) (CAOT, 2002; Townsend & Polatajko, 2007), the Person–Environment–Occupation–Performance (PEOP) (Christiansen & Baum, 1997) and the Person–Environment–Occupation (PEO) (Law, Cooper, Strong, Rigby, & Letts, 1996) provide a basis for understanding the scope of occupational therapy practice. These theoretical models discuss the interaction between people, their occupations and their environments, and the influence of each of these factors on occupational performance. However, none of these models explicitly articulates the role of ATs in enabling occupational performance.

There are a number of non-occupation-centred models that underpin AT practice, such as the Matching Person to Technology (MPT) model (Scherer, 2005) and the Human Activity Assistive Technology (HAAT) model (Cook & Hussey, 2002; Cook et al., 2008). Based on the use and non-use of AT by adults with physical disabilities, the MPT model seeks to explain the psychosocial aspects of technology use (Scherer, 2005). This model highlights the importance of understanding the person, technology and environmental context (milieu) in order to make a good match. It focuses on the user's personality, temperament and preferences, the salient characteristics of the technology, as well as the expectations, support and opportunities afforded by the environment, and how these impact potential technology use.

The HAAT model fits well with occupation-centred models as it seeks to explain the interrelationship between the *activity*, the AT user (*human*), the *AT* and the environment (*context*) (Cook & Hussey, 2002; Cook et al., 2008), illustrated in Figure 14.3. Rather than focusing specifically on the technology (AT), the HAAT model (Cook et al., 2008) describes all the elements in the *AT system* which represents 'someone (person with a disability) doing something (an activity) somewhere (within a context)' (p. 35). In common with occupation-centred models, the HAAT model focuses on enabling the person to participate rather than focusing on remediation of a physical, sensory or cognitive impairment. However, this model views AT as the means by which the person is enabled. The model consists of four elements: the *activity*, the *human*, the *assistive device* and the *context* (see Figure 14.3), each of which plays a unique but integral part in enabling the person to do what he/she wants or needs to be able to do.

Enabling the person to engage in *the activity* is the overall goal of an assistive or augmentative technology system (Cook et al., 2008). As with occupational therapy models, activities are categorised within three basic performance areas, namely: activities of daily living, work and productive activities, and play and leisure activities as demonstrated in Figure 14.4 (CAOT, 2002; Cook et al., 2008). However, whether an activity is defined as being self-care, productivity or leisure is determined by the meaning the individual gives to it. For example, reading may be considered in some contexts as a productive activity but viewed by the same person in another situation as a leisure activity.

The human performance component of the HAAT model conceptualises the human as the operator of the system who comes to the interaction

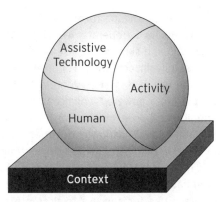

Figure 14.3 The HAAT model. Reproduced with permission from Elsevier (Cook et al., 2008, p. 36, Copyright 2008, 2002, 1995 by Mosby, Inc., an affiliate of Elsevier Inc.)

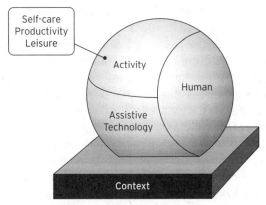

Figure 14.4 The HAAT model demonstrating link with occupations. Adapted from the HAAT model. Reproduced with permission from Elsevier (Cook et al., 2008, p. 36, Copyright 2008, 2002, 1995 by Mosby, Inc., an affiliate of Elsevier Inc.)

with experience, skills and abilities. It describes experience on a continuum between novice and expert. Novice users are more likely to use technologies in prescribed ways, and use conscious effort and soft technologies to support their effective use. Expert users, on the other hand, extend the use of their technologies, are more independent and exert less conscious effort when operating them. The model encourages therapists to recognise where the user is on the continuum and to assist him/her to become a proficient/expert user. Within this model, a distinction is made between the person's skills and abilities. *Abilities* are described as innate traits that a person brings to a new task while *skill* refers to the level of proficiency with which the task is undertaken. Consistent with occupational therapy models (e.g. CMOP; CAOT, 2002), human abilities comprise three elements, physical (e.g. motor and sensory), cognitive and affective (e.g. emotional).

These abilities influence the performance and successful completion of activities and the ability to operate AT. The model also recognises the importance of developing skills in the use of the technology as an enabler to engage successfully in activities. For example, a child would need to develop skills in the use of a joystick in order to be able to navigate within the environment using a powered wheelchair. This model cautions against selecting technologies based only on an understanding of the person's *current* level of ability as it acknowledges that skills can be further developed through the use of the technology over time. It draws on information processing, motor control and social learning theories to highlight the importance of engaging people fully in meaningful activities and providing them with opportunities for success to promote the effective use of AT (Cook et al., 2008).

AT is described as an extrinsic enabler that provides the mechanisms for a person with impairment to engage in the activity. The AT interfaces with the human, the environment and the activity and may or may not include a *processor* which translates information and forces received by or from the human into signals that control the activity output. The *human-technology interface* includes the positioning or postural support systems, the *control interface* and the display. Specific hardware is needed to fit the user's body and support posture and movement effectively to optimise performance. The *control interface* is the link that allows users to control the device and therefore needs to fit well with their experience, as well as their current and anticipated skills and abilities. The display provides feedback and information to the user. Some devices have processors that allow the device to control and process forces or data to produce required actions. The AT may provide one or more *outputs* which facilitate engagement in meaningful activity. For example, a communication device may provide voice, text or printed output. The *environment interface* is the link between the device and the external world or context. This interface has two facets, the first being the capacity to acquire environmental information and translate it into a form that can be accessed by the user. The second aspect to this interface is the capacity of the AT to respond to the demands of the environment (Cook et al., 2008). For example, a powered wheelchair may need to be able to move over a range of terrains and negotiate different gradients and spaces as well as a range of weather conditions. Although the HAAT model specifically identifies AT as an explicit component in the model, the model would work equally well for alternative strategies or personal assistance designed to enable the user. Using the HAAT model permits an evaluation of how these alternative strategies interface with the person, activities and environment. This would require that the AT section of the diagram (Figure 14.3) be replaced with an AT mechanism or system (de Jonge, Scherer, & Rodger, 2007).

The final aspect of the HAAT model is the *context*, described in terms of physical, social, cultural and institutional contexts. The *physical context* includes natural and built surroundings and physical parameters that enable, hinder or affect a person's performance with or without AT. It is therefore important to ensure the device is compatible with the environment. Some devices will need to work across a number of environments while others work under specific environmental conditions. For example, communication devices need to work in noisy, quiet, bright, dark, hot and cold environments while voice recognition technology works best in quiet conditions. The *social context* includes the people who interact directly or indirectly with the person using AT. The attitudes and capacity of family, teachers and peers to support the AT determine whether the AT is accepted, supported and used, or rejected, neglected and abandoned (Cook et al., 2008). The educational context is extremely important for children; not only do they spend on average 6–8 h at school, but these environments are also where students learn, and develop relationships with their peers through play, as well as manage self-care. Hence, ATs need to enable not only the child's access to educational materials, but also the development of friendships where appropriate.

The degree to which the AT can be supported by and supports other people within the user's *social context* also impacts on its acceptability. For example, technology that is complex to operate and/or difficult to maintain can become problematic for those in the application environment who support its use. Similarly, a piece of positioning equipment may not be used if it is too heavy for the person who supports the child (the parent) by transporting him/her to various application environments (McDonald, Surtees, & Wirz, 2003). Research has shown that AT improves participation and quality of life (Day & Jutai, 1996; Jutai, Fuhrer, Demers, Scherer, & DeRuyter, 2005; McDonald & Surtees, 2007); however, there is very little research about the effect of AT on the parents/caregivers/other family members or outcomes of AT use for care-giving (Henderson et al., 2008).

The *institutional context* includes the organisations in society responsible for policy, decision making and procedures that ensure children have access to devices and services to fund and support their use (Cook et al., 2008). The institutional context is complex with funding and services fragmented across resource and service systems, and often restricted to specific locations or application environments (Cowan & Turner-Smith, 1999; Wallace, Hayes, & Bailey, 2000). Universally, funding and provision of devices and access to adequate support is limited (McLaughlin, 2007). Within an educational setting, for example, a communication device may be funded to ensure the child can access the curriculum, but a positioning or seating system may not, even though the child requires a seating system to use his/her hands effectively to access the communication device and participate in classroom activities.

Information gathering for augmentative and assistive technologies

The occupation-centred practice process (Rodger, in press) was described in Chapter 2. The first aspect of this process, namely information gathering, is to identify the child's occupational concerns and strengths, as well as his/her occupational and life roles. In this context, our interest is in those roles and occupations that can be enhanced through AT as a basis for determining child- and family-centred goals. See Figure 14.5.

Goal setting

Sometimes children and their families come to see therapists with a vision of what they would like to achieve; however, often this vision evolves slowly. It may be difficult for the child and family to identify goals as an understanding of what technology can provide is often required in order to envisage the child's potential (Alliance for Technology Access, 2005). A vision for a child's future is largely affected by a perception of what he or she is capable of, a hope for what may be possible, as well as an understanding of what other children have achieved. With an understanding of technological developments and access to an ever-expanding range of technological possibilities, children and families can broaden their horizons and extend their vision of what is possible. Therapists need to embrace children's and families' visions of what they want to be able to do and provide them with information on technologies that can enable them to realise this vision. Alternatively, if the family has not yet developed a vision of what is possible, therapists can assist them in creating one by providing information on what technology can offer.

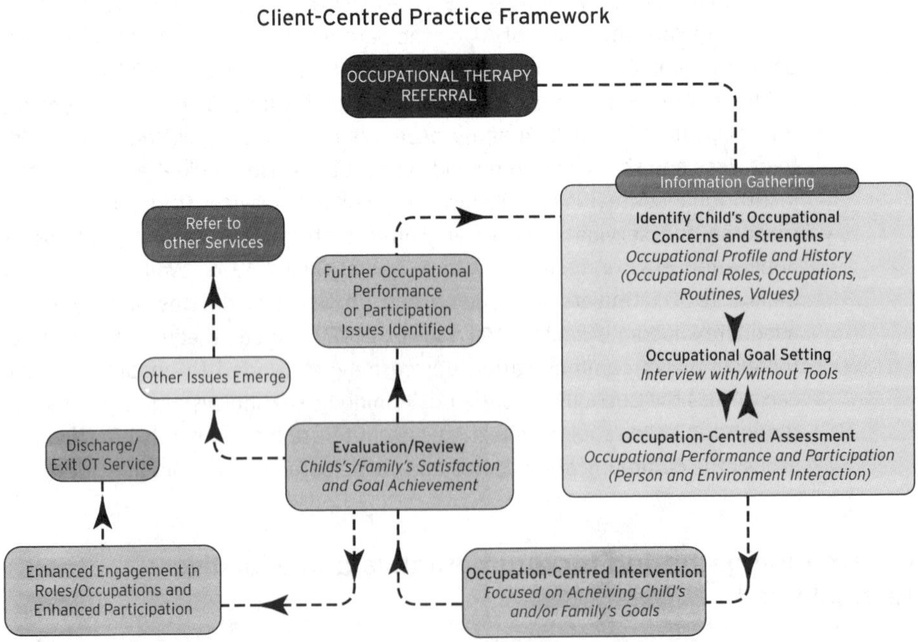

Figure 14.5 Occupation-centred practice process for children (Rodger, 2010). Reproduced with permission

Further, they can expand their horizons by introducing them to other families who are successfully using technology to achieve their goals.

Goal-setting tools

As addressed in detail in Chapter 6, a generic occupation-centred goal-setting tool such as the Canadian Occupational Performance Measure (COPM) (Law et al., 2005) can be utilised as an interview with parents and/or with the child to assist with occupation-based goal setting. In addition, based on the MPT Model, Scherer (2005) developed a suite of AT-specific tools designed to ensure that AT users' goals and preferences drive the selection process. The suite includes the Matching AT and CHild (MATCH) (Scherer, 1997), intended for infants to 5-year-olds, the Survey of Technology Use (SOTU) (Scherer, 1994) for infants to adults and the Educational Technology Device Predisposition Assessment (ETPA) (Scherer, 2004).

The MATCH assessment process uses a progression of instruments to assist the AT team work collaboratively with the parents to achieve the most appropriate AT match given the characteristics of the child, technology and environment as well as to decide on the best training strategies to ensure optimal AT use. This tool prompts parents to review the child's development and skills in a range of areas, including sleep/wake patterns, grasping and holding, hearing, understanding communication, expressing communication, physical strength/stamina, physical comfort and well-being, social and play skills, pre-academic development (size, shape and colour concepts), rate of learning, emotional well-being (tolerates changes and temper) and overall development (Institute for Matching Person & Technology, Inc., n.d.). The SOTU examines users' perspectives and experiences of technologies and activity limitations typically assisted with the use of technologies, while the ETPA specifically examines educational goals and aspects of the person, technology experience and environment that are likely to impact on technology selection (Scherer, 1994, 2004). Goal setting related to AT is not a discrete event but rather an ongoing potentially life-long process (Cook et al., 2008). Goals often need to be re-visited regularly as the child's skills develop and expectations about his/her performance will change with age and development. Long-term goals need to be established early so that the child's technology skills can be developed over time. For example, a preschool child with a severe visual impairment and limited hand function may be just beginning to require access to the school curriculum. While his or her immediate goals might be met using a range of simple technologies, it is likely that eventually he or she will require a Braille notetaker[1] to access higher levels

---

[1] Braille notetakers are Braille writing devices used as portable personal organisers and notebooks. They compartmentalise key information such as meeting notes, calendar events, personal contact information or general entries. Users have a choice between a standard keyboard configuration and a standard six-key Braille configuration. Many Braille notetakers are combined with Braille displays. Some of these devices are stand-alone while others interface with computers (http://www.techready.co.uk/Assistive-Technology/Braille-Notetakers, retrieved 24 April 2009).

of education. Consequently, early technologies and skill development will focus on developing the child's familiarity and skill in using Braille to ensure he or she is able to use Braille-based technologies in the longer term.

Occupation-centred assessment

Selection of the most appropriate ATs requires all aspects of the HAAT model (Cook et al., 2008) to be considered, namely the *human, the AT, the activity and the context*. A HAAT model-based assessment would first identify the occupation- or goal-related activities the child needs or desires to perform. Particular attention is given to: (1) analysing the specific features of the occupation (*activity*) including the unique meaning and purpose of the activity for the child and his or her family; (2) the distinctive way the activity is performed, depending on its purpose; (3) the experience and preferences of the child; and (4) the demands and structure of the occupation and environment (*context*).

The fit of the activity with the child's existing abilities (*human*) is then examined. The *child-activity fit* is assessed by observing the child performing the activity and identifying the specific difficulties being experienced. In some situations, assessing children's 'naked abilities' does not provide a clear indication of their capacity because they may require technologies to demonstrate what they can do. The technology (AT) then becomes an integral part of an iterative assessment process. If required, a deeper understanding of the child's specific skills and abilities can be gained by undertaking formal and/or informal assessment of performance components such as motor, sensory and perception, cognition, communication and psychosocial (Swinth, 2005).

For example, as a student (*life role*), schoolwork (*occupation*) requires the child to undertake writing (*activity*). Writing requires the child to communicate thoughts by producing and recording a series of symbols in a readable format to demonstrate knowledge, take notes, email friends and tell stories. Children have different preferences in terms of the process of planning and writing such as using a concept map, writing bulleted points and developing thinking and ideas through writing. At different stages of schooling, the frequency and volume of writing required and the style and quality of the finished product will vary. Students will need to write in a variety of environments including in the classroom, the library, on excursions and at home or under a range of conditions (e.g. note taking versus exam) (*context*).

By observing the child undertake various writing activities in the naturalistic environment, the therapist can examine the child's performance and determine points of activity breakdown. While a child might be able to take fractured notes, writing under exam conditions when a volume of text needs to be generated quickly may not be possible. A formal assessment of sitting posture, pencil control and writing speed may also be undertaken to identify possible reasons for performance breakdown and points of intervention. When a child is not physically able to produce written output but has independent thoughts and understands symbols, a range of technologies can be systematically employed to harness his/her existing abilities and determine the best means of production and output.

Assessments of ability and caregiver support

A number of occupation-centred assessments discussed in Chapter 7, as well as AT-specific assessment tools, can be used to provide an overview of the children's occupational performance and level of assistance required. One particular assessment that may be useful in identifying areas where assistance may be helpful for children is the *Pediatric Evaluation of Disability Inventory* (PEDI) (Haley, Coster, Ludlow, Haltiwanger, & Andrellos, 1992). This assessment, completed via parent report/interview, provides important information about the child's performance in mobility, self-care (basic and instrumental activities of daily living) and communication/social functioning, as well as the level of caregiver assistance required in completing these tasks. The information gained enables therapists to think about assistive devices which may help enhance the child's performance of activities as well as to consider the implications of the child's difficulties on the caregivers.

The *School Function Assessment* (SFA) (Coster, Deeney, Haltiwanger, & Haley, 1998), completed via teacher interview or report, is another standardised assessment that provides information about the child's participation in the educational environment, the supports required to enable performance on school-related tasks and the child's level of performance. The SFA has a freely available AT supplement (Silverman & Smith, 2006) specifically designed for children who use AT on a daily basis. The AT supplement may help to determine which extra supports or technologies the child needs at school and to evaluate the outcomes of equipment utilisation.

AT-specific assessments

To date, there are few published AT-specific assessment tools. The *Lifespace Access Profile* (Williams, Stemach, Wolfe, & Stanger, 1992), a team-based observational assessment for evaluating children with severe physical disabilities and the environment related to AT use, was used extensively from the mid-1990s to mid-2000s; however, it is no longer commercially available.

A more recently available and referenced tool, the *Student, Environment, Tasks and Tools (SETT) Framework* (Cook et al., 2008; Zabala, 1995; Zabala, n.d. in Swinth, 2005), is a tool that helps teams gather and organise information that can be used to guide collaborative decisions about services that foster the educational success of students with disabilities. The SETT framework is based on the premise that in order to develop an appropriate system of tools or supports, teams must first develop a shared understanding of the *student*, the school *environments* and the *tasks* required for active participation in the curriculum and for educational success. When the needs, abilities and interests of the student, the details of the environments and the specific tasks required are identified, teams are able to consider possible AT options that are student-centred, environmentally useful and tasks-focused.

Table 14.1 provides a list of SETT questions to assist teams to create student-centred, (self) environmentally useful and tasks-focused tool systems that foster participation and achievement (Zabala, Bowser, & Korsten, 2004/2005). Tools include devices, services, strategies, training, accommodations and modifications needed to help the student succeed. Some parts of the tool system address student needs, while other parts address environmental issues, such as classroom access, accessibility of instructional materials, as well as staff supports. In order to utilise the SETT framework, Zabala (n.d.) identified some critical elements that must be included, namely: shared knowledge across the team; collaboration, active and respectful communication; respect of multiple perspectives including those of student and parents; use of pertinent information; flexibility and patience on the

Table 14.1 Questions used in the student, environments, tasks and tools framework

The student
- What is (are) the functional area(s) of concern?
- What does the student need to be able to do that is difficult or impossible to do independently at this time?
- Special needs (related to area of concern)
- Current abilities (related to area of concern)
- Expectations and concerns
- Interests and preferences

The environments
- Arrangement (instructional, physical)
- Support (available to both the student and the staff)
- Materials and equipment (commonly used by others in the environments)
- Access issues (technological, physical, instructional)
- Attitudes and expectations (staff, family, other)

The tasks
- What specific tasks occur in the student's natural environments that enable progress towards mastery of Individualised Education Plan (IEP) goals and objectives?
- What specific tasks are required for active involvement in identified environments (related to communication, instruction, participation, productivity, environmental control)?

Overall questions
- Is it expected that the student will not be able to make reasonable progress towards educational goals without assistive technology devices and services?
- If yes, describe what a useful system of supports, devices and services for the student would be like if there were such a system of tools
- Brainstorm specific tools that could be included in a system that addresses student needs
- Select the most promising tools for trials in the natural environments
- Plan the specifics of the trial (expected changes, when/how tools will be used, cues, etc.)
- Collect data on effectiveness

Source: Zabala (n.d.).

part of team members so as not to rush in to suggesting possible solutions before the concerns have been adequately identified; and establishment of ongoing team processes for decision making throughout all stages of assessment and intervention. While there is as yet no empirical research validating the SETT framework, it appears to have considerable clinical utility and is worthy of consideration by teams to enhance the process of decision making regarding AT, compensations, modifications and accommodations, trial and evaluation.

Utilising assistive technology for children as an occupation-centred intervention

Provision of equipment alone is not sufficient to guarantee that children will be able to use their technology to successfully participate (McDonald, 2008; Verza, Carvalho, Battaglia, & Uccelli, 2006). As noted in the HAAT model, in addition to needing to fit with the person, the AT also interfaces with the activity and the physical and social environment. Hence, intervention has a dual focus. First, attention needs to be given to ensuring a good fit between the person and the technology with due consideration for the activity and context in which these are to be used to enhance participation. This often requires that time be dedicated to ensuring the child understands the technology and has developed the skills required to use it effectively. Depending on the sophistication of the technology and the child's level of experience and skill in using it, training the child to use the technology may initially be the sole focus of intervention. For example, many children need to spend time focused on learning to use a switch or to select options from a scanning display. Second, once the child has become proficient in using the technology, intervention will focus on the use of the AT in context. For example, a child can use a switch and scanning array to communicate via a speech-generating device or write via a computer. Of course, good skill training should also incorporate meaningful activities; however, these should be timed and graded to ensure success.

As the importance of using technology in context has become recognised, an increasing number of devices have been developed to allow staged contextual use of technology. For example, transitional mobility devices using a range of control mechanisms allow very young children to mobilise and explore their environments. Two such devices are:

- the Smart Wheelchair (http://callcentre.education.ed.ac.uk/Smart_WheelCh/What_is_it_SWA/what_is_it_swa.html)
- the Mobility 4 Kids range (http://www.mobility4kids.com/main/newsts.html)

Communication devices have been used in the context of real communication interactions for many years (Goossens, Crain, & Elder, 1999) to enhance the development of communication and technology skills and optimise social interaction and develop relationships.

To support the effective use of technology in context, attention needs to be given to how the social or people supports within the environment can promote active engagement and participation using technology. People in the application environment need to:

- Understand the purpose of the technology;
- Know how, when and where the child needs to be able to use the technology;
- Know how to structure the environment and activities to optimise the child's participation using technology;
- Be able to monitor the effectiveness of the technology in achieving its outcome and enabling participation;
- Know how the technology operates, and to troubleshoot difficulties if encountered;
- Know where and how to access expertise to assist in the use, updating and replacement of the technology.

Specific assistive technology interventions for children

Supporting leisure and play occupations

Active leisure and play are much neglected areas for children with significant disabilities who tend to engage in more passive leisure pursuits. Play and leisure can be supported using a range of means (Dietz & Swinth, 2008) such as commercially available toys, for example, activity centres/boards, themed mobiles, talking books, and light and sound projectors that with little adaptation afford play opportunities. Commercial toys can also be modified using Velcro® or extending handles or adapted for use with a switch or alternative control device such as a battery-operated bubble blower or any other battery-operated toy and remote control vehicles. Specialised play devices such as multisensory rooms are also available for children with significant physical and developmental disabilities.

As children grow older, play and leisure activities often become increasingly technology based (e.g. computer games, PlayStations®, music and video games) (Johnson & Klaas, 2007). This technology often requires modification for some children to access it. Examples include accessing an Apple iPod® via a sip and puff switch (Jones, Grogg, Anschutz, & Fierman, 2008) and adaptations to the methods of activating a PlayStation®. Children can also be provided with alternative access methods and displays to enable them to play computer games. Virtual reality also provides children with disabilities with increasing play opportunities. For example, children with limited mobility and upper limb control can participate in a range of activities such as yoga, tennis, skiing and playing the guitar using Wii® technology. There are also a growing number of virtual environments for children such as Tippy Tales (http://www.tippytales.com), Disney's Toontown Online (http://play.toon-town.com/webHome.php) or Habbo Hotel (http://www.habbohotel.com).

It is important that children with disabilities experience a broad range of play experiences and that technology does not define their play experience. Technology can sometimes alienate and distance children from regular play opportunities and encounters. Children's play experiences can be extended by providing them with positioning supports to enable them to play on the floor side lying or sitting positions. Lack of stability results in difficulty in using hands and eyes together during play, self-care or school activities; therefore, children can benefit from external positioning devices or adaptive seating systems to help them to access these activities (Hartley & Thomas, 2003). Customised mobility devices can also enable children to access a range of terrains such as the beach, park and walking tracks. Standing devices enable children to participate in activities with their peers such as ball games, cooking and fence painting. Some playgrounds provide accessible play experiences such as swings, and roundabouts. Similarly, from a very early age, communication is essential for participation for play and most other occupations. Augmentative and alternative communication (AAC) technologies provide children with communication impairments with a means of relaying their thoughts and feelings to others. When introduced early, communication systems can assist children to request toys, choose between play options, engage in imaginary and pretend play and interact with their peers during social and other play activities.

Supporting productive occupations

Children with or without disabilities spend a substantial amount of time in the school environment engaging in productive occupations. Initially, access to the physical school environment is required to enable the child to participate in school activities. Modifications such as ramps, space to move around the school and classrooms and appropriate work areas for schoolwork are essential for children with mobility and other impairments. Reading and recording are two of the key ways that children engage in schoolwork. Adapted books can enable children to engage in literacy tasks such as spelling and reading as seen in Figure 14.6. Computer-based technologies provide the foundation for translating any standard hard copy or electronic print document into alternative formats such as enlarged print, speech and Braille. Children who are not yet literate can also access print material that has been translated into symbols.

Children who experience difficulty recording their work often fall behind their peers at school. If children have difficulty holding pens or pencils, low-tech solutions such as built-up handles can be trialled. Children who are not able to use writing implements effectively can record thoughts and ideas using a computer or communication device. Children who are unable to access a

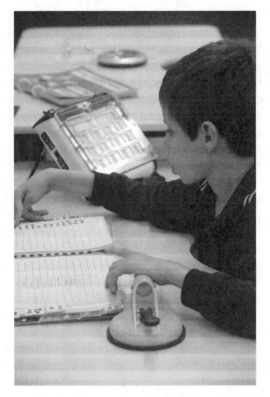

Figure 14.6 Using adapted book to participate in class, while stabilised using bar. Reproduced with permission

computer or communication device may be able to dictate to a person, or use voice recognition software (such as Dragon Naturally Speaking®) to record information.

Children need to be able to access technology in order to use it. Access can be provided to technologies such as computers and communication and mobility devices directly using a keyboard, mouse alternative or joystick or indirectly using a switch or switch array in combination with a scanning display. Keyboards and displays can be alphabet or symbol based. Accessing technology directly via a keyboard, mouse or mouse alternative is almost always preferable to using indirect access via a switch (Rosto, 2003). While direct access requires greater motor demands, it is often faster and has fewer cognitive demands than indirect access (Light & Drager, 2007).

Supporting everyday occupations

Children with disabilities often experience difficulty undertaking activities of daily living. Although children may experience problems performing specific aspects of these activities, it is important that they develop autonomy and are afforded opportunities to direct and/or undertake any aspect of the activity that they can manage. Everyday utensils such as spoons, cups, plates, keys and hair brush can be modified by enlarging or extending the handles to enable children to take a more active role in their self-care. Electric devices such as a toothbrush or shaver can allow children and adolescents with poor hand function to manage their personal hygiene. Environmental modifications may also be required to allow children to access various areas of the house and fixtures and fittings such as light switches, door handles, etc.

Special-purpose devices such as electronic feeders and page turners can also provide children with autonomy and control during eating and reading. Environmental control units (ECUs) allow children with limited physical ability to control appliances and fittings within the home environment (Cook et al., 2008). This simplest ECU allows an individual to use a switch to turn an appliance on or off. Some of these devices allow the duration to be preset so that an appliance such as food processor can be activated to run for a specified time. Programmable devices, which can be accessed via an enlarged keypad or a switch, can be used to control numerous devices in the home such as televisions, DVD players, fans and lights, which are controlled using infrared remote controls. More sophisticated ECUs allow a number of devices within the home to be controlled or pre-programmed from one location using voice, switch or computer interface.

There are a number of activities, however, that children with severe disabilities may always require assistance with such as bathing, dressing and toileting. Hence, AT devices such as hoists and mobile shower chairs can be very helpful to carers to ensure their comfort and safety for transfers and physical caretaking activities, particularly as children become older and heavier to lift and handle.

Evaluating AT outcomes

The impact of AT devices on the user and his/her family has been increasingly recognised. Consistent with the occupation-centred practice figure, evaluation of outcomes in terms of satisfaction and specific goal achievement is a critical step in the service delivery process. It is now understood that using technology to enable function positively impacts the health, well-being and identity of the individual (Jutai, Ladak, Schuller, Naumann, & Wright, 1996). The *Quebec User Evaluation of Satisfaction with Technology* (QUEST 2.0) (Demers, Weiss-Lambrou, & Ska, 2002) can be used to evaluate the user's satisfaction with the AT device itself, as well as the way the device was provided. This has primarily been used with adults, but can be used by parent report. The MPT tools (Scherer, 1997) discussed earlier such as the MATCH also provide the opportunity to evaluate satisfaction with the child's skills and development after the technology has been introduced and compare this with pre-intervention satisfaction.

Still under development at time of writing is the *Family Impact of Assistive Technology (FIATS) Scale* (Ryan et al., 2006; Ryan, Campbell, & Rigby, 2007). This scale was developed to detect change in the adaptability of families who have young children who are unable to sit without support as 'Assistive technologies may have a role in mitigating caregiver stress and burden by improving functional performance, social interaction and autonomy in children with physical disabilities' (Ryan et al., 2006, p. 165). The revised version of FIATS has 89 items covering nine unique domains, each of which taps into the perceived impact of technology use on families. The domains include: *autonomy* or the degree to which the child needs help to perform activities; *disposition* or the degree to which the child is content during the day; *effort*, that is, the degree of exertion needed to assist the child; *function* or the degree to which the child has voluntary control over his/her own actions; *respite*, that is, the degree to which parent needs relief from care-giving; *social and family interaction* or the degree to which the child interacts with others; *supervision*, that is, the degree to which the child requires attention from family members; *well-being/safety* or the degree to which parent is worried about the child's well-being and safety; and finally *technology acceptance*. FIATS can be used to study the effect of postural control devices and other AT may help healthcare professionals, parents and third-party payers to understand how these technologies may be used to support and improve child performance and family life.

Conclusion

AT is a very exciting and constantly evolving area of occupation-centred practice as it requires the practitioner to integrate his/her understanding of the person, the environment, the technology and the children's occupation to enhance their participation in meaningful life roles. AT if correctly prescribed, supported and used has the potential to change the lives of children and to significantly decrease the care-giving burden for parents. The AT device is only one part of the picture in enabling children with disabilities to participate in their daily occupations. In order to optimise children's participation, therapists need to view the AT within the context of the child's abilities and skills, meaningful occupations and his/her multiple naturalistic environments. The HAAT model and the occupation-centred practice process for children (Rodger, in press) together provide a framework for understanding how AT options can assist children and families to fully participate in meaningful child and family occupations.

References

Alliance for Technology Access. (2005). *Computer and web resources for people with disabilities*. Berkeley, CA: Hunter House.

Canadian Association of Occupational Therapists. (CAOT). (2002). *Enabling occupation: An occupational therapy perspective* (2nd ed.). Ottawa, ON: CAOT Publications.

Christiansen, C. H., & Baum, C. M. (1997). Person–environment occupational performance: A conceptual model for practice. In C. H. Christiansen, & C. M. Baum (Eds.), *Occupational therapy: Enabling function and well-being* (2nd ed., pp. 46–71). Thorofare, NJ: CB Slack Incorporated.

Cook, A. M., & Hussey, S. M. (2002). *Assistive technologies principles and practice* (2nd ed.). St. Louis, MO: Mosby.

Cook, A. M., Polgar, J. M., & Hussey, S. M. (2008). *Cook & Hussey's assistive technologies: Principles and practice* (3rd ed.). St. Louis, MO: Mosby Elsevier.

Coster, W. J., Deeney, T., Haltiwanger, J. T., & Haley, S. M. (1998). *School Function Assessment*. San Antonio, TX: Psychological Corporation.

Cowan, D. M., & Turner-Smith, A. R. (1999). The user's perspective on the provision of electronic assistive technology: Equipped for life? *British Journal of Occupational Therapy, 62*(1), 2–6.

Day, H., & Jutai, J. (1996). Measuring the psychosocial impact of assistive devices: The PIADS. *Canadian Journal of Rehabilitation, 9*(3), 159–168.

de Jonge, D., Scherer, M., & Rodger, S. (2006). *Assistive technology in the workplace*. St. Louis, MO: Mosby Elsevier.

Demers, L., Weiss-Lambrou, R., & Ska, B. (2002). The Quebec User Evaluation of Satisfaction with Assistive Technology (QUEST 2.0): An overview and recent progress. *Technology & Disability, 14*, 101–105.

Dietz, J. C., & Swinth, Y. (2008). Accessing play through assistive technology. In L. D. Parham, & L. S. Fazio (Eds.), *Play in occupational therapy for children* (2nd ed., pp. 395–425). St. Louis, MO: Mosby Elsevier.

Goossens, C., Crain, S., & Elder, P. (1999). *Engineering the preschool environment for interactive symbolic communication* (4th ed.). Birmingham, AL: Southeast Augmentative Communication Conference Publications.

Haley, S. M., Coster, W. J., Ludlow, L. H., Haltiwanger, J. T., & Andrellos, P. J. (1992). *Pediatric Evaluation of Disability Inventory*. San Antonio, TX: Psychological Corporation.

Hartley, H., & Thomas, J. E. (2003). Current practice in the management of children with cerebral palsy: A national survey of paediatric dieticians. *Journal of Human Nutrition and Dietetics, 16*(4), 219–224.

Henderson, S., Skelton, H., & Rosenbaum, P. (2008). Assistive devices for children with functional impairments: Impact on child and caregiver function. *Developmental Medicine & Child Neurology, 50*, 2.

Institute for Matching Person & Technology, Inc. (n.d.). *Matching person & technology*. Retrieved 19 June 2009 from http://matchingpersonandtechnology.com/.

Johnson, K. A., & Klaas, S. J. (2007). The changing nature of play: Implications for pediatric spinal cord injury. *Journal of Spinal Cord Medicine, 30*(Suppl. 1), S71–S75.

Jones, M., Grogg, K., Anschutz, J., & Fierman, R. (2008). A sip-and-puff wireless remote control for the apple iPod. *Assistive Technology, 20*(2), 107–110.

Jutai, J., Ladak, N., Schuller, R., Naumann, S., & Wright, V. (1996). Outcomes measurement of assistive technologies: An institutional case study. *Assistive Technology, 8*(2), 110–120.

Jutai, J. W., Fuhrer, M. J., Demers, L., Scherer, M. J., & DeRuyter, F. (2005). Towards a taxonomy of assistive technology device outcomes. *American Journal of Physical Medicine & Rehabilitation, 84*(4), 294–302.

Law, M., Baptiste, S., Carswell, A., McColl, M. A., Polatajko, H., & Pollock, N. (2005). *The Canadian Occupational Performance Measure* (4th ed.). Ottawa, ON: CAOT Publications ACE.

Law, M., Cooper, B., Strong, S., Rigby, P., & Letts, L. (1996). The person–environment–occupation model: A transactive approach to occupational performance. *Canadian Journal of Occupational Therapy, 63*, 9–23.

Light, J., & Drager, K. (2007). AAC technologies for young children with complex communication needs: State of the science and future research directions. *Augmentative and Alternative Communication, 23*(3), 204–216.

McDonald, R. (2008). Adaptive seating interventions for children and young people with severe and complex disabilities: Evidence, research and proposed model for future research practice. Paper presented at the *24th International Seating Symposium*, 24–28 March 2008, Vancouver, Canada.

McDonald, R., & Surtees, R. (2007). Changes in postural alignment when using kneeblocks for children with severe motor disorders. *Disability and Rehabilitation: Assistive Technology, 2*(5), 287–291.

McDonald, R., Surtees, R., & Wirz, S. (2003). A comparison between parent and therapists' views of their child's individual seating systems. *International Journal of Rehabilitation Research, 26*(3), 235–243.

McLaughlin, J. (2007). My child needs a piece of adaptive equipment: Now what? Well, it depends! *Exceptional Parent, 37*(11), 46–47.

Rodger, S. (in press). Becoming more occupation centred when working with children. In S. Rodger (Ed.), *Occupation-centred practice for children: A practical guide for occupational therapists*. Oxford: Wiley Blackwell.

Rodger, S. (2010). Becoming more occupation centred when working with children. In S. Rodger (Ed.), *Occupation-centred practice for children: A practical guide for occupational therapists*. Oxford, UK: Wiley Blackwell.

Rosto, L. (2003). Designing for life: Universal design addresses the needs and abilities of all people throughout the life span. *Advance for Directors in Rehabilitation, 12*(1), 59–60.

Ryan, S., Campbell, K. A., Rigby, P., Germon, B., Chan, B., & Hubley, D. (2006). Development of the new family impact of assistive technology scale. *International Journal of Rehabilitation Research, 29*(3), 195–200.

Ryan, S. E., Campbell, K. A., & Rigby, P. J. (2007). Reliability of the family impact of assistive technology scale for families of young children with cerebral palsy. *Archives of Physical Medicine and Rehabilitation, 88*(11), 1436–1440.

Scherer, M. J. (1994). *Matching person and technology*. Webster, NY: Institute for Matching Person and Technology.

Scherer, M. J. (1997). *Matching Assistive Technology and CHild (MATCH) assessment process*. Webster, NY: Institute for Matching Person and Technology.

Scherer, M. J. (2004). *Matching person and assistive technology process and accompanying assessment instruments*. Webster, NY: Institute for Matching Person & Technology.

Scherer, M. J. (2005). *Living in a state of stuck: How technology impacts the lives of people with disabilities* (2nd ed.). Cambridge, MA: Brookline Books.

Silverman, M. K., & Smith, R. O. (2006). Consequential validity of an assistive technology supplement for the school function assessment. *Assistive Technology, 18*(2), 155–165.

Swinth, Y. (2005). Assistive technology: Low technology, computers, electronic aids for daily living and augmentative communication. In J. Case-Smith (Ed.), *Occupational therapy for children* (5th ed., pp. 615–656). St. Louis, MO: Elsevier Mosby.

Townsend, E., & Polatajko, H. (2007). *Enabling occupation II: Advancing an occupational therapy vision for health, well-being & justice through occupation.* Ottawa, ON: Canadian Association of Occupational Therapists.

Verza, R., Carvalho, M. L., Battaglia, M. A., & Uccelli, M. M. (2006). An interdisciplinary approach to evaluating the need for assistive technology reduces equipment abandonment. *Multiple Sclerosis, 12,* 88-93.

Waldron, D., & Layton, N. (2008). Hard and soft assistive technologies: Defining roles for clinicians. *Australian Occupational Therapy Journal, 55,* 61-64.

Wallace, J. F., Hayes, M., & Bailey, M. N. (2000). Assistive technology loan financing: A status of program impact and consumer satisfaction. *Technology and Disability, 13,* 17-22.

Williams, W. B., Stemach, G., Wolfe, S., & Stanger, C. (1992). *Lifespace Access Profile.* Irvine, CA: Assistive Technology Systems.

World Health Organization (WHO). (2004). A glossary of terms for community health care and services for older persons, Ageing and Health Technical Report, Volume 5, Kobe City, Japan: WHO.

Zabala, J. S. (n.d.). *Using the SETT framework to level the learning field for students with disabilities.* Retrieved 27 April 2009 from www.letsgoexpo.com/viewfile.cfm?LCID=1135&eID=80000093.

Zabala, J. S. (1995). The SETT framework: Critical areas to consider with making informed assistive technology decisions. Houston, TX: Region 5 Education Service Centre (ERIC Document reproduction Service No. ED381962).

Zabala, J. S., Bowser, G., & Korsten, J. (2004/2005). SETT and ReSETT: Implications for AT implementation. *Closing the Gap, 23*(5), 1-4.

Chapter 15

Decision Making for Occupation-centred Practice with Children

Jodie Copley, Sally Bennett, and Merrill Turpin

Learning objectives

Specifically, this chapter aims to:

- Describe decision making and decision-making processes.
- Identify the information that therapists need in order to make informed decisions and the sources of this information.
- Describe how a clinician might examine, evaluate and synthesise this information when considering alternatives and dealing with uncertainties.
- Discuss the shared nature of decision making.

Introduction

Occupational therapists working with children make professional decisions all the time, for example, deciding what assessment to use, what intervention approach to take, how to set up the environment for a session or how to respond to the child on a moment-by-moment basis. Most of these decisions are made without an awareness of their underlying thought processes; however, the nature of decision making in occupational therapy is complex. Because of the diversity of clients accessing occupational therapy services, decisions about how best to intervene in any one situation are multi-faceted and based on the integration of diverse information sources. This chapter explores the process of making decisions in the context of working with children and their families.

Decision making and information sources

What is decision making? Put simply, it is the process of making informed choices among possible alternatives. As such, it is a process whereby information is collected, evaluated, sifted and synthesised in order to make choices between different options. It is a concept used across countless disciplines and in everyday life. Decision making, whether in healthcare or other areas of life, requires an individual to choose between alternatives, sometimes requiring multiple decisions at the same time. Understanding the possible consequences of each choice and the values and preferences of those affected by those consequences is paramount. Therefore, in order to make choices about options, a range of information is required. People who have experience in a particular field have a well-developed understanding of the type of information that is needed to make decisions in that specific area. They also understand how to evaluate information, given the source it was derived from; what information needs to be emphasised; and how information from a range of sources might be synthesised.

Professional decision making shares many of the same principles of decision making used in other areas of life, albeit often with greater uncertainties, complexities and more stakeholders contributing to and affected by the decisions made. These decisions not only are dependent on the therapist's professional knowledge and experience, but are also the result of a dynamic interaction of multiple sources of information, from both within the therapist and outside the therapist (i.e. information from the child and family, the service, etc.).

Certainty is a rare commodity in clinical practice. Decisions often need to be made without a clear understanding of the whole situation or of all their potential consequences. Useful and trustworthy information is not always available to support occupational therapists' decisions and the likelihood of dealing with unexpected situations or outcomes is high and needs to be expected in clinical practice. For these reasons, many decisions are neither 'right nor wrong' in an absolute sense, but might be made with a view to modifying or refining them after reflecting on observations of progress or outcomes (Higgs, Burn, & Jones, 2001). In the face of uncertainty, clear foundations for decision making become more obvious. These include the importance of expertise and the art of practice (Hinojosa & Kramer, 2009).

Access to trustworthy, comprehensive and relevant information is essential for effective decision making. Many types of information from a range of sources need to be considered when making decisions. Four important sources and types of information therapists commonly use when making decisions will be considered (Rycroft-Malone et al., 2004). These include information: (1) about clients, their families and their contexts; (2) about the practice context and available resources; (3) from research; and (4) from clinical experience.

Information about clients, families and their contexts

Preceding chapters have provided a comprehensive account of the occupation-centred tools and processes available for information gathering about children and families (see Chapters 3, 6 and 7). Here we will explore the types of client- and family-related information gathered by therapists that impact on their decisions.

Research studies investigating the factors that occupational therapists working with children consider when making intervention decisions have identified that the 'needs of the child' are paramount (Copley, Nelson, Turpin, Underwood, & Flanigan, 2008; Feder, Majnemer, & Symes, 2000; Storch & Eskow, 1996). But what information is required to determine the needs of the child and family?

In a qualitative study exploring the factors influencing choice of intervention approach among experienced occupational therapists, Copley et al. (2008) found that a wide range of information about the child and family is collected not only through the initial assessment, but also as intervention progresses. This information may be collected on an ongoing basis using assessment tools and through interviews with parents, teachers and others involved with different aspects of the child's life. It may emerge from informal discussions with parents or from observations of children in their natural environments. Information gathering is cumulative, as it helps the therapist to build 'a picture' of the child's and family's occupations. It is within this context that therapists make decisions.

Key information gathered about the child and his/her family may include:

- the child's age and developmental stage (including occupational development)
- the nature of and reasons for the child's difficulties
- the child's personal characteristics and interests
- the child's health and history of previous intervention
- the child's family constellation and functioning
- what the family wants and expects from the service

The child's age and developmental stage

Along with motor and social development and occupations such as school, play and self-care abilities, children develop cognitively and emotionally and develop self-awareness. Their daily lives become more structured as they attend formal education at school. Expectations of what they can achieve and their efficiency in achieving new skills increase, while expectations of the help required for success decrease. Foundational skills – such as learning to hop and jump, learning to form letters and words, learning to look after/ arrange their possessions or being able to concentrate on an adult-chosen task – may or may not be sufficient to support achievement. However, children are expected to participate in school, play, self-management and home life regardless of their underlying skills. Hence, occupational therapists must consider varied implications of a child's age when making decisions. The ways in which therapists apply interventions appears to change as the child gets older (Copley et al., 2008).

For example, therapists reported being more likely to work with younger children (e.g. under 5 years of age) on skills that might have wide application as they develop. Depending on their level of emotional and social maturity, younger children may have less capacity for insight into their task difficulties and therefore may be less likely to engage in and persist with difficult tasks. For these reasons, therapists were less likely to use problem-solving approaches or to work directly on specific tasks with younger children (Copley et al., 2008). Instead, they tended to address elements of the task often out of context. For example, therapists may choose to work on letter formation by using a water gun to 'write' the letters on concrete, or help the child form the letters with a finger in shaving cream.

As the child becomes older (e.g. 9 or 10 years), however, therapists in our study perceived a growing urgency to facilitate occupational task achievement within the child's natural environments. However, a characteristic of occupation-centred practice is contextual relevance which should be encouraged, irrespective of age (see Chapter 2). In addition, older children are often more motivated to achieve specific occupational tasks that are meaningful to them. Many therapists, through their clinical expertise, know that improvement in skills may not occur fast enough or to the level required to meet the rapidly increasing demands for independent learning and self-management placed on older children at school. Task-related and compensatory strategies (e.g. use of specific equipment and changing the way in which the task is done) may be needed to enable participation and progress in learning in a more immediate way. Hence, therapists might think about such questions as:

- Can the child present his/her work in an alternative manner and still achieve his learning goals?
- Can information be provided in a different way to assist learning?
- How can the child be assisted to meet expectations for task performance at home and school by changing the environment, the task or the way the child performs it?

In addition, therapists reported that they may be more likely to engage older children collaboratively in the intervention process as they are perceived to be more able to analyse and evaluate their own performance than younger children (Copley et al., 2008). In making decisions, however, concepts of 'older' and 'younger' should *not* be limited to chronological age. While the child's developmental age and social-emotional maturity are highly relevant, children as young as 4 years may be able to collaborate in addressing occupational tasks *if* the therapist uses child-centred language and goal-setting tools. Whatever the child's age, information gathering can be used to gradually gain a clearer view of task performance within the child's natural environments, allowing occupationally relevant tasks to be addressed as early as possible.

The nature of and reasons for the child's difficulties

We have previously discussed the need to understand both the child's difficulties with task performance and the underlying reasons (Copley et al., 2008; Wurth, Hindman, Copley, & Nelson, 2006). As discussed in previous chapters, identifying the breakdown in task performance from a person-environment-occupation perspective is often needed to guide intervention (e.g. Chapters 8–10). Hence, therapists frequently need to observe the child performing the task, or a simulation of the task, and understand the context within which it usually occurs. They ask themselves questions such as:

- How is the environment set up when this task is done?
- What are the environmental facilitators and inhibitors?
- What is the developmental level of the child?
- How is the child positioned?
- How is the task presented?
- What instructions are given?
- What equipment is used by the child?
- How does he/she approach the task?
- What assistance is available?
- What is happening around him/her as they complete the task?
- Is there a time pressure to complete the task?
- What are the expected outcomes?

This information helps the therapist to decide what type of intervention might be needed.

In addition to gathering information relating to task performance, therapists often seek information about any background or underlying causes of performance difficulties that could guide intervention decisions. For example, a child who is disruptive in class may be doing so for a variety of reasons. The therapist may identify that the child has anxiety about task performance, resulting in task-avoidance behaviours. In this case, the therapist may draw upon psychosocial intervention approaches (Olson, 1999, 2009), using anxiety management and behavioural strategies.

Alternatively, information gathering may reveal that the child presents with a sensory modulation disorder (Kimball, 1999; Schaaf et al., 2009). In this case, behaviours such as tapping the desk or verbalising constantly would be interpreted as seeking sensory information in an effort to control and keep the sensory input experienced predictable. From this perspective, the therapist might choose to employ a sensory processing framework (Schaaf et al., 2009) to help the child understand their sensory responses (e.g. The Alert Program; Williams & Shellenberger, 1994) and might aim to reduce the behaviour by modifying the class environment and the teacher's interaction with the child to better meet his/her sensory needs.

In some cases, the characteristics of the child may preclude certain intervention approaches. For example, where difficulties with speech and language are contributing problems, approaches requiring extensive verbal discussion and problem-solving such as CO-OP (Polatajko & Mandich, 2004) may be more difficult to employ. In other situations, underlying difficulties may result in secondary problems for which the therapist might use a particular intervention. As one therapist described regarding children with learning difficulties:

> Sometimes you can identify that a child has low muscle tone when they walk in the door by the fact that their shoulders are up around their ears somewhere, and for years they have been stabilising in that way. The fatigue they get from the tensing they do means that you have to come from a biomechanical perspective because otherwise they will end up with shoulder and neck problems. (Copley et al., 2008, p. 109)

Personal characteristics and interests of the child

Some intervention approaches and techniques may be more suited to some children than others, based on their individual characteristics and personality traits. For example, a child who enjoys moving and being physically active may not respond well to seated activities that are very verbal in nature. A child who is shy and unsure of himself may engage better in quiet verbal tasks with the therapist than action-oriented 'performing' in front of a group of other children. A child who likes to sing may find that singing him/herself through his/her morning routine keeps him/her on task better than a wall chart. A child who is motivated to master specific tasks may engage well in problem-solving-based teaching and learning approaches, while a less motivated child may benefit from time spent investigating his personal interests and the use of therapy techniques that build self-efficacy by providing control and success. Hence, therapists use information about a range of personal characteristics including: the child's learning style, level of motivation, cognitive abilities, strengths and talents to guide their decisions.

Health and history of previous intervention

A specific medical diagnosis may lead the therapist to consider certain intervention approaches particularly if there is research evidence to support the use of a specific intervention for that condition. For example, interventions such as Relationship Development Intervention (RDI) and Social Stories® have been developed specifically for children with autistism spectrum disorder (Gray, 2000; Gutstein & Sheely, 2002). In the case of both these interventions, evidence about their efficacy while positive in small samples is still being accrued (Ali & Frederickson, 2006; Gutstein & Sheely, 2002). However, whether or not a child has been provided with a specific diagnosis, therapists collect a range of information regarding the child's health and developmental history that may be relevant to intervention decisions. Information about the child's vision, hearing, language skill development, auditory processing, medications, diet and sleep patterns are also important in determining the reasons for the child's difficulties, as well as relevant interventions.

Information about any previous interventions may influence current decisions. It is useful to know how the child has responded to particular interventions in the past, although these responses may change over time.

Home environment and family functioning

Since families have an important influence on children, the therapist seeks to understand the way family members interact. For example, a home environment in which there is frequent conflict and habitual negative interactions may impact on the child's motivation and self-concept, as well as the family's ability to generalise intervention strategies to home and school. Alternately, a family in financial difficulty may be struggling to meet the child's basic needs for shelter, food, clothing and education. Understanding the daily priorities and interactions of the family is critical to supporting the child's meaningful participation in social and occupational roles. For example, in a family where a single mother is frequently incapacitated by morning stiffness associated with rheumatoid arthritis, it may be more realistic and valued for a child to learn how to make his/her own breakfast and help his/her younger brother dress for school rather than to do his/her homework.

What the family wants and expects from the service

The child's family comes to occupational therapy with particular expectations about what will be achieved. These expectations are considered when making decisions. For instance, therapists may find that it is more difficult to engage parents in working on occupational tasks with their child if they expect the therapist to 'fix' their child's underlying problem (e.g. low muscle tone or balance issues). Later in this chapter, we emphasise that collaborative decision making and clear communication with the child and family about intervention choices can help to modify these expectations and assumptions.

Information about the practice context

The characteristics of the service in which therapists work also impact on decision making (Feder et al., 2000). The culture and structure of service provision in the therapist's workplace may facilitate or hinder occupational therapists' application of occupation-centred practice. When working in the public sector, the assumed role of the occupational therapist within the multi-disciplinary team can steer therapists towards certain interventions or limit their ability to address particular occupational goals (Copley et al., 2008). For instance, whether the child sees the occupational therapist will depend on the organisation's view of the occupational therapy role, particularly where an administrator makes such decisions at the point of intake into the service or responds to the mandate of the funding body. This will influence the types of client difficulties or goals the occupational therapist is able to address. Conversely, absence of other professions in the team may create the situation where the occupational therapist will be expected to address issues that are usually managed by other professionals (Wurth et al., 2006).

Other organisation- or service-related factors include the resources required to implement specific interventions, and the structure, timing and location of service provision (Copley et al., 2008). Different interventions have varying space, resource and equipment requirements. For example, therapists have cited a lack of access to occupation-centred assessment tools as a reason for using performance component assessments (Copley et al., 2008). Physical resources such as space and equipment are required for certain interventions, for example, addressing motor-based goals or using sensory integration (Bundy, Lane, & Murray, 2002). The duration and regularity of therapy contact may also be determined by client waiting lists and service timetables that are not always within therapists' control.

Direct costs of service provision to clients can be financial as well as related to time, effort and inconvenience. Limited resources force therapists to make value-based decisions about the services offered as well as who will benefit and who will miss out. These constraints may affect the therapist's ability to engage with the client and family frequently and/or long enough to deliver particular interventions. Access to the child's daily environments such as home and school, the key factor supporting occupation-centred interventions, may be limited by the service organisation.

The core business, expectations and service delivery practices of any organisation relate to a number of factors such as its history, service provision focus, mission statement, values and funding sources. While some of these are beyond therapists' control, others may be within his or her sphere of influence. The characteristics of the practice context may lead the therapist to make clinical decisions that fit within the organisation's service provision philosophy. Often this is done without conscious awareness on the part of the therapist. However, if therapists feel restricted in their choice of appropriate intervention options, the need to educate service managers and teams and promote the role and methods of occupational therapy may be required to enable occupation-centred practice.

Information from empirical research

Research is a structured process for developing and testing theories and practice models. Research can be used to develop further knowledge about occupational therapy, assess needs for services, evaluate the effectiveness of interventions, standardise assessment tools, provide information about client's experiences and examine the process of therapy, allowing further refinement of practice. There are many different types of research, all of which can provide therapists with useful information to inform clinical decisions.

To get the most from research information, understanding the different types of research and their strengths and weaknesses is essential.

In this section, we will emphasise that the type of research used by therapists to inform practice should match the therapist's information needs because different types of research produce different types of knowledge (Bennett & Bennett, 2000). *Qualitative research* might provide information about how clients generally experience a disability or how they perceive the usefulness of therapy recommendations (Taylor, 2007). For example, qualitative research has recently been employed to consider the experience of children living with juvenile idiopathic arthritis and how they perceive home exercise regimes (De Monte, Rodger, Broderick, & Jones, in press). If therapists want to know about the likely course of a medical condition or disability, *cohort or longitudinal studies* can provide useful information since they track changes over time (Sackett, Richardson, Rosenberg, & Haynes, 2000).

Randomised controlled trials (RCTs) test the effectiveness of specific interventions used in a particular way because they control for factors that might influence the results, which ensures that any changes observed can be attributed to the intervention being tested (Sackett et al., 2000). *Systematic reviews* of RCTs pool information from many trials, aiming to overcome the limitations of any one study and maximising the sample sizes from which conclusions about the effectiveness of specific interventions can be drawn (Glanville & Lefebvre, 2000). Due to the highly individualised nature of the interventions that are often delivered by occupational therapists, and the heterogeneity in the client groups examined, RCTs may not always be appropriate (Nelson & Mathiowetz, 2004).

Instead, many questions concerning the effectiveness of occupational therapy interventions are more suited to *quasi-experimental* studies in which there is no random allocation and not all extraneous variables are controlled *or single case experimental designs* in which the child acts as his/her own control (Johnston, Ottenbacher, & Reichardt, 1995). There are texts devoted to research methods and applicability of the resulting knowledge for various clinical decisions (e.g. Sackett et al., 2000; Taylor, 2007). However, it is important that therapists use the right type of information for the required decisions.

Is it applicable to my practice?

Research findings may not always be applicable to the context of clinical service, and in some cases may not have high clinical utility (Carpenter, 2004). Therapists may see a difference between the interventions investigated in research studies and authentic practice, in that research investigates interventions implemented in a standardised manner, whereas in clinical practice a wider variety in implementation occurs due to factors such as the therapist's skill level and the client's individual situation. However, this variation introduces elements of bias, extraneous influences and difficulty in determining the 'true' benefit of an intervention provided. Clinicians use reasoning to adapt interventions based on the environment, the family situation, the individual characteristics of the client and goals. It is difficult, although not impossible, to capture these contextual and responsive aspects of practice in controlled research. In addition, published studies (Hinojosa & Kramer, 2009; Nelson, Copley, Flanigan, & Underwood, 2009) and research in progress by the authors have found that occupational therapists combine different inter-vention approaches in practice, whereas research studies frequently inves-tigate 'pure' interventions so as to determine the efficacy of one approach over another.

Does it tell me all I need to know?

While therapists believe they need to consider research findings when making clinical decisions, they feel they cannot depend solely on this information as their clinical questions cannot always be answered by existing research (Bennett et al., 2003). Therapists have cited a lack of available research regard-ing specific techniques or intervention approaches and particular client groups that may be difficult to categorise (e.g. children with learning diffi-culties) as problematic in translating research to practice (Copley & Allen, in review). Where there is a lack of research to draw from or competing research findings, therapists nonetheless have a responsibility to consider broader information to make decisions and apply the best evidence available.

Structures and supports for accessing, interpreting and applying research

Sackett, Rosenberg, Gray, Haynes, and Richardson (1996) developed a model of evidence-based healthcare that includes the systematic retrieval of the best evidence available, and the critical appraisal of this evidence for valid-ity, clinical relevance and applicability. To use research information in prac-tice, therapists identify the need for a structure and supports within their own organisation that allows ready access to relevant research information, as well as guidance in interpreting and applying it to their practice (Caldwell, Whitehead, Fleming, & Moes, 2008). In research being undertaken by the first author, therapists suggested the following:

(1) Create a system to collect and disseminate research information that includes the following steps:
   ● Identify and prioritise topics.
   ● Identify the resources available to the organisation to collect the information (e.g. searching OT Seeker (http://www.otseeker.com), a database of RCTs and systematic reviews relevant to occupational therapy, share with staff from other organisations providing similar services and access professional association interest groups).
   ● Create a database to classify and store the information using a structure that is relevant to the service (e.g. information on specific interventions

and techniques such as sensory integration, CO-OP or Social Stories®, information on models of practice such as family-centred therapy or inter-professional service provision).

- Establish systems of communication among staff to share the information gained (e.g. journal clubs, dedicated staff meetings, newsletters and monthly email updates).

(2) Create a framework to appraise the clinical applicability of the research that includes the following steps:

- Develop a service-based hierarchy of evidence that is relevant to their clinical practice. Identify the characteristics of research studies most valued by that organisation or therapist.
- Develop clinical criteria for appraising the research using questions such as:

Is it applicable to our service? (Do we see those clients? Do we deal with those problems? Do we use the intervention in that way?)

Does it have utility in our service? (Could we do that?)

Does it add value to our service? (Would doing this achieve more than we already are?)

Information from clinical experience

Professionals use their prior experiences to deal with the complexity of practice. Socio-cultural theories of learning suggest that professional expertise is developed through interaction with communities of practice (Lave & Wenger, 1991; Walker, 2001). Professionals learn the practices, activities and ways of thinking and knowing about their profession through participation in their communities of practice. Expertise develops 'as an individual gains greater knowledge, understanding and mastery' (Walker, 2001, p. 24) in his/her practice area. Clinicians' experiences in the use of assessments, interventions and communication with clients and other health professionals help them decide what approach to use for any given situation. Because knowledge developed through clinical experience may never have been put into words, it is often difficult to describe or teach to others, except through demonstration, direct supervision or by telling clinical stories. Novices become socialised with the values, roles, expectations and body of knowledge through engagement with more experienced members of their practice communities.

Therapists' personal clinical experiences remain the biggest influence on their practice decisions. A survey of Australian occupational therapists found that the source of information most frequently relied upon for making clinical decisions was the use of clinical experience (Bennett et al., 2003). This finding is further supported by a qualitative decision-making study undertaken by the authors (King, Copley, & Turpin, 2008).

Clinical experience is a source of information for therapists and influences whether, how and to what extent information is integrated into practice (Craik & Rappolt, 2003). A study describing the information used by an experienced paediatric occupational therapist illustrates how clinical experience is used when making clinical decisions (King et al., 2008). Commenting on her use of a particular handwriting technique with her clients, the therapist reflected on how previous experiences of success using a particular technique influence further clinical decisions:

> I have found some of the interventions I use very successful with those populations and the "magic c" is one that I find really successful with kids who have a level of dyspraxia or motor planning difficulty. That is one that I tend to use across the board for a lot of those children. Obviously if they are struggling with letter formation I would consistently use it because I've had success doing it. (King et al., 2008)

Integrating information despite alternatives and uncertainties

The previous section of this chapter discussed the various types of information required for making professional decisions. However, gathering information is only one step in the process. Once relevant data have been obtained, therapists need to make sense of this varied and, at times, contradictory information in order to make decisions for particular clients in particular service contexts. A number of different bodies of knowledge can be useful for informing the process of combining information in order to make clinical decisions. These are evidence-based practice (Sackett et al., 2000), clinical reasoning (Higgs, 2007) and literature on the use of theories and practice models with children (Dunbar, 2007; Hinojosa & Kramer, 2009).

Evidence-based practice and decision making

The definition of evidence-based medicine most often quoted was written by Sackett et al. (1996) and reads, 'evidence based medicine is the conscientious, explicit, and judicious use of current best evidence [research] in making decisions about the care of individual patients' (p. 71). This definition acknowledges that research information is an important source of evidence for health practitioners when making clinical decisions. However, when only this first part of the definition is used, attention is quickly focused on the *type* of information, rather than *how* this information might be used in practice. Importantly, the rest of the definition reads as follows:

> The practice of evidence based medicine means *integrating* individual clinical expertise with the best available external clinical evidence from systematic research. By individual clinical expertise we mean the proficiency and judgement that individual clinicians acquire through *clinical experience and clinical practice*. Increased expertise is reflected in many ways, but especially in more effective and efficient diagnosis and in the more

thoughtful identification and compassionate use of individual patients' predicaments, rights, and preferences in making clinical decisions about their care. (p. 71, emphasis added)

Informed by this broader description, occupational therapists are able to conceptualise their practice as requiring the integration of information from the various sources already discussed. In particular, this description suggests that evidence-based practice is *not* purely a cognitive process, but also requires an understanding of the children and families with whom therapists work and the practice context (Rycroft-Malone et al., 2004).

Occupational therapy has been described as a 'research emergent' profession (Ilott, 2004, p. 347). This means that insufficient research has been undertaken to provide an adequate foundation for *all* of the practices of the profession. Therapists have reported that the extent to which they utilise research information depends on whether they see it as applying to their particular practice context and whether it answers their clinical questions (Bennett et al., 2003; Copley & Allen, in review).

There is also a growing appreciation of the need to consider how 'practice evidence' or clinical narrative and experience can be included as a legitimate means of generating healthcare evidence (Pearson, Wiechula, Court, & Lockwood, 2005). Copley and Allen (in review) found that occupational therapists identified two types of practice evidence that can be generated. First, *individual-level practice evidence* refers to individual therapists evaluating client outcomes on a case-by-case basis while second, *whole service-level practice evidence* involves evaluation of service processes and outcomes. Therapists further identified that standards and processes are needed for the generation and use of practice information at both the individual and whole service levels.

Other possibilities identified included the creation of a systematic peer review process allowing therapists to observe each others' practice and discuss the clinical decisions they made for specific clients. This discussion could also provide a way of evaluating client outcomes in a forum that allowed for systematic consideration of various explanations for the outcomes achieved.

Craik and Rappolt (2003) summarised the way in which therapists integrate different pieces of information as follows:

Through structured reflection on past, current and possible future clinical encounters, occupational therapists can uncover tacit knowledge from their clinical experience and use these insights to evaluate and integrate new research evidence into their practice. Using a client-centred practice paradigm, structured reflection, case application and peer consultation may facilitate occupational therapists' evaluation and integration of research evidence along with client preferences, values, and beliefs. (p. 272)

Thus, a range of different types of information need to be combined by the occupational therapist in order to make clinical decisions. Increasingly, information from sources such as clinical narrative and experience are being explored as legitimate sources of evidence and the importance of reflection on practice is being acknowledged.

Clinical reasoning

The second body of literature that can contribute to understanding how therapists integrate diverse information is clinical reasoning. This has been defined as 'a context-dependent way of thinking and decision making in professional practice to guide practice actions' (Higgs, 2007, p. 1). Therapists may start their decision-making process by considering information from research, but they are also responsive to context and may often 'change course' based on the child's responses, the child's and parents' goals and opinions, and additional insights as intervention progresses.

A number of terms have been used to describe the general reasoning processes used by occupational therapists. These include narrative, interactive, scientific, ethical, procedural, pragmatic and conditional reasoning (Chapparo & Ranka, 2000; Mattingly & Fleming, 1994; Neistadt, 1998; Schell & Cervero, 1993) as well as interpersonal reasoning (Taylor, 2008). Each describes a different focus for reasoning. While clinical reasoning has been described in a variety of different ways, the literature does not suggest that one kind of reasoning is used exclusively by therapists at any one time. Fleming (1991) used the term 'the three-track mind' to label how therapists switch so quickly between different ways of thinking that it appears almost simultaneous. She observed that a therapist might be assessing a person's muscle tone by moving a part of the person's body (procedural reasoning) while simultaneously asking the person about some aspect of his or her life (interactive reasoning) and thinking about the person in the future (conditional reasoning). Of note, different reasoning styles elicit different types of information, which in turn can inform practice in different ways.

Berry and Ryan (2002) suggested that throughout the process of integrating information, the therapist is 'thinking on two different levels' (p. 424). This refers to a 'hands-on' level that relates to actually working with the child, and a conceptual level that relates to using theoretical knowledge to decide on how intervention should proceed. 'Hands-on' level thinking begins as soon as the therapist has contact with the child, while the conceptual level may take longer (Copley et al., 2008). This is because decision making at the conceptual level is informed by the information being gathered over time by therapists as they develop a relationship with the child and family, understand the family's context and expectations, and form meaningful occupational goals (Copley et al., 2008).

The 'hands-on' level of thinking described by Berry and Ryan (2002) is exemplified by the concept of embedded practices. These are core practices that experienced therapists use with all children no matter which interventions they choose to apply. Embedded practices are automatic ways of working that allow the therapist to develop rapport with and be responsive to the child. Embedded practices include the therapist's ways of engaging and motivating the child (often known as therapeutic use of self) (Taylor, 2008), a focus on mastery of occupational tasks, home and school application of therapy strategies and the continuous evolution of interventions in response to the needs of the child (Copley et al., 2008). While therapists automatically set their embedded practices in motion to establish a positive relationship with the child and to focus on task mastery and participation in daily contexts, they are simultaneously starting the process of identifying the child's unique needs and selecting appropriate interventions.

Choosing and combining intervention approaches

The third concept useful for highlighting how occupational therapists integrate information is their choice and combination of intervention approaches. In recent years, it has been identified that, when practicing with children, occupational therapists draw from a range of different theoretical models, frames of reference and intervention approaches (Brown, Rodger, Brown, & Roever, 2005; Hinojosa & Kramer, 2009; Rodger, Brown, & Brown, 2005), combining these to create their own 'theory of practice' (Copley et al., 2008). While therapists will, at times, use particular approaches such as sensory integration, neuro-developmental treatment or CO-OP in a 'purist' manner, they more often use a combination of techniques, drawn from various intervention approaches, and tailor these to address the unique needs of each child, family and service context (Brown et al., 2005; Hinojosa & Kramer, 2009; Nelson et al., 2009; Rodger et al., 2005).

Experienced occupational therapists cite a number of reasons for combining intervention approaches. These include the ability to address the multiple needs of each child and the difficulty of separating some approaches used (Nelson et al., 2009). For example, the technique of multi-sensory cueing is used widely but does not appear to belong to any one approach (Copley et al., 2008). Depending on the way in which it is applied, it could be used from a cognitive mediation perspective (e.g. verbal self-cueing using the child's own words) or a sensory-motor perspective (e.g. adding visual start and stop points to letter formation and tracing the letter on a textured surface before using a pencil).

The decisions made about which intervention techniques to apply and combine are a factor of the occupational performance areas being targeted and the features of task performance that are assumed to contribute to goal achievement (Copley et al., 2008). If, for example, the therapist assumes that a comfortable, upright sitting posture is important to prevent the child from wriggling in his seat and becoming distracted, then this therapist may use biomechanical techniques (Colangelo, 1999; Colangelo & Shea, 2009) and employ forward tilt cushions and desk slopes, as well as upper body strengthening activities, to increase the child's postural stability. The same therapist may assume that completing class tasks requires focused attention in the classroom environment and that this child's difficulty with screening out unimportant background sensory information impacts on his application to the task. The therapist may, therefore, use a sensory processing perspective (Kimball, 1999; Schaaf et al., 2009) incorporating strategies such as the use of ear plugs, a quieter position in class and frequent opportunities for movement to manage the child's limited attention to task. In the interests of developing the child's self-management of classroom tasks, this therapist may further use techniques from an acquisitional frame of reference (Luebben & Brasic Royeen, 2009; Royeen & Duncan, 1999). An example would be having the child identify when he does his 'best listening', identify what helps him to stay on task, and then use strategies and techniques drawn from CO-OP (Polatajko & Mandich, 2004) such as guided discovery and problem-solving to generate child-chosen strategies to achieve a series of plans for 'getting work done quickly'.

Shared decision making

Shared decisions require a partnership between the therapist, the child and his/her family. Communication is focused on achieving shared understanding of treatment goals and plans (Trevena & Barratt, 2003). Consistent with client-centred practice (see Chapter 3), a client may be involved in the decision-making process by helping to identify and clarify the issue, identifying and evaluating possible solutions as well as choosing treatment options (Entwistle & Watt, 2006).

Shared decision making can be facilitated by determining the extent to which clients want to be involved in decision making, developing a respectful and empowering relationship in which clients can participate, providing clear information, attending to the clients' expectations, feelings and ideas, and valuing the clients' life experiences. A health professional's ability to communicate effectively is crucial to successful client involvement in these decisions.

A key aspect of shared decision making is the formulation of intervention goals. Therapists working with children are often heard to lament: 'But some parents don't have any goals'. The overall approach and communication processes used by either an individual therapist or the organisation as a whole to formulate goals is worth consideration. In many situations, service users trust the expertise of health professionals. Hence, the parent and child are provided with recommendations to follow without much discussion or collaboration with the practitioner as to what aspects of performance should be addressed and how this might occur. To promote shared decision making in both goal formulation and intervention selection, the occupational therapist may need to consider the following:

- Is it clear to the family what expectations the therapist/organisation has for their involvement in decisions?
- Does the initial information received by the family when they first become involved with the service include how they might be involved in the therapy process?

- Does it explicitly state the following:
  (a) Goals are made collaboratively;
  (b) The therapist would like to address issues or concerns that are relevant in the child's and family's daily life;
  (c) The therapist will be gathering information about these issues and together with the child and family setting goals to address them;
  (d) The therapist would like the parent to stay for all therapy sessions so that strategies discovered might be used at home or school.

This type of information can help to prepare the family to think about what is of most importance to them and how they might like the situation to change, preparing them to contribute their ideas and giving a clear invitation for close communication with the therapist throughout the process. The involvement of other significant people, such as the child's teacher, could also be explicitly invited at this stage. Other considerations include:

- Is the service structured to prioritise time for discussion, goal setting and evaluation with the child and parents?
- Do appointments allow time for initial discussion to establish concerns, the use of goal-setting tools with both parents and children, and regular opportunities to talk about the child's progress and make new decisions?
- Are specific processes needed to facilitate goal formulation and evaluation?

As covered in earlier chapters (e.g. Chapter 6), formal goal-setting tools can be employed to provide a structure for goal setting with parents and children. However, even when using these tools, skill is required in tailoring the questioning process to the family and their individual situation. It should not be assumed that families have a clear idea of their goals at the outset. They may not be aware of which goals the occupational therapist may be able to address, nor what might be realistic to hope for regarding their child's progress. They may not know about the usual development and expectations of a child at a particular age or school grade level. They may not be able to specifically identify the next steps that their child needs to achieve in order to participate in daily tasks. Therefore, the process of goal formulation is a two-way interaction. The therapist will gather specific information about the child's current performance in the current situation and provide this information along the way to the parents and child in order to help them envisage the next step to aim for (knowing what is possible and clarifying what they want) and participate reciprocally in the goal-setting process. If the goal is homework completion, the therapist may use open-ended questioning such as:

- Tell me what happens at homework time now?
- Where does she do her homework?
- Who else is around?
- How long does it take?
- What kind of help do you give?

The therapist must also have a clear idea of the context surrounding and expectations placed on the child:

- What would be the usual educational expectations for the child at this grade level in terms of homework completion?
- What are the skills required for the child to complete their homework?
- What does the task involve in terms of steps, process, timing, etc.?

As discussed earlier, the therapist combines information from many different sources to make clinical decisions, including information from research and clinical experience. To be truly collaborative in decision making, it is necessary for therapists to communicate with the family how they are using this information to decide, for example, to use one intervention over another. To explain this reasoning in a user-friendly manner, the therapist should match the style and content of the explanation to the parents' or child's level of understanding and information needs.

For example, a parent may request that the therapist work on the pencil grip of their 12-year-old child when handwriting. The therapist's assessment has indicated that while the child's pencil grip looks unusual, there are a number of other issues contributing to his slow handwriting. His planning of pencil strokes appears effortful and he needs to concentrate carefully to write neatly with even sizing and spacing, so that he can later read and edit his work. His teacher is more concerned that the child is able to express his ideas than maintain neat writing. Rather than simply respond to the parent's request, it may be important for the therapist to provide an explanation such as:

> From the research that has been done as well as my experience with other children, it may be difficult to change his pencil grip at this stage. Also, I don't have enough information to tell me that even if he changes his grip, his writing will get faster. What we do know is that the amount of handwriting he needs to do will increase pretty quickly over the next year or two, so it will be important that the effort he is using for handwriting doesn't get in the way of showing what he knows and getting his ideas out. For some children I have seen, learning how to type and using other ways of presenting their work like oral presentations has been quite useful so they can pay more attention to the content and the language rather than using all their effort on just producing the handwriting.

Conclusion

We have seen that decision making is a complex process that involves integration of different types of information from clients, their families, practice context, research and clinical experience. Therapists need to make sense of this varied information in order to make decisions for particular clients in *particular* service contexts. Frequently, this decision making must be managed despite a level of uncertainty due to lack of evidence or best practice protocols. This requires a process of constantly evaluating and integrating information. Clinical reasoning skills are essential for sorting though this information in order to optimise professional decision making. Ultimately decisions are made in collaboration with clients; hence, attention to processes that might facilitate shared decision making is crucial.

References

Ali, S., & Frederickson, N. (2006). Investigating the evidence base of social stories. *Educational Psychology in Practice, 22*(4), 355-377.

Bennett, S., & Bennett, J. (2000). The process of evidence-based practice in occupational therapy: Informing clinical decisions. *Australian Occupational Therapy Journal, 47*(4), 171-180.

Bennett, S., Tooth, L., McKenna, K., Rodger, S., Strong, J., Ziviani, J., et al. (2003). Perceptions of evidence based practice: A survey of Australian occupational therapists. *Australian Occupational Therapy Journal, 50*, 13-22.

Berry, J., & Ryan, S. (2002). Frames of reference: Their use in paediatric occupational therapy. *British Journal of Occupational Therapy, 65*, 420-427.

Brown, G. T., Rodger, S., Brown, A., & Roever, C. (2005). A comparison of Canadian and Australian paediatric occupational therapy practice: Theory, assessments, and interventions. *Occupational Therapy International, 12*, 137-161.

Bundy, A., Lane, S., & Murray, E. (2002). *Sensory integration: Theory and practice.* Philadelphia, PA: F.A. Davis.

Caldwell, E., Whitehead, M., Fleming, J., & Moes, L. (2008). Evidence-based practice in everyday clinical practice: Strategies for change in a tertiary occupational therapy department. *Australian Occupational Therapy Journal, 55*(2), 79-84.

Carpenter, C. (2004). The contribution of qualitative research to evidence-based practice. In K. W. Hammell, & C. Carpenter (Eds.), *Qualitative research in evidence-based rehabilitation* (pp. 1-13). Edinburgh, UK: Churchill Livingstone.

Chapparo, C., & Ranka, J. (2000). Clinical reasoning in occupational therapy. In J. Higgs, & M. Jones (Eds.), *Clinical reasoning in the health professions* (2nd ed., pp. 128-137). Oxford, UK: Butterworth & Heinemann.

Colangelo, C. A. (1999). Biomechanical frame of reference. In P. Kramer, & J. Hinojosa (Eds.), *Frames of reference for pediatric occupational therapy* (2nd ed., pp. 257-322). Philadelphia, PA: Lippincott Williams & Wilkins.

Colangelo, C. A., & Shea, M. (2009). A biomechanical frame of reference for positioning children for functioning. In P. Kramer, & J. Hinojosa (Eds.), *Frames of reference for pediatric occupational therapy* (3rd ed., pp. 489-567). Philadelphia, PA: Lippincott Williams & Wilkins.

Copley, J., & Allen, S. (2009). Using all the available evidence: Perceptions of paediatric occupational therapists about how to increase EBP. *International Journal of Evidence Based Healthcare.*Published Online: Aug 20 2009 11:59PM DOI: 10.1111/j.1744-1609.2009.00137.

Copley, J., Nelson, A., Turpin, M., Underwood, K., & Flanigan, K. (2008). Factors influencing therapists' interventions for children with learning difficulties. *Canadian Journal of Occupational Therapy, 75*(2), 105-113.

Craik, J., & Rappolt, S. (2003). Theory of research utilization enhancement: A model for occupational therapy. *Canadian Journal of Occupational Therapy, 70*(5), 266-275.

De Monte, R., Rodger, S., Broderick, S., & Jones, F. (2009). Living with juvenile idiopathic arthritis: Children's experiences of participating in home exercise programmes. *British Journal of Occupational Therapy, 72*(8), 357-365.

Dunbar, S. B. (2007). Theory, frame of reference and model: A differentiation for practice considerations. In S. B. Dunbar (Ed.), *Occupational therapy models for intervention with children and families* (pp. 1-10). Thorofare, NJ: CB Slack Incorporated.

Entwistle, V., & Watt, I. (2006). Patient involvement in treatment decision-making: The case for a broader conceptual framework. *Patient Education and Counselling, 63*, 268-278.

Feder, K., Majnemer, A., & Symes, A. (2000). Handwriting: Current trends in occupational therapy practice. *Canadian Journal of Occupational Therapy, 67*, 197-204.

Fleming, M. H. (1991). The therapist with the three track mind. *American Journal of Occupational Therapy, 45*, 1007-1014.

Glanville, J., & Lefebvre, C. (2000). Identifying systematic reviews: Key resources. *Evidence-based Medicine, 5*, 68-69.

Gray, C. (2000). *The new social story book*. Arlington, TX: Future Horizons.

Gutstein, S. W., & Sheely, R. K. (2002). *Relationship development intervention with young children*. London, UK: Jessica Kingsley Publishers.

Higgs, J. (2007). The complexity of clinical reasoning: Exploring the dimensions of clinical reasoning expertise as a situated, lived phenomenon. *Collaborations in practice and education advancement*. Sydney, NSW: The University of Sydney (CPEA, Occasional Paper 6).

Higgs, J., Burn, A., & Jones, M. (2001). Integrating clinical reasoning and evidence-based practice. *AACN Clinical Issues, 12*(4), 482-490.

Hinojosa, J., & Kramer, P. (2009). Frames of reference for the real world. In P. Kramer, & J. Hinojosa (Eds.), *Frames of reference for pediatric occupational therapy* (3rd ed., pp. 571-581). Philadelphia, PA: Lippincott Williams & Wilkins.

Ilott, I. (2004). Challenges and strategic solutions for a research emergent profession. *American Journal of Occupational Therapy, 58*(3), 347-352.

Johnston, M. V., Ottenbacher, K. J., & Reichardt, C. S. (1995). Strong quasi-experimental designs for research on the effectiveness of rehabilitation. *American Journal of Physical and Medical Rehabilitation, 74*, 383-392.

Kimball, J. G. (1999). Sensory integration frame of reference: Theoretical base, function/dysfunction continua, and guide to evaluation. In P. Kramer, & J. Hinojosa (Eds.), *Frames of reference for pediatric occupational therapy* (2nd ed., pp. 119-168). Philadelphia, PA: Lippincott Williams & Wilkins.

King, T., Copley, J., & Turpin, M. (2008). *Exploring information used by a paediatric occupational therapist when making clinical decisions*. The University of Queensland, St. Lucia, Queensland, Australia: Unpublished manuscript.

Lave, J., & Wenger, E. (1991). *Situated learning: Legitimate peripheral participation*. Cambridge, UK: University Press.

Luebben, A. J., & Brasic Royeen, C. (2009). An acquisitional frame of reference. In P. Kramer, & J. Hinojosa (Eds.), *Frames of reference for pediatric occupational therapy* (3rd ed., pp. 461-488). Philadelphia, PA: Lippincott Williams & Wilkins.

Mattingly, C., & Fleming, M. H. (1994). *Clinical reasoning: Forms of inquiry in a therapeutic practice*. Philadelphia, PA: F.A. Davis.

Neistadt, M. (1998). Teaching clinical reasoning as a thinking frame. *American Journal of Occupational Therapy, 52,* 221-229.

Nelson, A., Copley, J., Flanigan, K., & Underwood, K. (2009). Occupational therapists prefer combining multiple intervention approaches for children with learning difficulties. *Australian Occupational Therapy Journal, 56*(1), 51-62.

Nelson, D. L., & Mathiowetz, V. (2004). Randomized controlled trials to investigate occupational therapy research questions. *American Journal of Occupational Therapy, 58*(1), 24-34.

Olson, L. J. (1999). Psychosocial frame of reference. In P. Kramer, & J. Hinojosa (Eds.), *Frames of reference for pediatric occupational therapy* (2nd ed., pp. 323-376). Philadelphia, PA: Lippincott Williams & Wilkins.

Olson, L. J. (2009). A frame of reference to enhance social participation. In P. Kramer, & J. Hinojosa (Eds.), *Frames of reference for pediatric occupational therapy* (2nd ed., pp. 306-348). Philadelphia, PA: Lippincott Williams & Wilkins.

Pearson, A., Wiechula, R., Court, A., & Lockwood, C. (2005). The JBI model of evidence-based healthcare. *International Journal of Evidence-based Healthcare, 3,* 207-215.

Polatajko, H. J., & Mandich, A. (2004). *Enabling occupation in children: The Cognitive Orientation to Daily Occupational Performance (CO-OP) approach.* Ottawa, ON: CAOT Publications.

Rodger, S., Brown, G. T., & Brown, A. (2005). Profile of paediatric occupational therapy practice in Australia. *Australian Occupational Therapy Journal, 52,* 311-325.

Royeen, C. B., & Duncan, M. (1999). Acquisition frame of reference. In P. Kramer, & J. Hinojosa (Eds.), *Frames of reference for pediatric occupational therapy* (2nd ed., pp. 377-400). Philadelphia, PA: Lippincott Williams & Wilkins.

Rycroft-Malone, J., Seers, K., Titchen, A., Harvey, G., Kitson, A., & McCormack, B. (2004). What counts as evidence in evidence-based practice? *Journal of Advanced Nursing, 47*(1), 81-90.

Sackett, D. L., Richardson, W. S., Rosenberg, W., & Haynes, R. B. (2000). *Evidence-based medicine: How to practice and teach EBM* (2nd ed.). Edinburgh, UK: Churchill Livingstone.

Sackett, D. L., Rosenberg, W. M., Gray, J. A. M., Haynes, R. B., & Richardson, W. S. (1996). Evidence based medicine: What it is and what it isn't. *British Medical Journal, 312,* 71-72.

Schaaf, R. C., Schoen, S. A., Smith Roley, S., Lane, S. J., Koomar, J., & May-Benson, T. A. (2009). A frame of reference for sensory integration. In P. Kramer, & J. Hinojosa (Eds.), *Frames of reference for pediatric occupational therapy* (3rd ed., pp. 99-186). Philadelphia, PA: Lippincott Williams & Wilkins.

Schell, B. A., & Cervero, R. M. (1993). Clinical reasoning in occupational therapy: An integrative review. *American Journal of Occupational Therapy, 47,* 605-610.

Storch, B. A., & Eskow, K. G. (1996). Theory application by school-based occupational therapists. *American Journal of Occupational Therapy, 50,* 662-668.

Taylor, M. C. (2007). *Evidence-based practice for occupational therapists* (2nd ed.). Oxford, UK: Blackwell Science.

Taylor, R. (2008). *The intentional relationship: Occupational therapy and use of self.* Philadelphia, PA: F.A. Davis.

Trevena, L., & Barratt, A. (2003). Integrated decision making: Definitions for a new discipline. *Patient Education and Counselling, 50,* 265-268.

Walker, R. (2001). Social and cultural perspectives on professional knowledge and expertise. In J. Higgs, & A. Titchen (Eds.), *Practice knowledge and expertise in the health professions* (pp. 22-29). Oxford, UK: Butterworth Heinemann.

Williams, M. S., & Shellenberger, S. (1994). *How does your engine run? A leader's guide to the alert program for self-regulation*. Albuquerque, NM: Therapy Works, Inc.

Wurth, T., Hindman, N., Copley, J., & Nelson, A. (2006). *How occupation-based are occupational therapists working with children with learning difficulties?* The University of Queensland, St. Lucia, Queensland, Australia: Unpublished manuscript.

Index